THE LATIN ALEXANDER TRALLIANUS

THE LATIN ALEXANDER TRALLIANUS

THE TEXT AND TRANSMISSION OF A LATE LATIN MEDICAL BOOK

D. R. LANGSLOW

SOCIETY FOR THE PROMOTION OF ROMAN STUDIES
JOURNAL OF ROMAN STUDIES MONOGRAPH NO. 10
2006

First published in 2006 by
The Society for the Promotion of Roman Studies
Senate House, Malet Street, London WC1E 7HU

The monograph is published with the aid of a grant from the Hugh Last Fund

British Library Catalogue in Publication Data
A catalogue record for this book is available
from the British Library

ISBN 0 907764 32 0
978 0 907764 32 8

Cover picture: Paris, BN, lat. 9332 (early 9th century), f. 140r

Produced by Alden Press

CONTENTS

LIST OF PLATES

The author and publishers gratefully acknowledge the following for providing the illustrations:

Archivio storico di Montecassino (II)
Bibliotheca apostolica vaticana (IX)
Bibliothèque nationale de France (Cover, I, VI, VII)
The Bodleian Library, University of Oxford (VIII)
Centre National de la Recherche Scientifique, Institut de Recherche et d'Histoire des Textes (III, IV, X), and the Bibliothèques municipales of Angers (III), Orléans (IV) and Vendôme (X)
Special Collections Department, Glasgow University Library (V)
Stiftsbibliothek St. Gallen (XI).

LIST OF TABLES

PREFACE AND ACKNOWLEDGEMENTS

One does not have to work for long on Latin medical texts before being referred, by the *Thesaurus linguae Latinae* or another work, to 'Alex. Trall.', only to find that, while the passage is obviously relevant and important, its precise form is obscure or meaningless. This is because the only available 'edition' of the Latin version of Alexander of Tralles, an early printing of 1504, contains numerous errors and (as I hope to show in Chapter 4 below) is based anyway on a late recension at many removes from the earliest reconstructable version. Only the excerpts (in Latin translation) from the lost Greek works of Philumenus (first century A.D.) and Philagrius (fourth century A.D.) contained in the second book of the Latin Alexander have been the object of critical editions.

I began an early paragraph of a grant-application to the UK Arts and Humanities Research Board (as it then was), one of this project's two principal sponsors, with the words, 'It is, frankly, astonishing that the Latin Alexander has never been critically edited, especially in view of the long-standing interest of scholars in Latin (and Greek) medical texts; the importance of Alexander in the history of Byzantine medicine; and the significance of the Latin version of his *Therapeutica* and *On fevers* in the history of medicine in the medieval West.' Having now a much better appreciation of the scale of the undertaking, in terms not only of the sheer size of the text but of the complexity of the tradition, I find it now much less astonishing that no classicist or medievalist has yet taken on the task of editing this medical book. On the other hand, I am now even more confident than I was then that it is a worthwhile endeavour, and that — quite apart from being a prerequisite to addressing the fundamental questions regarding the origin of the Latin text, who? when? where? and why? — an edition of the Latin Alexander stands to make an important contribution to the history of the transmission of medical (and medico-magical) knowledge in the West in late antiquity and the early Middle Ages.

The present volume may be regarded as a set of prolegomena to a first critical edition. It begins with an introduction (Chapter 1) to Alexander's life and his works, and their influence and echoes, and an outline account (Chapter 2) of his works in Greek and some comparisons and contrasts with the Latin version, in broad terms and in detail. Chapter 2 includes some discussion of the tradition of the Greek original, and makes clear the far-from-straightforward and sometimes distant relationship between the Latin version and the Greek text, in particular in its most recent edition, by Theodor Puschmann (2 vols, Vienna, 1878–9). It emerges that the Greek text used by the maker(s) of the Latin Alexander was much superior to that printed by Puschmann and is now mostly lost in Greek, so that the reconstructed Latin text promises to be a much more important witness to the Greek text than the Greek is to the Latin (a situation comparable with that of the respective Greek and Latin traditions of (e.g.) Hippocrates and Oribasius). There follows a description (Chapter 3) of the Latin manuscript copies, and a proposed reconstruction (Chapter 4) of the genetic relations between them. Chapter 3 considers not only the 'mainstream' tradition (of complete or near-complete copies of the Latin text) but also the principal strands of the rich 'secondary', excerpting tradition of substantial parts of the work. I began work on the excerptors of the Latin Alexander for the sake of completeness and with the essentially historical purpose stated at the end of the last paragraph; I did not expect that it would yield findings of significance for editorial purposes. However, the archetype of at least one of the sets of excerpts (that *On gout*) is higher in the stemma than the archetype of the mainstream manuscripts, which both facilitates characterization of the latter, and offers a series of correct readings otherwise lost from the Latin tradition. Chapter 4 presents and tries to explain and justify my first attempt at a *stemma codicum* (illustrated in Plate XII). This turned out to be a much more difficult and complicated undertaking than I had expected, and I do not pretend to have sorted everything out satisfactorily. I have deliberately left alternative possibilities open, and I have signalled a number of loose ends which I am as yet unable to tie up. This is one of the principal places where I hope for constructive criticism from interested readers with more experience than I of reconstructing traditions. Finally, in Chapter 5, I offer some preliminary remarks on the Latinity of the Latin Alexander, and a sample edition — with translation, critical apparatus, and philological and linguistic notes — of the chapters on coughing at the start of Book 2. Here, too, I shall be particularly grateful for readers' comments and advice as the work of preparing the complete edition proceeds.

I owe many debts of gratitude and more for being helped to this point. The project was born in a conversation with Jim Adams (in the bar of the Northern Lawn Tennis Club, West Didsbury, Manchester, in March 1992) about those Latin medical texts in most urgent need of a critical edition, and it and I have benefited from his generous support and invaluable advice and learning ever since, especially in 1994/5, when he and I were able to meet regularly in Oxford to discuss the reconstruction of miscellaneous chapters of the Latin Alexander — on one memorable occasion, Harry Jocelyn and Cloudy Fischer joined us — (parts of Chapter 5 have their origin in those meetings), and in recent months, when he kindly read, corrected, and made many valuable comments on Chapter 5 in proof.

In spite of its inception more than fourteen years ago, the bulk of the work on this book was done in two short periods of funded research leave, June–September 1998 and January–May 2002, both of them at the Medizinhistorisches Institut (as it then was) of the Johannes Gutenberg-University of Mainz, both of them hosted by Cloudy Fischer, of whom more in a moment. They were happy and productive times, under near-optimal conditions, and I am profoundly grateful to the then Director, Werner Kümmel, and to all the staff of the Institute in those years for their welcome, support and friendship, and for sharing with me the valuable research assistance of Olaf Schneiß. The earlier visit was funded by the Alexander von Humboldt-Stiftung, which had previously supported the groundwork for my book *Medical Latin in the Roman Empire* (Oxford, 2000), and which has since funded further work on the Latin Alexander (again in Mainz), allowing me to prepare a provisional electronic text of the first two of the three books, on which I have been able to draw for some of the notes in Chapters 4 and 5. The more recent visit to Mainz, in 2002, vital for finishing this stage of the project, was made possible by an award from the Arts and Humanities Research Board under its Research Leave Scheme. Smaller but still important pieces of funding had been provided by the University of Oxford for the purchase of microfilm copies of manuscripts in the period 1992–8, and for the excellent research assistance of Iveta Mednikarova in 1997/8, and since 1999 have been available for expenses incurred in travelling to autopsy manuscripts from a grant awarded by the University of Manchester. For information about or access in person to most of the Latin Alexander manuscripts I am indebted to staff of the Koninklijke Bibliotheek van België/Bibliothèque Royale de Belgique, Brussels; the

Bibliothèque publique et universitaire in Geneva; the Stiftsbibliothek in St Gall; the Bayerische Staatsbibliothek, Munich; the Bibliothèque nationale de France, Paris; the Bibliothèques municipales of Angers, Chartres, Orléans, and Vendôme; the British Library, London; the libraries of Gonville and Caius College, Cambridge, and Pembroke College, Oxford; to Alan Piper, Archives and Special Collections, Durham University Library; to Don Faustino Avagliano, Archivio di Montecassino. Frequently in my hands (and I hope constantly in my mind), as I worked with the manuscripts and my collations of them towards Chapters 3 and 4, was Martin West's superlative *Textual Criticism and Editorial Technique* (Stuttgart, 1973).

Since 1998, various aspects of the project have been presented in research seminars in the universities of Mainz (twice), Manchester (twice), Helsinki (twice), Munich, Birmingham, Lausanne, A Coruña and London (at the Warburg Institute), and have benefited from the questions and comments voiced on each occasion. In 2002 Barbara Zipser generously shared with me the findings of her work on the manuscript tradition of the Greek Alexander. David Ganz answered with tremendous speed and authority a series of questions on the dating and provenance of some of the Latin manuscripts, and I profited also from comments and information offered by Monica Green. Then and on numerous occasions since, Eliza Glaze has very kindly allowed me sight of her notes and writings prior to publication, and helped me at many points, especially in Chapter 3, with information on manuscripts and bibliography. In the summer of 2002, Michael Reeve read virtually the whole typescript and made numerous insightful comments, especially on Chapter 4. In 2003, Peter Wiseman, the then Editor of the *JRS* Monographs Series, to whom I am grateful also for his part in the accepting of the present work into the series, made further substantial improvements to the shape and arrangement of every chapter. The conceiving of the new University of Manchester, and the birth of Lucy Langslow in February 2004, further delayed the submitting of the final typescript until August of that year. Since then, Lynn Pitts has achieved in difficult circumstances (to say nothing of the author she had to deal with!) an extraordinarily good job of copy-editing and seeing the book through (in various ways difficult) proof stages. Most recently, a number of people have contributed to the provision of a sample of illustrations of the Latin Alexander manuscripts, and the permission to reproduce them: in addition to the formal acknowledgements after the List of Plates above, I should like to thank in particular for their speed and kindness the staff of the Special Collections Department of Glasgow University Library, especially David Weston and Niki Pollock; Don Faustino Avagliano, direttore dell'Archivio di Montecassino and Luigi Giannetti, photographer of Montecassino; and John Bothwell of the Marine Biological Association. I am very grateful also to the University of Manchester for a grant towards the costs of obtaining the images and the permissions to publish them.

By far the largest debt, however, I owe to Cloudy Fischer, who ever since we first spoke of the Latin Alexander more than ten years ago has been a tireless and unstinting source of advice, encouragement, and information on all subjects, from points of Latinity to quantities of medicinal ingredients, and above all in the matters of the secondary tradition of the text and bibliography. He read and corrected Chapters 1–4 in proof, the whole of the typescript, and numerous drafts of especially Chapters 3–5 between 1998 and 2002. I hope he will not object too strongly if I remind him of part of my toast to the Institute on my last evening in Mainz. Zweite Voraussetzung eines von Humboldt geförderten Forschungsaufenthaltes: ein Gastgeber, der für das Verhalten des

Stipendiaten haftet. In dieser Hinsicht bin ich zutiefst verschuldet: hier will ich nur sagen, ich hoffe sehr, daß Herr Fischer es mir glaubt, daß ich mir dessen bewußt bin, was ich ihm zu verdanken habe — es wird auf praktisch jeder Seite der aus dem Projekt entstandenen Monographie deutlich — und daß er die vielen Stunden nicht bereut, die wir zusammen in dem — angesichts der vielen grundlegenden, mir von ihm dort vermittelten Einsichten — passenderweise 123 genannten Zimmer verbracht haben.

I alone am responsible for all remaining errors and imperfections in the present work, but each of the colleagues and institutions named above has helped to improve it out of all recognition, and I am profoundly and eternally grateful to them all.

I dedicate this book to my family, and especially to the memory of Ama Karin.

DRL
Manchester, May 2006

CONVENTIONS AND ABBREVIATIONS

References to the Greek text of Alexander of Tralles are to *volume*, *page*, *line* of the edition of Theodor Puschmann (2 vols, Vienna, 1878–9), and are sometimes prefixed with 'Greek' or 'Gk' for 'the Greek Alexander'.

For the text of the Latin Alexander, I refer to *book.chapter.section* (or 't.', for 'chapter title') in those chapters which I edit in the present work, otherwise simply to *book.chapter* of the early printed edition (Lyons, 1504; my '*ed.*'), although I divide longer chapters informally into *init.*, *med.*, and *fin.*; except in the chapters on coughing (edited in Chapter 5), I retain the 1504 chapter divisions and numbers, even where these are plainly or probably wrong.

References to Philumenus and Philagrius (cf. especially Section 2.4.2 below) are to the edition of Petre Mihăileanu (Bucharest, 1910).

Abbreviations of and references to all other Latin texts follow the conventions of the *OLD* or, for the later period, the *ThLL*. Greek authors and works are cited according to the conventions of LSJ or more explicitly.

In addition the following abbreviations are used in reference to these late antique/early medieval Latin texts:

Pod.	*De podagra* (cf. especially Section 3.2.5 below)
Lib. diaet.	*Liber diaetarum diuersorum medicorum* (Section 3.2.4 below)
Lib. pass.	*Liber passionalis* (Section 3.2.2)
Pass.	*Passionarius Garioponti* (Section 3.2.6)
Ter.	*Tereoperica* (Section 3.2.3)

In quotations of Greek and Latin texts:

[ ] enclose material presumed to be secondary;

< > enclose material presumed to be original and requiring to be restored;

italics signal material presumed to have become corrupted;

+– and –+ in the Latin/Greek text enclose material absent from the corresponding portion of the Greek/Latin version, respectively; conversely, +– –+ alone in the middle of a Greek/Latin quotation indicates the presence at that point of additional material (unspecified) in the Latin/Greek counterpart.

( ) are used within word-forms in some quotations from manuscripts to indicate graphic abbreviations. Abbreviations are completed (e.g. 'p(er)', 'c(aus)a', 'sp(iritu)s'), unless there is doubt as to the scribe's intention (e.g. 'ad dolor( )' indicates that I am uncertain between 'ad dolor(em)' and 'ad dolor(es)').

The sigla of manuscripts employed in the present work are listed at the start of Chapter 3, pp. 38–9 below. Not very subtly, I have used as sigla the first one or two letters of the name of the city where the manuscript rests today, upper case for complete copies (e.g. A for Angers), lower case for excerpting manuscripts (e.g. ba for Barcelona), with an additional numeral to distinguish two or more copies preserved in the same city (e.g. P1, P2, P3 for the three complete copies in Paris; vat1, vat2, vat3, vat4 for the four Vatican manuscripts of the secondary tradition). Lost copies are denoted by Greek letters; closely-related lost copies are sometimes distinguished by means of the complement sign $'$ (e.g. η' is a daughter of η, θ' and θ'' are both close relatives of θ). The same sign is used with sigla of surviving copies (e.g. P3$'$) to mean 'this manuscript before it was corrected at this point'.

The conventions used in the presentation of the sample edition of the chapters on coughing are described at the start of Chapter 5, pp. 175–6 below.

BIBLIOGRAPHY

The following list includes all abbreviated references to modern scholarly literature used in the present work. The titles of periodicals and journals are abbreviated after the manner of *L'Année philologique* (Paris, 1928–) or more explicitly.

Adams, *Paul. Aeg.* = F. ADAMS, *The Seven Books of Paulus Aegineta Translated from the Greek with a Commentary*, 3 vols (London, 1844–1847)

Adams, *Sexual Vocabulary* = J. N. ADAMS, *The Latin Sexual Vocabulary* (London, 1982)

Adams, *Bilingualism* = J. N. ADAMS, *Bilingualism and the Latin Language* (Cambridge, 2003)

Adams and Deegan = J. N. ADAMS and M. DEEGAN, 'Bald's *Leechbook* and the *Physica Plinii*', *Anglo-Saxon England* 21 (1992), 87–114

Allen = P. ALLEN, 'The Justinianic plague', *Byzantion* 49 (1979), 1–20

Andersson-Schmitt = M. ANDERSSON-SCHMITT, H. HALLBERG and M. HEDLUND, *Mittelalterliche Handschriften der Universitätsbibliothek Uppsala. Katalog über die C-Sammlung* VI (Mss. C 551-935), Acta Bibliothecae R. Univ. Ups. 26: 6 (Stockholm, 1993)

André, *Plantes* = J. ANDRÉ, *Les noms de plantes dans la Rome antique* (Paris, 1985)

André, *Anatomie* = J. ANDRÉ, *Le vocabulaire latin de l'anatomie* (Paris, 1995)

ANRW = H. TEMPORINI and W. HAASE (eds), *Aufstieg und Niedergang der römischen Welt* (Berlin/New York, 1972–)

Aubert, *Notices ... Genève* = H. AUBERT, *Notices sur les manuscrits Petau conservés à la Bibliothèque de Genève* (Paris, 1911)

Avril and Załuska = F. AVRIL and Y. ZAŁUSKA, *Manuscrits enluminés de la Bibliothèque Nationale. Manuscrits d'origine italienne*, 2 vols (Paris, 1980–1984)

Baader, 'Phill. 1790' = G. BAADER, 'Der Berliner Codex Phillipp. 1790, ein frühmittelalterliches medizinisches Kompendium', *Med.-Hist. Journal* 1 (1966), 150–5

Baader, 'Überlieferung' = G. BAADER, 'Zur Überlieferung der lateinischen medizinischen Literatur des frühen Mittelalters', *Forschung Praxis Fortbildung* 17 (1966), 139–41

Baader, 'Die Anfänge' = G. BAADER, 'Die Anfänge der medizinischen Ausbildung im Abendland bis 1100', in *Settimane di studio del Centro italiano di studi sull'altomedioevo XIX: La scuola nell'occidente latino dell'alto medieovo, Spoleto, 15–21 aprile 1971* (Spoleto, 1972), 669–718; 724–42

Baader, 'Adaptations' = G. BAADER, 'Early medieval Latin adaptations of Byzantine medicine in Western Europe', in Scarborough, *Symposium*, 251–9

Barbillion = L. BARBILLION, *Études critiques d'histoire de la médecine* (Paris, 1930) (Ch. 8. 'Alexandre de Tralles et sa lettre sur les helminthes, VIe siècle après J.-C.')

Bariéty and Coury = M. BARIÉTY and Ch. COURY, *Histoire de la médecine* (Paris, 1963)

Beccaria, *Codici* = A. BECCARIA, *I codici di medicina del periodo presalernitano (secoli IX, X e XI)* (Rome, 1956)

Beccaria, 'Sulle tracce' = A. BECCARIA, 'Sulle tracce di un antico canone latino di Ippocrate e di Galeno', (I.–III.) *Italia medioevale e umanistica* 2 (1959), 1–56; 4 (1961), 1–75; 14 (1971), 1–23

Behrends = F. BEHRENDS, 'Two poems by Fulbert among photographs of Chartres mss.', *Scriptorium* 31 (1977), 295–6

Biraben = J.-N. BIRABEN, *Les hommes et la peste en France et dans les pays européens et méditerranéens*, 2 vols (Paris/The Hague, 1975–1976)

Bischoff, *Studien* = B. BISCHOFF, *Mittelalterliche Studien. Ausgewählte Aufsätze zur Schriftkunde und Literaturgeschichte*, 3 vols (Stuttgart, 1966–1981)

Bischoff, 'Italienische Hss.' = B. BISCHOFF, 'Italienische Handschriften des 9.–11. Jahrhunderts in frühmittelalterlichen Bibliotheken außerhalb Italiens', in *Il libro e il testo* (Urbino, 1985), 171–94

Bischoff, *Nachlaß* = B. BISCHOFF, *Handschriftenarchiv Bernhard Bischoff*, Bibliothek der Monumenta Germaniae Historica, Hs. C 1, C 2 — Microfiche-Edition, ed. A. Mentzel-Reuters (Munich, 1997)

Bischoff, *Katalog* = B. BISCHOFF, *Katalog der festländischen Handschriften des neunten Jahrhunderts (mit Ausnahme der wisigotischen). Teil 1: Aachen–Lambach* (Wiesbaden, 1998)

Bloch = I. BLOCH, 'Alexandros von Tralles', in M. Neuburger and J. Pagel (eds), *Handbuch der Geschichte der Medizin (begründet von Theodor Puschmann)*, 3 vols (Jena, 1902–1905), I, 535–45

Böhner = K. BÖHNER, *Geschichte der Cecidologie. Ein Beitrag zur Entwicklungsgeschichte naturwissenschaftlicher Forschung und ein Führer durch die Cecidologie der Alten* (Mittenwald, 1933)

Bond = C. U. FAYE and W. H. BOND, *Supplement to the Census of Medieval and Renaissance Manuscripts in the United States and Canada* (New York, 1962)

Bracciotti = A. BRACCIOTTI, 'L'Apporto della tradizione indiretta per la costituzione di un testo critico delle *Curae herbarum*', *Rivista di cultura classica e medioevale* 42 (2000), 61–102

Brunet, *Alexandre* = F. BRUNET, *Oeuvres médicales d'Alexandre de Tralles*, 4 vols (Paris, 1933–1937)

Brunet, *Médecine* = F. BRUNET, *Alexandre de Tralles et la médecine byzantine* (Paris, 1933)

Brunet and Miéli = P. BRUNET and A. MIÉLI, *Histoire des sciences: Antiquité* (Paris, 1935)

BTML = G. SABBAH, P.-P. CORSETTI and K.-D. FISCHER, *Bibliographie des textes médicaux latins: Antiquité et haut Moyen Age*, Centre Jean Palerne Mémoires 6 (Saint-Étienne, 1987)

BTML Suppl. = K.-D. FISCHER, *Bibliographie des textes médicaux latins: Antiquité et haut Moyen Age: premier supplément*, Centre Jean Palerne Mémoires 15 (Saint-Étienne, 2000)

Buck = A. H. BUCK, *The Growth of Medicine: from the Earliest Times to about 1800* (New Haven, 1917)

Burnett, 'Flavours' = C. BURNETT, '*Sapores sunt octo*: the medieval Latin terminology for the eight flavours', *Micrologus* 10 (2002), 99–112

Calcoen = R. CALCOEN, *Inventaire des manuscrits scientifiques de la Bibliothèque royale Albert Ier*, 3 vols (Brussels, 1965–1975)

Cameron, 'Bald's *Leechbook*' = M. L. CAMERON, 'Bald's *Leechbook*: its sources and their use in compilation', *Anglo-Saxon England* 12 (1983), 153–82

Cameron = M. L. CAMERON, *Anglo-Saxon Medicine*, Cambridge Studies in Anglo-Saxon England 7 (Cambridge, 1993)

Castiglioni = A. CASTIGLIONI, *Histoire de la médecine* (trans. J. Bertrand and F. Gidon) (Paris, 1931) [cf. *A History of Medicine* (translated from the Italian and edited by E. B. Krumbhaar), 2nd edn (New York, 1947)]

Cat. Casin. = *Codicum Casinensium manuscriptorum catalogus*, cura et studio monachorum S. Benedicti Archicoenobii Montis Casini, I/1 (Codd. 1-100) (Monte Casino, 1915)

Cat. Escorial = G. ANTOLÍN, *Catálogo de los códices latinos de la Real Biblioteca del Escorial*, 5 vols (Madrid, 1910–1923)

Cat. gén. Arsenal = *Catalogue général des manuscrits des Bibliothèques publiques de France: Paris, Bibliothèque de l'Arsenal*, 9 vols (Paris, 1885–1899)

Cat. gén. Dép. = *Catalogue général des manuscrits des Bibliothèques publiques de France: Départements*, numerous vols

Cat. Harley = *A Catalogue of the Harleian Manuscripts in the British Museum*, 4 vols + indexes (London, 1808–1812)

Cat. Monac. = *Catalogus codicum Latinorum Bibliothecae Regiae Monacensis*, I/1 (Codd. 1-2329) (Munich, 1892^2)

Cavallo, 'Libri' = G. CAVALLO, 'Libri e continuità della cultura antica in età barbarica', in *Magistra Barbaritas. I Barbari in Italia* (Milan, 1984), 603–62

Cavallo, 'Cultura scritta' = G. CAVALLO, 'La cultura scritta tra antichità e alto medioevo', in A. Carile (ed.), *Storia di Ravenna. II. 2 Dall'età bizantina all'età ottoniana* (Venice, 1992), 79–125

Corlieu = A. CORLIEU, *Les médecins grecs, depuis la mort de Galien jusqu'à la chute de l'Empire d'Orient (210–1453)* (Paris, 1885)

Corner = G. W. CORNER, 'On early Salernitan surgery and especially the "Bamberg Surgery", with an account of a previously undescribed manuscript of the Bamberg Surgery in the possession of Dr. Harvey Cushing', *Bull. Hist. Med.* 5 (1937), 1–32

Coxe = H. O. COXE, *Catalogus codicum mss. qui in collegiis aulisque Oxoniensibus hodie adseruantur*, 2 vols (Oxford, 1852)

Daremberg = Ch. DAREMBERG, *Histoire des sciences médicales*, 2 vols (Paris, 1870)

Delisle = L. Delisle, *Inventaire des manuscrits latins conservés à la Bibliothèque Nationale sous les numéros 8823–18613, I (Codd. 8823–14231)* (Paris, 1863)

De Lucia = R. DE LUCIA, 'Una redazione inedita del Περὶ ἑλμίνθων di Alessandro di Tralle', in A. Garzya and J. Jouanna (eds), *Trasmissione e ecdotica dei testi medici greci. Atti del IV Convegno Internazionale, Parigi, maggio 2001* (Naples, 2003), 53–63

De Renzi = S. DE RENZI (ed.), *Collectio Salernitana* (*Documenti inediti, e trattati di medicina appartenenti alla scuola medica salernitana, raccolti ed illustrati da G. E. T. Henschel, C. Daremberg, e S. De Renzi; premessa la storia della scuola*), 5 vols (Naples, 1852–1859)

Diels, *Handschriften* = H. DIELS, *Die Handschriften der antiken Ärzte*, Abhandlungen der königl. preuß. Akad. d. Wiss. 1905, 1906 (Berlin, 1906), II, 11–12

Diels, *Nachtrag* = H. DIELS, *Bericht über den Stand des interakademischen Corpus Medicorum Antiquorum und erster Nachtrag zu den in den Abhandlungen 1905 und 1906 veröffentlichten Katalogen: Die Handschriften der antiken Ärzte, I. und II. Teil*, Abhandlungen der königl. preuß. Akad. d. Wiss. 1907 (Berlin, 1908)

Diepgen = P. DIEPGEN, *Geschichte der Medizin*, 2 vols (Berlin, 1949–1951)

DKP = *Der Kleine Pauly: Lexikon der Antike* (ed. K. Ziegler and W. Sontheimer), 5 vols (Munich, 1964–1975)

DNP = *Der Neue Pauly: Enzyklopädie der Antike* (ed. H. Cancik, H. Schneider and M. Landfester), 18 vols + index (Stuttgart, 1996–2003)

Domínguez Bordona = J. DOMÍNGUEZ BORDONA, *Manuscritos con pinturas*, 2 vols (Madrid, 1933)

Dronke = P. DRONKE, 'New approaches to the School of Chartres', *Anuario de estudios medievales* 6 (1969), 117–40

DSB = *Dictionary of Scientific Biography* (ed. C. C. Gillispie), 14 vols + index (New York, 1970–1980)

Dubief = Marie-José IMBAULT-HUART, Lise DUBIEF and Bernard MERLETTE, *La médecine au moyen âge à travers les manuscrits de la Bibliothèque Nationale* (Paris, 1983)

Duffy = J. M. DUFFY, 'Byzantine medicine in the sixth and seventh centuries: aspects of teaching and practice', in Scarborough, *Symposium*, 21–7

Durling, *Guide*[1] = R. J. DURLING, 'A guide to the medical manuscripts mentioned in Kristeller's *Iter Italicum III*', *Traditio* 41 (1985), 341–65

Durling, *Guide*[2] = R. J. DURLING, 'A guide to the medical manuscripts mentioned in Kristeller's *Iter Italicum IV*', *Traditio* 46 (1991), 347–79

Fabricius, *Bibliotheca* = J. A. FABRICIUS, *Bibliotheca Graeca*, vol. 12 (Hamburg, 1724)

Fabricius, *Galens Exzerpte* = C. FABRICIUS, *Galens Exzerpte aus älteren Pharmakologen* (Berlin, 1972)

Fischer, 'Pseudo-Democritus' = K.-D. FISCHER, 'Der *Liber medicinalis* des Pseudo-Democritus', in M. E. Vázquez-Buján (ed.), *Tradición e innovación de la medicina latina de la antigüedad y de la alta edad media. Actas del IV Coloquio Internacional sobre los «Textos médicos latinos antiguos»* (Santiago de Compostela, 1994), 45–56

Fischer, '*Lib. Byz.*' = K.-D. FISCHER, 'Der *Liber Byzantii*, ein unveröffentlichtes griechisches therapeutisches Handbuch in lateinischer Übersetzung', in C. Deroux (ed.), *Maladie et maladies dans les textes latins antiques et médiévaux. Actes du Ve Colloque International «Textes médicaux latins», Bruxelles, 4–6 septembre 1995* (Brussels, 1998), 276–94

Fischer, 'Dr Monk' = K.-D. FISCHER, 'Dr Monk's Medical Digest', *Social History of Medicine* 13 (2000), 239–51

Fischer, 'Wer liest' = K.-D. FISCHER, 'Wer liest, der findet. Versprengte kleinere Stücke medizinischer Werke in mittelalterlichen Handschriften', in *Docente Natura (Mélanges ... Guy Sabbah)* (St Etienne, 2000), 69–90

Fischer, '*Lib. tert.*' = K.-D. FISCHER, 'Der pseudogalenische *Liber tertius*', in Garofalo and Roselli, 101–32

Fischer, *ed. pr.* Lib. tert. = K.-D. FISCHER, 'Galeni qui fertur Ad Glauconem liber tertius *ad fidem codicis Vindocinensis 109*', in Garofalo and Roselli, 283–346

Fischer and von Staden = K.-D. FISCHER and H. VON STADEN,'Ein angeblicher Brief des Herophilos an König Antiochus, aus einer Brüsseler Handschrift erstmals herausgegeben', *Sudhoffs Archiv* 80 (1996), 86–98

Fraisse = A. FRAISSE, *Cassius Felix, De la médecine. Texte établi, traduit et annoté* (Paris, 2002)

Fredriksson = M. FREDRIKSSON, *Esculapius*' De stomacho. *Edited with an Introduction, Translation, and Commentary*, unpub. diss. Uppsala (2002)

Gallardo = B. J. GALLARDO, *Ensayo de una biblioteca española*, 4 vols (Madrid, 1863–1889); *II, Apendice: Indice de Manuscritos de la Biblioteca Nacional* (1866)

Gameson = R. GAMESON, *The Manuscripts of Early Norman England (c. 1066–1130)* (Oxford, 1999)

García = Z. GARCÍA, *Bibliotheca Patrum Latinorum Hispaniensis (Nach den Aufzeichnungen Rudolf Beers), II. Band*, Sitzungsberichte der kaiserl. Akad. der Wissenschaften in Wien (Phil.-Hist. Klasse) 169, 2 (Vienna, 1915)

Gar. ed. (1536) = *Habes sincerioris medicinæ amator, iterum renatos VIII de morborum causis, accidentibus et curationibus libros Gariopontі medici, qui usu et successu artis nemini ex ueteribus cedit, testibus qui usi sunt eius remediorum ratione indicationeue* (Basileæ apud Henricum Petrum, 1536)

Garofalo and Roselli = I. GAROFALO and A. ROSELLI (eds), *Galenismo e medicina tardoantica: fonti greche, latine e arabe. Atti del Seminario Internazionale di Siena, Certosa di Pontignano, settembre 2002* (Naples, 2003)

Georges = K. E. GEORGES, *Ausführliches lateinisch-deutsches Handwörterbuch* (8th edn, rev. H. Georges), 2 vols (Hanover, 1913–19)

Glaze, *Medical Books* = F. E. GLAZE, *The Perforated Wall: The Ownership and Circulation of Medical Books in Medieval Europe, ca. 800–1200*, unpub. diss. Duke University (1999)

Glaze, 'Galen refashioned' = F. E. Glaze, 'Galen refashioned: Gariopontus in the later Middle Ages and Renaissance', in E. L. Furdell (ed.), *Textual Healing. Essays on Medieval and Early Modern Medicine* (Leiden, 2005), 53–75

Glaze, '*Passionarius*' = F. E. GLAZE, 'Gariopontus of Salerno's *Passionarius*: origins and influence', unpub. ms.

Gossen = H. GOSSEN, 'Rochen und Seedrachen', *PWRE, Suppl. 8* (Stuttgart, 1956), 641–8

Green, '*De genecia*' = M. H. GREEN, 'The *De genecia* attributed to Constantine the African', *Speculum* 62 (1987), 299–323

Green, 'Handlist I' = M. H. GREEN, 'A handlist of the Latin and vernacular manuscripts of the so-called *Trotula* texts (I)', *Scriptorium* 50 (1996), 137–75

Green, '*Trotula*' = M. H. GREEN, 'The development of the *Trotula*', *Revue d'Histoire des Textes* 26 (1996) (= eadem, *Women's Healthcare in the Medieval West. Texts and Contexts*, Variorum Collected Studies Series CS680 (Aldershot, 2000)), 119–203

Hecker = J. F. HECKER, *Geschichte der Heilkunde: nach den Quellen bearbeitet*, 2 vols (Berlin, 1822–1829)

Hoefer = F. HOEFER, 'Alexandre de Tralles', *Nouvelle biographie universelle générale*, 46 vols (Paris, 1852–1866), I, 915–18

Hofmann and Szantyr = J. B. HOFMANN and A. SZANTYR, *Lateinische Syntax and Stilistik* (Munich, 1965)

Homburger, *Bern* = O. HOMBURGER, *Die illustrierten Handschriften der Bürgerbibliothek Bern* (Bern, 1962)

Howald and Sigerist = E. HOWALD and H. SIGERIST (eds), *Antonii Musa De herba uettonica liber. Pseudoapulei Herbarius. Anonymi De taxone liber. Sexti Placiti Liber medicinae ex animalibus*, Corpus Medicorum Latinorum 4 (Leipzig, 1927)

Hunger = H. HUNGER, *Die hochsprachliche profane Literatur der Byzantiner*, 2 vols (Munich, 1978)

Ieraci Bio, 'Trasmissione' = A. M. IERACI BIO, 'La trasmissione della letteratura medica greca nell'Italia meridionale fra X e XV secolo', in A. Garzya (ed.), *Contributi alla cultura greca nell'Italia meridionale* (Naples, 1989), 133–257

Ieraci Bio, 'Interferenze' = A. M. IERACI BIO, 'Interferenze occidentali nella medicina bizantina', in *Dalla medicina greca alla medicina salernitana: percorsi e tramiti. Atti del Convegno Internazionale, Raito di Vietri sul Mare, giugno 1995* (Salerno, 1999), 279–97

Ieraci Bio, 'Centri' = A. M. IERACI BIO, 'Centri di trasmissione della letteratura medica in età tardoantica e bizantina', in A. Leone and G. Sangermano (eds), *Nel Mediterraneo medievale: la medicina. Atti della giornata di studio, Fisciano, maggio 2004* (Salerno, 2005), 23–44

Inventario = *Inventario General de Manoscritos de la Biblioteca Nacional*, 10 vols (Madrid, 1953–1984)

Jacquart, 'Transmission' = D. JACQUART, 'Principales étapes dans la transmission des textes de médecine (XIe–XIVe siècle)', in J. Hamesse and M. Fattori (eds), *Rencontres de cultures dans la philosophie médiévale: Traductions et traducteurs de l'antiquité tardive au XIVe siècle. Actes du Colloque International de Cassino, 15–17 juin 1989* (Louvain-la-Neuve/Cassino, 1990), 251–71

Jacquart and Micheau = D. JACQUART and F. MICHEAU, *La médecine arabe et l'occident médiéval*, Collection Islam-Occident 7 (Paris, 1990)

James = M. R. JAMES, *A Descriptive Catalogue of the Manuscripts in the Library of Gonville and Caius College, I (Mss. 1–354)* (Cambridge, 1907); *II (Mss. 355–721)*, (Cambridge, 1908); *Supplement* (Cambridge, 1914)

Ker II, III = N. R. KER, *Medieval Manuscripts in British Libraries. Vol. II: Abbotsford–Keele* (Oxford, 1977); *Vol. III: Lampeter–Oxford* (Oxford, 1983)

Kibre, 'Repertorium II' = P. KIBRE, 'Hippocrates Latinus: Repertorium of Hippocratic writings in the Latin Middle Ages (II)', *Traditio* 32 (1976), 257–92

Kibre, *Hipp.Lat.* = P. KIBRE, *Hippocrates Latinus. Repertorium of Hippocratic Writings in the Latin Middle Ages* (rev. edn, New York, 1985)

Krieger-Königsberg = KRIEGER-KÖNIGSBERG, 'Zur Parasitologie, Pathologie und Therapie der Helminthiasis bei Paulos Aiginetes', *Die medizinische Welt* 16 (1952), 542–6

Kristeller, 'School of Salerno' = P. O. KRISTELLER, 'School of Salerno', *Bull. Hist. Med.* 17 (1945), 138–94

Kristeller III, IV, V, VI = P. O. KRISTELLER, *Iter Italicum III* (*Alia Itinera I*) (London/Leiden, 1983); *Iter Italicum IV* (*Alia Itinera II*) (London/Leiden, 1989); *Iter Italicum V* (*Alia Itinera III and Italy III*) (London/Leiden, 1990); *Iter Italicum VI* (*Italy III and Alia Itinera IV*) (London/Leiden, 1992)

Kudlien, *DSB* = F. KUDLIEN, 'Alexander of Tralles' in C. C. Gillispie (ed.), *Dictionary of Scientific Biography* (New York, 1970–1980), I, 121

Landgraf = G. LANDGRAF (ed. and comm.), *Ciceros Rede für Sex. Roscius aus Ameria* (Erlangen, 1882)

Langslow, *Medical Latin* = D. R. LANGSLOW, *Medical Latin in the Roman Empire* (Oxford, 2000)

Langslow, 'Particles' = D. R. LANGSLOW, 'Latin discourse particles, "medical Latin" and "classical Latin"', *Mnemosyne* 53 (2000), 537–60

Langslow, 'Alex. Trall.' = D. R. LANGSLOW, 'Die lateinische Übersetzung der *Therapeutika* des Alexander von Tralles. Bemerkungen zur Textüberlieferung und zum Wortschatz', in S. Sconocchia and F. Cavalli (eds), *Testi medici latini antichi. Le parole della medicina: lessico e storia. Atti del VII Convegno Internazionale, Trieste, ottobre 2001* (Bologna, 2004), 177–92

Langslow, '*utique*' = D. R. LANGSLOW, 'Linguistic "highs" and "lows" in late Latin medical texts: Latin *utique* and the dangers of generalizing', in S. Kiss, L. Mondin and G. Salvi (eds), *Latin et langues romanes. Études ... József Herman* (Tübingen, 2005), 313–25

Löfstedt, *Coniectanea* = E. LÖFSTEDT, *Coniectanea. Untersuchungen auf dem Gebiete der antiken und mittelalterlichen Latinität* (Uppsala and Stockholm, 1950)

Loew, *Beneventan Script* = E. A. LOEW, *The Beneventan Script. A History of the South Italian Minuscule* (Oxford, 1914) (2nd edn prepared and enlarged by V. Brown, 2 vols, (Rome, 1980))

Loew, *Scriptura Beneventana* = E. A. LOEW, *Scriptura Beneventana* (Oxford, 1929)

Lowe, '*Membra disiecta*' = E. A. LOWE in 'Nouvelle liste de *membra disiecta*', *Rev. Bénéd.* 43 (1931), 5–8; 101–5 (at p. 103)

Lowe, *CLA* = E. A. LOWE, *Codices Latini Antiquiores*, 11 vols plus Supplement (Oxford, 1934–1971)

LSJ = H. G. LIDDELL, R. SCOTT and H. S. JONES, *A Greek-English Lexicon* (9th edn, Oxford, 1940); with the Revised Supplement ed. P. G. W. Glare (Oxford, 1996)

MacKinney, *Medicine* = L. C. MACKINNEY, *Early Medieval Medicine with Special Reference to France and Chartres* (Baltimore, 1937)

MacKinney, 'Ethics' = L. C. MACKINNEY, 'Medical ethics and etiquette in the early Middle Ages: the persistence of Hippocratic ideals', *Bull. Hist. Med.* 26 (1952), 1–30

MacKinney, *Illustrations* = L. C. MACKINNEY, *Medical Illustrations in Medieval Manuscripts* (London, 1965)

Madan and Craster = F. MADAN and H. H. E. CRASTER, *A Summary Catalogue of Western Manuscripts in the Bodleian Library at Oxford, Vol. II, Part 1 (Collections received before 1660 and miscellaneous MSS. acquired during the first half of the 17th Century) Nos. 1–3490* (Oxford, 1922)

Maire = B. MAIRE (ed.), *Gargilius Martialis. Les remèdes tirés des légumes et des fruits*, Collection Budé (Paris, 2002)

Manitius = M. MANITIUS, *Handschriften antiker Autoren in mittelalterlichen Bibliothekskatalogen*, Zentralblatt für Bibliothekswesen Beiheft 67 (Leipzig, 1935)

Masullo = R. MASULLO, *Filagrio: Frammenti* (Naples, 1999)

Mayerhoefer = J. MAYERHOEFER, *Lexicon der Geschichte der Naturwissenschaften*, 8 vols (Vienna 1959–[1996] [continued as *Archiv der G. d. N.*]) – 2 (1961), 181

Mazzini, 'secoli V e VI' = I. MAZZINI, 'Il latino medico in Italia nei secoli V e VI', in *La cultura in Italia fra tardo antico e alto medioevo. Atti del convegno tenuto a Roma, Consiglio nazionale delle ricerche, dal 12 al 16 novembre 1979* (Rome, 1981)

Mazzini and Palmieri = I. MAZZINI and N. PALMIERI, 'L'École médicale de Ravenne: programmes et méthodes d'enseignement, langue, hommes', in P. Mudry and J. Pigeaud (eds), *Les écoles médicales à Rome. Actes du IIe Colloque International sur les textes médicaux latins antiques, Lausanne, septembre 1986* (Geneva, 1991), 285–310

Meyer = E. H. F. MEYER, *Geschichte der Botanik. Studien*, 4 vols (Königsberg, 1854–1857; repr. Amsterdam, 1965)

Meyer-Steineg and Sudhoff = Th. MEYER-STEINEG and K. SUDHOFF, *Illustrierte Geschichte der Medizin* (5th edn revised and enlarged by R. Herrlinger and F. Kudlien; Stuttgart, 1965)

Mihăileanu = P. MIHĂILEANU, *Fragmentele latine ale lui Philumenus şi Philagrius* (Bucharest, 1910)

Milwards = E. MILWARDS, *Trallianus reviviscens, or An Account of Alexander Trallian, One of the Greek Writers that Flourished after Galenus, Shewing that these Authors are far from Deserving the Imputation of Mere Compilers* (London, 1734)

Molinier, *Oeuvres* = U. C. BUSSEMAKER, C. DAREMBERG and A. MOLINIER, *Oeuvres d'Oribase*, 6 vols (Paris, 1851–1876)

Mørland, *Oribasius* = H. MØRLAND, *Die lateinischen Oribasiusübersetzungen*, Symbolae Osloenses fasc. suppl. V (Oslo, 1932)

Mørland, 'Nachträge' = H. MØRLAND, 'Zu einer neuen Ausgabe der Nachträge zu Alexander Trallianus', *Symb. Osl.* 12 (1933), 91–3

Mostert = M. MOSTERT, *The Library of Fleury: A Provisional List of Manuscripts* (Hilversum, 1989)

Neuburger = M. NEUBURGER, *Geschichte der Medizin*, 2 vols (Stuttgart, 1906–1911)

Newton, *Monte Cassino* = F. NEWTON, *The Scriptorium and Library at Monte Cassino, 1058–1105*, Cambridge Studies in Palaeography and Codicology 7 (Cambridge, 1999)

Noßke = B. NOSSKE, *Alexandri (Tralliani?) liber de agnoscendis febribus et pulsibus et urinis*, unpub. Diss. med. Leipzig (1919)

Nutton, 'Alex. Trall.' = V. NUTTON, 'Alexander Trallianus', *DNP* 1 (1996), 483–4

Nutton, 'Galen to Alexander' = V. NUTTON, 'From Galen to Alexander, aspects of medicine and medical practice in late antiquity', in Scarborough, *Symposium*, 1–14

ODB = *Oxford Dictionary of Byzantium* (A. P. Kazhdan editor-in-chief), 3 vols (New York/Oxford, 1991)

OLD = P. G. W. GLARE (ed.), *Oxford Latin Dictionary* (Oxford, 1968–82)

Ongaro, 'epatica' = G. ONGARO, 'La patologia epatica nel pensiero di Alessandro di Tralle', *Rivista della società italiana di storia di medicina* 10 (1966), 58–73

Önnerfors, *Stud. phil.* = A. ÖNNERFORS, *In* Medicinam Plinii *studia philologica* (Lund, 1963)

Önnerfors, *Med. Plin.* = A. ÖNNERFORS (ed.), *Plinii Secundi Iunioris qui feruntur De medicina libri tres* (*CML*, 3) (Berlin, 1964)

Önnerfors, *Phys. Plin.* = A. ÖNNERFORS (ed.), *Physica Plinii Bambergensis* (Hildesheim, 1975)

Orofino = G. OROFINO, *I codici decorati dell' Archivio di Montecassino* (Rome, 1994–1996)

Pellegrin, 'Fragments' = E. PELLEGRIN, 'Fragments et membra disiecta', in *Bibliothèques retrouvées: Manuscrits, bibliothèques et bibliophiles du moyen age et de la Renaissance (Recueil d'études publiées de 1938 à 1985)* (Paris, 1988), 343–64 (reprinted from *Codicologica* 3 (1980), 70–95)

Pellegrin *et al.*, *Vaticane* = E. PELLEGRIN, J. FOHLEN, C. JEUDY, Y.-F. RIOU, and A. MARUCCHI, *Les manuscrits classiques latins de la Bibliothèque Vaticane, I* (Paris, 1975); *II.1* (Paris, 1978); *II.2* (Paris, 1982); *III.1* (Paris, 1991)

Politzer = A. POLITZER, *Geschichte der Ohrenheilkunde*, 2 vols (Stuttgart, 1907–1913)

Puschmann = Th. PUSCHMANN, *Alexander von Tralles. Original-Text und Übersetzung nebst einer einleitenden Abhandlung. Ein Beitrag zur Geschichte der Medicin*, 2 vols (Vienna, 1878–1879; reprinted Amsterdam, 1963)

Puschmann, *Nachträge* = Th. PUSCHMANN, *Nachträge zu Alexander Trallianus* (Berlin, 1887)

PWRE = A. PAULY, G. WISSOWA and W. KROLL (eds), *Real-Encyclopädie der classischen Altertumswissenschaft* 66 vols + indices (Stuttgart, 1893–2000)

REW = W. MEYER-LÜBKE, *Romanisches etymologisches Wörterbuch* (3rd edn, Heidelberg, 1935)

Riché = P. RICHÉ, *Education et culture dans l'Occident barbare, VIe–VIIIe siècles*, Patristica Sorbonensia 4 (Paris, 1962)

Rose, *Anecdota* = V. ROSE, *Anecdota graeca et graecolatina: Mitteilungen aus Handschriften zur Geschichte der griechischen Wissenschaft*, 2 vols (Berlin, 1864–1870; reprinted Amsterdam, 1963)

Rose, *Verzeichnis ... Berlin* = V. ROSE, *Verzeichnis der lateinischen Handschriften der Kgl. Bibliothek zu Berlin, vol. I* (Berlin, 1893)

Sabbah, 'Cassius Felix' = G. SABBAH, 'Le *De medicina* de Cassius Felix à la charnière de l'Antiquité et du Haut Moyen Age', in M. E. Vázquez-Buján (ed.), *Tradición e innovación de la medicina latina de la antigüedad y de la alta edad media. Actas del IV Coloquio Internacional sobre los «Textos médicos latinos antiguos»* (Santiago de Compostela, 1994), 11–28

Sarton = G. A. L. SARTON, *Introduction to the History of Science* (Baltimore, 1927–1948)

Scarborough, *Symposium* = J. SCARBOROUGH (ed.), *Symposium on Byzantine Medicine (Dumbarton Oaks 1983)*, Dumbarton Oaks Papers 38 (Dumbarton Oaks, 1985)

Schanz = M. SCHANZ, C. HOSIUS and G. KRÜGER (eds), *Geschichte der römischen Literatur bis zum Gesetzgebungswerk des Kaisers Justinian*, 4 vols (Munich, 1914–1935)

Schenkl = H. SCHENKL, *Bibliotheca patrum latinorum britannica. II, 3: Die schottischen Bibliotheken* (Vienna, 1896)

Scherer = V. SCHERER, *Die* Epistula de ratione ventris vel viscerum. *Ein Beitrag zur Geschichte des Galenismus im frühen Mittelalter*, Diss. med. dent. der Freien Universität Berlin (1977)

Schmalzbauer = G. SCHMALZBAUER, 'Medizinisch-diätetisches über die Podagra aus spätbyzantinischer Zeit', *Jahrbuch der Österreichischen Byzantinistik* 23 (1974), 229–43

Schmid, *Caelius Aurelianus* = P. SCHMID *Contributions à la critique du texte de Caelius Aurelianus*, Diss. Neuchâtel (1942)

Schuba = L. SCHUBA, *Die medizinischen Handschriften der Codices Palatini Latini in der Vatikanischen Bibliothek*, Kataloge der Universitätsbibliothek Heidelberg 1 (Wiesbaden, 1981)

Schubring, 'Epistula' = K. SCHUBRING, 'Epistula Paraxagorae', *Sudhoffs Archiv* 46 (1962), 295–310

Schubring, 'Petrizoneli' = K. SCHUBRING, 'Johann Petrizoneli und die Urheberschaft der "Practica"', *Sudhoffs Archiv* 46 (1962), 364–6

Schwyzer and Debrunner = E. SCHWYZER, *Griechische Grammatik*, vol. 2 suppl. and ed. A. Debrunner (Munich, 1950)

Seidler = E. SEIDLER, *Die Heilkunde des ausgehenden Mittelalters in Paris: Studien zur Struktur der spätscholastischen Medizin*, Sudhoffs Archiv Beiheft 8 (Wiesbaden, 1967)

Septier = A. SEPTIER, *Manuscrits de la bibliothèque d'Orléans* (Orléans, 1820)

Sezgin = F. SEZGIN, *Geschichte des arabischen Schrifttums. III. Medizin – Pharmazie – Zoologie – Tierheilkunde bis ca. 430 H.* (Leiden, 1970)

Sigerist, *Rezeptliteratur* = H. E. SIGERIST, *Studien und Texte zur frühmittelalterlichen Rezeptliteratur*, Studien zur Geschichte der Medizin 13 (Leipzig, 1923)

Sigerist, 'Maße und Gewichte' = H. E. SIGERIST, 'Maße und Gewichte in den medizinischen Texten des frühen Mittelalters', *Kyklos* 3 (1930), 439–44

Sigerist, 'A summer' = H. E. SIGERIST, 'A summer of research in European Libraries', *Bulletin of the Institutes of the History of Medicine* 2 (1934), 559–610

Sigerist, 'Italy' = H. E. SIGERIST, 'The medical literature of the early Middle Ages. A program – and a report of a summer of research in Italy', *Bulletin of the Institutes of the History of Medicine* 2 (1934), 26–50

Sigerist, 'The Sphere' = H. E. SIGERIST, 'The *Sphere of Life and Death* in early mediaeval manuscripts', *Bull. Hist. Med.* 11 (1942), 292–303

Sigerist, 'Vendôme' = H. E. SIGERIST, 'Early mediaeval medical texts in manuscripts of Vendôme', *Bull. Hist. Med.* 14 (1943), 68–113

Sigerist, 'Latin med. lit.' = H. E. SIGERIST, 'The Latin medical literature of the early Middle Ages', *JHM* 13 (1958), 127–45

Silverstein = Th. SILVERSTEIN, *Medieval Scientific Writings in the Barberini Collection. A Provisional Catalogue* (Chicago, 1957) (review by C. J. Ermatinger, *Manuscripta* 2 (1958), 100–1)

Silvestre = H. SILVESTRE, 'Incipits des traités médiévaux de sciences expérimentales dans les manuscrits latins de Bruxelles', *Scriptorium* 5 (1951), 145–60

Souter = A. SOUTER, *A Glossary of Later Latin to 600 A.D.* (Oxford, 1949)

von Staden, *Herophilus* = H. VON STADEN, *Herophilus. The Art of Medicine in Early Alexandria* (Cambridge, 1989)

Stauber = R. STAUBER, *Die Schedelsche Bibliothek: Ein Beitrag zur Geschichte der Ausbreitung der italienischen Renaissance, des deutschen Humanismus und der medizinischen Literatur* (ed. O. Hartig) (Nieuwkoop, 1908)

Steudel = J. STEUDEL, 'Medizinische Ausbildung in Deutschland 1600–1850', in S. Schwenk, G. Tilander and C. A. Willemsen (eds), *Et multum et multa* (Fs. K. Lindner) (Berlin, 1971), 393–420

Stoffregen = M. STOFFREGEN, *Eine frühmittelalterliche lateinische Übersetzung des byzantinischen Puls- und Urintraktats des Alexandros*, Diss. med. dent. der Freien Universität Berlin (1977)

Stok = F. STOK, 'I prologhi del *De pulsis et urinis* di "Alessandro"', in C. Santini, N. Scivoletto and L. Zurlì (eds), *Prefazioni, prologhi, proemi di opere tecnico-scientifiche latine*, 3 vols (Rome, 1990–1998), III, 259–83

Strohmaier = G. STROHMAIER, 'Die Rezeption und die Vermittlung: die Medizin in der byzantinischen und in der arabischen Welt', in M. D. Grmek (ed.), *Die Geschichte des medizinischen Denkens. Antike und Mittelalter* (Munich, 1996) (orig. *Storia del pensiero medico occidentale. I. Antichità e medioevo* (Rome/Bari, 1993)), 151–81

Sudhoff, *Chirurgie* = K. SUDHOFF, *Beiträge zur Geschichte der Chirurgie im Mittelalter: graphische und textliche Untersuchungen in mittelalterlichen Handschriften*, 2 parts, Studien zur Geschichte der Medizin 10 & 11/12 (Leipzig, 1914–1918)

Sudhoff, 'Unterricht' = K. SUDHOFF, 'Medizinischer Unterricht und seine Lehrbehelfe im frühen Mittelalter', *Archiv f. Gesch. der Medizin* 21 (1929) [= *KS/Fs. Sudhoff*], 28–37

Svennung, *Wortstudien* = J. SVENNUNG, *Wortstudien zu den spätlateinischen Oribasiusrezensionen* (Uppsala, 1932)

Svennung, *Palladius* = J SVENNUNG, *Untersuchungen zu Palladius und zur lateinischen Fach- und Volkssprache* (Uppsala, 1935)

Talbot = C. H. TALBOT, 'Some notes on Anglo-Saxon medicine', *Medical History* 9 (1965), 156–69

Temkin, 'Hippokratismus' = O. TEMKIN, 'Geschichte des Hippokratismus im ausgehenden Altertum', *Kyklos* 4 (1932), 1–80

Temkin, *Galenism* = O. TEMKIN, *Galenism. Rise and Decline of a Medical Philosophy* (Ithaca/London, 1973)

Thorndike, *History* = L. THORNDIKE, *A History of Magic and Experimental Science*, 8 vols (New York, 1923–1958)

Thorndike and Kibre = L. THORNDIKE and P. KIBRE, *A Catalogue of Incipits of Mediaeval Scientific Writings in Latin* (2nd edn, London, 1963)

ThLL = *Thesaurus Linguae Latinae* (Leipzig, 1900–)

Ullmann = M. ULLMANN, *Die Medizin im Islam* (Leiden, 1970)

Ullmann, *Islamic Medicine* = M. ULLMANN, *Islamic Medicine*, Islamic Surveys 11 (Edinburgh, 1978)

Väänänen, *Lat. vulg.* = V. VÄÄNÄNEN, *Introduction au latin vulgaire* (3rd edn, Paris, 1981)

Vázquez Buján = M. E. VÁZQUEZ BUJÁN, 'Problemas generales de las antiguas traducciones médicas latinas', *Studi medievali* 25 (1984), 641–80

Verzeichnis ... St. Gallen = *Verzeichnis der Handschriften der Stiftsbibliothek von St. Gallen* (Halle, 1875)

Vezin = J. VEZIN, *Les* scriptoria *d'Angers au XIe siècle* (Paris, 1974)

Vineis, *Itala* = E. VINEIS, *Studio sulla lingua dell' Itala* (Pisa, 1974)

Warner and Gilson = G. F. WARNER and J. P. GILSON, *Catalogue of Western Manuscripts in the Old Royal and King's Collections in the British Museum*, 4 vols (London, 1921)

Wellmann, 'Alex. Trall.' = M. WELLMANN, 'Alexandros aus Tralles', *PWRE* 1 (1894), 1460–1

Wellmann, 'Neue Schrift' = M. WELLMANN, 'Eine neue Schrift des Alexander von Tralles', *Hermes* 42 (1907), 533–41

Wickersheimer, 'Un manuscrit' = E. WICKERSHEIMER, 'Un manuscrit médical de l'époque carolingienne ayant appartenu à l'Abbaye d'Echternach [Par. lat. 11219]', *T'Hémecht, Zeitschrift für Luxemburger Geschichte* 6 (1953), 173–89

Wickersheimer, *Manuscrits* = E. WICKERSHEIMER, *Les manuscrits latins de médecine du haut moyen âge dans les bibliothèques de France* (Paris, 1966)

World Who's Who = *World Who's Who in Science: A Biographical Dictionary of Notable Scientists from Antiquity to the Present* (ed. A. G. Debus) (Chicago, 1968)

Wust = S. WUST, 'Bibliographie Johann Winters von Andernach', in *Johann Winter aus Andernach (Ioannes Guinterius Andernacus) 1505–1574. Ein Humanist und Mediziner des 16. Jahrhunderts*, Andernacher Beiträge 6 (Andernach, 1989), 52–85

Young and Aitken = J. YOUNG and P. HENDERSON AITKEN, *A Catalogue of the Manuscripts in the Library of the Hunterian Museum in the University of Glasgow* (Glasgow, 1908)

Zipser = B. ZIPSER, *Pseudo-Alexander Trallianus*, De oculis: *Einleitung, Text, Übersetzung und Kommentar*, Diss. Heidelberg (2003) (microfiche edition)

CHAPTER 1. ALEXANDER OF TRALLES AND THE *THERAPEUTICA*

1.1. Alexander of Tralles

The author of the Greek *Therapeutica* is identified with the Alexander mentioned by the contemporary Byzantine historian Agathias 'Scholasticus' of Myrina, writing of the year A.D. 557 (*Hist.* 5.6.5 Keydell), as one of the brothers of Anthemius, native of the city of Tralles (above modern Aydın) in the valley of the River Meander (modern Menderes) in the border region between ancient Lydia and Caria. According to Agathias, Alexander was one of five brothers,[1] each of whom achieved high distinction in his chosen profession.[2] Probably most notable of the five — and Agathias' main subject at this point — was the architect Anthemius (d. before A.D. 558), who was responsible for the building (A.D. 532–7) of the second Hagia Sophia in Constantinople, the first having been burnt down in the 'Nika' revolt of January A.D. 532.[3] The other brothers were Metrodorus the grammarian and teacher (who was summoned with Anthemius to Justinian's court), Olympius the jurist, and Dioscorus, who like Alexander became a doctor. While Dioscorus lived out his life in Tralles, practising medicine there with great success, Alexander in old age received an honourable summons to Rome and settled there.[4]

This seems to be all the external evidence that we have on Alexander of Tralles. It is unclear to me on what grounds his dates are commonly given as A.D. 525–605.[5] It is impossible to deduce from Agathias the chronological relation between Alexander's move to Rome and the events of the main narrative at this point (A.D. 557), although Agathias writes as if Alexander is no longer alive. The latest sources cited in the *Therapeutica* are Aëtius of Amida (sixth century, first half) and Jacobus Psychrestus (fifth to sixth century). Aëtius is cited once only, in the very last section of the book on fevers, which looks suspiciously like a later addition.[6] Jacobus is referred to three times, twice on gout and once on coughing, where Alexander includes a brief eulogy of the man.[7] These references are also

[1] Perhaps the youngest, as Agathias mentions him last, although this is stated as fact in many of the handbooks.

[2] This prompts Agathias to congratulate their mother, *Hist.* 5.6.5: μακαρίσαιμι ἂν ἔγωγε αὐτῶν τὴν μητέρα, οὕτω ποικίλης παιδείας ἀνάπλεων γονὴν ἀποκυήσασαν.

[3] See Mango's article in the *ODB*, with further references. Meyer, II, 379 ventures the view that Alexander's *Therapeutica* rivals his brother's church in endurance and brilliance(!).

[4] Agath., *Hist.* 5.6.5: ἅτερος δὲ ἐν τῇ πρεσβύτιδι Ῥώμῃ κατῴκησεν ἐντιμότατα μετακεκλημένος. Cf. J. R. Martindale (ed.), *The Prosopography of the Later Roman Empire*, Vol. IIIA (Cambridge, 1992), 44–5.

[5] These dates are given (confidently and consistently, but without being documented) by among others Sarton, 453; Ullmann, 85; Hunger, II, 297; Cameron, 69; Jacquart and Micheau, 22, 92; Scarborough in the *ODB*, s.v. 'Alexander of Tralles'. Alexander is perhaps the object of a tralaticious 'handbook-mythology', which includes as standard the statement that he travelled widely (see below) and flimsier pieces of embroidery, for example, that he travelled with the army, that he travelled in his early years, that he studied in Alexandria, that he was called to Rome because of the plague, perhaps by Pope Gregory the Great: for none of these is there a shred of evidence. Unfortunately, the soberest account of Alexander's life, that in Meyer's history of botany of all places (II, 379–80), was not taken as a model.

[6] I, 437–9 Puschmann = Aëtius 5.89 (p. 69, 14–70, 23 Olivieri). Puschmann (I, 437 n. 2) questions the authenticity of this chapter.

[7] On gout, II, 565, 11ff. (= 2.267 of the Latin version; also in the *De podagra*: see 3.2.5 below) and 570, 13ff.; on coughing, II, 163, 6ff.: τοῦτο τὸ φάρμακον Ἰακώβου τοῦ ψυχρηστοῦ ὀνομάζουσι, μεγάλου ἀνδρὸς καὶ θεοφιλεστάτου περὶ τὴν τέχνην γενομένου. ἐκαλεῖτο δὲ ψυχρηστὸς ὅτι ὑγραινούσῃ τροφῇ ἐκέχρητο. καὶ τοῦτο ποιεῖν ἐφαίνετο, ἐπειδὴ τοὺς πολλοὺς ἑώρα τῶν ἀνθρώπων φιλοπράγμονας ὄντας καὶ φιλαργύρους καὶ ἀεὶ ἐν λύπαις καὶ φροντίσιν ὅλον αὐτῶν ζῶντας τὸν βίον (= 2.12: 'Hoc enim medicamen ipsius Iacobi $\overline{\text{xpi}}$ [*sic*] esse nominatur magnifici uiri. Vocatus est autem ipse xps quia humidis cibis utebatur. Et hoc facere uidebatur quoniam multos uidebat hominum amicos rerum existentes et amatores esse pecuniarum et semper in tristiciis et sollicitudine in tota uita sua uixisse' [text of A]).

in the Latin tradition of the *Therapeutica*, and are certainly genuine. If Jacobus had reached the pinnacle of his career as personal doctor to the Emperor Leo I (d. A.D. 474),[8] a mid- or even early sixth-century date for Alexander becomes feasible,[9] rather than the usual very late sixth-/very early seventh-century date (above and n. 5). If it is possible that Alexander wrote the *Therapeutica* before A.D. 542, we need no longer wonder at his silence on the plague that reached Constantinople and Italy in that year.[10] An earlier dating of the completion of the Greek *Therapeutica* may have the further advantage of allowing time for the Latin version to be more closely associated with the late sixth-century translations of Oribasius and Rufus — if, that is, this traditional dating is correct, and if the association of the Latin Alexander with one or more versions of the Latin Oribasius seems on other grounds desirable (we shall return to this last question in 5.3.2 below).

The text of the *Therapeutica* itself offers very little additional information about the life of Alexander (on the information that it provides on Alexander as a doctor, see below, pp. 6–8). The short preface (I, 289 Puschmann) to the book on fevers transmitted in Greek and Latin traditions alike (see 1.2 below) as the last book of the *Therapeutica* represents the author as an aged doctor, no longer able to practise,[11] who at the behest of one Cosmas, the dedicatee,[12] is setting down the fruits of his experience of many years of medical practice,[13] and in plain and simple layman's language;[14] he is bound to accede to Cosmas' request among other reasons because Cosmas' father was one of his first teachers.[15] In addition, if we may trust the headings of the respective recipes, we learn that Alexander's father was named Stephanus and was also a doctor,[16] and that Alexander had picked up new remedies in person in Corfu, Gaul, and Spain.[17] The latter point has been taken to indicate that Alexander travelled widely,[18] perhaps with the army,[19] although there is no evidence for a military connection,[20] and it is noticeable and perhaps

[8] cf. Hunger, II, 290; Nutton, *DNP*, s.v. 'Iakobos Psychrestos'.

[9] Meyer, II, 380, argues from Agathias' dates that Alexander was writing *c.* A.D. 565. Riché, 185, who cites only Schanz and Brunet, *Alexandre*, has Alexander in Rome *c.* A.D. 560.

[10] Puschmann, I, 83 (followed by Thorndike, *History*, I, 575) has noted that the *Therapeutica* is curiously silent on the plague of A.D. 542. Indeed, the bubonic plague pandemics of A.D. 541–4, 557–61, 570–4, all of which affected Tralles, Constantinople, Rome, and Ravenna, cannot have escaped Alexander's attention, wherever he was living at the time; but it is striking that our sources on the many outbreaks of the Justinianic plague are rarely if ever medical writers, so this silence need not be indicative of date. See Biraben, I, 25–48, and Allen.

[11] I, 289, 8–9: γέρων ... καὶ κάμνειν οὐκέτι δυνάμενος.

[12] Identified, but purely speculatively, with Cosmas Indicopleustes, the author of *Cosmographia Christiana* (Puschmann, I, 83 n. 1; Bloch, 535 n. 2; Brunet, *Alexandre* I, 34–5).

[13] I, 289, 9–10: τοῦτο τὸ βιβλίον ἔγραψα συντάξας τὰς μετὰ πολλῆς τριβῆς ἐν ταῖς τῶν ἀνθρώπων νόσοις καταληφθείσας πείρας.

[14] I, 289, 12–14: ἐσπούδασα γὰρ, ὡς ἐνδέχεται, κοιναῖς καὶ μᾶλλον εὐδήλοις χρήσασθαι λέξεσιν, ἵνα καὶ τοῖς τυχοῦσιν ἐκ τῆς φράσεως εὔλυτον εἴη τὸ σύνταγμα.

[15] I, 289, 4–6: ὁ γὰρ [i.e. Cosmas' father] ἐξ ἀρχῆς εὐθὺς οὐ μόνον ἐν τοῖς ἔργοις τῆς τέχνης, ἀλλὰ καὶ τῶν κατὰ βίον πραγμάτων ἁπάντων δεξιὸς ὑπουργὸς ἐγένετο.

[16] cf. II, 139, 17: ἀναγαργάρισμα συναγχικοῖς ᾧ ἐχρήσατο Στέφανος ὁ πατήρ μου κἀγὼ καλόν.

[17] cf. I, 565, 1: ἄλλο ὅπερ ἔλαβον παρὰ Κερκυραίου ἀγροίκου, ... 565, 4: ἕτερον ὅπερ ἔλαβον ἐν Γαλλίᾳ, ... 565, 16: ἐν δ'Ἰσπανίᾳ πρὸς ἐπιληπτικοὺς τοῦτ' ἔμαθον (ἔλαβον Mf). Note also a few lines earlier I, 563, 11: ἔλαβον καὶ τοῦτο ἐν Τουσκίᾳ (Τουρκὶᾳ 2201 2202 L C, ἐν γῇ Περσῶν 2203 M) παρὰ ἀγροίκου τινός, which is taken to refer to Tuscany. The reading of Mf is slightly unclear, but Τουσκίᾳ would seem to be borne out by *Tuscia* in the Latin version. Some of the handbooks have North Africa instead of Corfu, presumably reading Κυρηναίου instead of Κερκυραίου at I, 565, 1 quoted above.

[18] Uncritically retailed by Langslow, *Medical Latin*, 70.

[19] For a particularly fanciful reconstruction (which has perhaps fed the handbook tradition), see Brunet, *Alexandre*, I, 14ff.

[20] The second part of the recommendation at 1.72: 'Hoc enim experimentatum est a multis, maxime autem a militibus' is hard to evaluate, as it is not in the Greek text (I, 565, 10). 2.134: 'scis enim a me curatum fuisse militem' is in the chapters from Philagrius (cf. 2.4.2 below).

suspicious that extensive travels should yield just three mentions of foreign remedies, all within the space of a single page, and all for the treatment of a single disease — epilepsy. On the other hand, seven references to 'in Rome', 'among the Romans'/'in Latin',[21] together with the mention in the preface to Cosmas of the author's old age, are at least consistent with Agathias' statement that Alexander moved to Rome late in life, and with the view that the *Therapeutica* was composed during Alexander's time in Rome.[22]

Alexander is held to have been a Christian. This is in itself perfectly plausible, although the evidence cited by Puschmann (I, 84) — the calling of the holy Old Testament names and the mention of Lot's wife in an incantation at the very end of the book on gout (II, 585, 9ff.) — is not compelling, as this material may easily be a later addition. The Latin version contains at 2.15 an allusion to the book of *Proverbs* (26:11) in the words 'like a dog returning to its own vomit' ('quemadmodum canis iterum ad uomicam reuertitur' [text of γ]). The Greek text, however, has only 'like dogs' (II, 245, 21, ὥσπερ οἱ κύνες), so that, as things stand, the biblical reference would bear only on the background of the translator, and not on that of Alexander himself.[23]

We may infer that Alexander's patients included the well-to-do from the wide range of hard-to-obtain and expensive ingredients that his remedies often call for (e.g. II, 37, 11, crocodile droppings),[24] and from occasional pieces of circumstantial evidence regarding the means and way of life of his patients, such as a reference to one sufferer from brain-fever (φρενῖτις) with a large number of servants in his house (I, 515, 20–1), or the fact that Alexander prescribes, for the treatment of certain stomach ailments, visits to hot springs, sea-voyages, and long spells overseas (II, 249, 23–5).[25]

Puschmann (followed by Bloch, 536, and Neuburger, II, 110) states that those parts of the *Therapeutica* which are in the form of academic lecture-notes indicate that Alexander must have taught medicine — where, he does not say — but he gives no references to the passages that he has in mind. A phrase of the sort 1.129 *init.*, 'tempus autem mutari nos cogit ad . . . ' is at first glance suggestive of the context of a lecture, but the Latin appears to overtranslate the Greek at this point, which has nothing corresponding to *cogit* (II, 123, 23f., μεταβαίνειν ἤδη καιρὸς πρὸς . . .), and καιρός

[21] I, 327, 17–18: διόπερ οὐδὲ τοὺς ἔχοντας ἀσθενῆ πάνυ τὴν δύναμιν δεῖ σκαφολουτρεῖν, ὅ ἐστι παρὰ Ῥωμαίοις εἰς τίναν ἐμβαλεῖν; I, 373, 24–5: εὗρον δ' ἐγὼ πολλοὺς τῶν ἐν Ῥώμῃ ἰατρῶν οὐδ' ὄνομα τολμῶντας ὀνομάσαι τῶν πεπόνων ὡς χολὴν τικτόντων αὐτῶν (not in the Latin); I, 457, 1–2: θαψίας, ᾗτινι οἱ βαφεῖς χρῶνται, ἣν οἱ Ῥωμαῖοι ἐρβαρυβίαν καλοῦσι (1.13: 'herba rubea'); II, 191, 21: κεχρήσθω τῷ παρὰ Ῥωμαίοις καλουμένῳ φαριχύλῳ (2.164: 'suco uteris farris'); II, 261, 19: καὶ ἡ παρὰ Ῥωμαίοις καλουμένη μέλκα (2.27: 'melca'); II, 513, 20–2: λαμβανέτωσαν ἢ ῥοσάτου ἢ ἀψινθάτου ψυχρίζοντες ὡσαύτως, καθάπερ εἰώθασι ποιεῖν οἱ Ῥωμαῖοι τὸ καλούμενον ῥεκεντάτον = 2.242 *ad fin.*: 'bibant rosatum aut absintiatum infrigdatum in aqua frigida quemadmodum Rome facere consueuer(unt) q(uo)d appellant recentatum' (text of A). II, 541, 33–543, 1: ἐγὼ γοῦν οἶδα τῶν πάνυ διαφανεστάτων ἀνδρῶν τινα ἐν τῇ Ῥώμῃ τῇ διὰ τῶν ἁλῶν ἀεὶ χρώμενον πυρίᾳ = 2.259: 'Ego igitur scio q(ue)ndam nobilissimum uirum Rome de salibus fom(en)tationibus semp(er) usum fuisse' (text of A).

[22] Brunet, *Alexandre* I, 46–7, insists that the references to Rome/Latin (see n. 21) make it absolutely clear that Alexander did not write the *Therapeutica* in Rome.

[23] cf. Wellmann, 'Neue Schrift', 541.

[24] Note, however, that Alexander states at II, 205, 12–15 (on those spitting blood) that he has often treated patients successfully without recourse to costly drugs.

[25] cf. Duffy, 26 n. 36, who notes also the injunction to carry a sneezing-ointment in a box made of horn (I, 493, 19–20). Cf. also II, 541, 33: ἐγὼ γοῦν οἶδα τῶν πάνυ διαφανεστάτων ἀνδρῶν τινα ἐν τῇ Ῥώμῃ τῇ διὰ τῶν ἁλῶν ἀεὶ χρώμενον πυρίᾳ = 2.259: 'Ego igitur scio quendam nobilissimum uirum Romae de salibus fomentationibus semper usum fuisse' (text of A), but note that Alexander does not say that he treated this man, nor even that he knew him (Puschmann's 'ich kenne einen . . . , bei dem' is misleading; cf. the Latin *scio* with acc. + inf.). Note also 1.9 (in Greek only in ms. Mf): 'Cogimur saepius ab amicis... et maxime a potentibus aut regibus'.

ἐστι is elsewhere used expressly of composing a written work (I, 535, 4, οὐ νῦν ἐστι καιρὸς γράφειν = 1.60 *fin.*, 'non est nunc tempus scribere').[26]

1.2. Works Ascribed to Alexander of Tralles

In addition to the *Therapeutica* (introduced below) several other works of more or less doubtful authenticity are ascribed to Alexander. Transmitted under his name in the Greek tradition are shorter works on, respectively, fevers, intestinal worms, the eyes, and the pulse and the urine in diagnosis. If Alexander appears to refer to works of his own on head-wounds and fractures, no other trace of these survives.[27]

The work Περὶ πυρετῶν, preceded by the dedication to Cosmas already mentioned (and printed by Puschmann (I, 289–439) at the front of the *Therapeutica*), may safely be regarded as genuine. There is probably a reference to it in the *Therapeutica* (II, 313, 11–12; not in Latin), and moreover it is transmitted as Book 12 of the *Therapeutica* in all the non-fragmentary Greek manuscripts (and in the Latin tradition). In terms of style, it is much more carefully written than the *Therapeutica*, but in terms of its medical approach it is very much of a piece with the longer work, and numerous linguistic and structural agreements between the two works strongly support the traditional attribution.[28] Failing indication to the contrary, references to the *Therapeutica* in the present work should be taken to include the book on fevers.

The Περὶ ἑλμίνθων, which takes the form of a letter addressed to a certain Theodorus,[29] is generally accepted as genuine. The manuscripts are unanimous in ascribing it to Alexander, and the style and content are perfectly consistent with Alexander's authorship (see Puschmann, I, 105).

A work Περὶ ὀφθαλμῶν in two books is interpolated in some of the Greek manuscripts of the *Therapeutica*, although the preface to the two books interpolated in Greek manuscript M states that the work was originally in three books.[30] Now, Alexander refers (II, 3, 2 = 1.85 in the Latin) to an earlier work of his own on the eyes in three books, and there are references in the Arabic tradition to a translation of Alexander's work on the eyes in three books. Nevertheless, on grounds of form, style, and content, the Περὶ ὀφθαλμῶν is regarded as spurious by Puschmann, Hirschberg,[31] and now Zipser.

Also rejected as spurious is the diagnostic work on the pulse and the urine in fever ascribed to 'the doctor Alexander', transmitted in Greek in Par. gr. 2316 (fifteenth

[26] cf. also II, 283, 3–4: ὧν οὐκ ἔστι καιρὸς μνημονεύειν νῦν = 2.37.11: 'de quibus nunc tempus non est ad commemorandum'.

[27] Alexander alludes to a discussion (written rather than oral) of wounds to the head and other parts of the body at I, 485, 11–12: τελεώτερον δὲ λεχθήσεται,ἡνίκα περὶ τῶν ἐν κεφαλῇ τραυμάτων καὶ τῶν ἐν τοῖς ἄλλοις μορίοις συνισταμένων τὸν λόγον ποιούμεθα (the Latin translation is poor, to say the least! 1.33: 'Perfectius scilicet dictum est de uulnerato capite quod in aliis locis consistente libro fecimus' (text of A)). The reference to a work on fractures is not unequivocal: I, 535, 5–6: ἐν τῷ (ἔνθα Mf) περὶ καταγμάτων (λόγῳ 2203 M) = 1.60 *fin.*: 'ubi de fracturis conuenit [contigit *ed.*] loqui'. On a putative work of Alexander on poisons, see Wellmann, 'Neue Schrift'.

[28] See Puschmann's discussion, I, 102–4.

[29] Edited by Puschmann at the end of the *Therapeutica* (II, 586–99). There is a French translation and a bland appraisal by Barbillion, 71–9. De Lucia has recently published a hitherto unknown redaction of the work, from Par. Suppl. gr. 631 (I owe this reference to Cloudy Fischer).

[30] Edited by Puschmann in the *Nachträge*, 130–79.

[31] Puschmann, I, 107, is prepared to entertain the possibility that it is a work of Alexander's youth, but clearly favours alien authorship. Hirschberg (apud Bloch, 536) sees the treatise as the work of a novice from a very late date.

century) and (in two versions) in numerous Latin manuscripts (see below). Puschmann even opines (I, 105–6) that the Greek is a translation of the Latin, although he is apparently alone in this view.[32]

Of the above-mentioned works we have in Latin the *Therapeutica* together with the work on fevers, and the treatise on the pulse and the urine. In the Latin tradition the connection between the *Therapeutica* and the *De febribus* is as close as it is in the Greek: in virtually all the Latin manuscripts the *Therapeutica* constitutes Books 1 and 2, the work on fevers the third and final book of what I am calling (in shorthand) throughout the present work 'the Latin Alexander'.[33] This is introduced systematically below (2.3).

The Latin *De pulsibus et urinis* ascribed to 'Alexander' survives in numerous manuscripts in not one but two early medieval translations made separately from Greek copies deriving from a single Greek archetype.[34] Stoffregen reports that his comparisons of the Latin *De pulsibus* with the Latin Alexander yielded only negative results,[35] but the two works are nonetheless bound together in that the *De pulsibus* is transmitted either with the Latin Alexander proper (notably in Angers 457, my A; see p. 40) or, much more commonly, with the (pseudo-)Galenic early medieval ensemble of medical texts (Galen, *Ad Glauconem de medendi methodo*; the '*Liber tertius*'; Theodorus Priscianus; Aurelius; Esculapius) which frequently contains the reworking of the Latin Alexander on gout.[36]

While apt to be confused with Alexander of Aphrodisias, Alexander of Tralles is also well represented in the Arabic medical tradition from the tenth century onwards, although his works survive here only in citations.[37] Together with Oribasius, Aëtius, and especially Paul of Aegina, Alexander enjoyed considerable prestige in early medieval Arab scientific circles, where he is known as the author of separate works on intestinal worms, the eyes, and fevers, and of a 'compendium' or 'handbook' (*kunnāš*) in a longer and a shorter version, known from an early date in an Arabic translation which has not survived but which is much cited. If the last can refer to longer and shorter versions of the *Therapeutica*, this list of treatises matches exactly that of the genuine works in the Greek tradition. Other books on various other particular diseases, ascribed by Arabic writers to Alexander Trallianus, may, if genuine, be separately transmitted parts of the *Therapeutica*.[38]

Excerpts from one or more of Alexander's works are reported to exist also in Hebrew in a medical compendium composed in the year 1199. The basis of the Hebrew translation is said to be a Latin version, but one containing numerous Arabic words (not a feature of the extant Latin Alexander).[39]

[32] cf. Baader, 'Latin adaptations', 253–6.

[33] On the other hand, in contrast to the Greek tradition, the *De febribus* is transmitted separately in Latin, if (to my knowledge) in only one manuscript, namely Barcelona, Ripoll 181 (early thirteenth century), described in 3.3 below, p. 90. On the book-divisions of the Latin Alexander in Paris, lat. 6882 (my P3), see 2.3.3 and 3.1.1 below, pp. 18–20, 51.

[34] On the transmission, see Stoffregen, 7–71 (on the two versions and their relations to the Greek original, especially 30–2) and Stok, 259–83. On the *De pulsibus et urinis*, note also Noßke; *BTML*, 31–2, nos 2–5; *BTML Suppl.*, 13, no. A-3; and Nutton's judicious article in *DNP*, s.v. 'Alexandros' [30].

[35] Stoffregen, 147.

[36] This may account for the ascription of the work in some manuscripts to Galen. Stoffregen notes that the *De pulsibus* enjoys a secondary tradition in the Latin Galen, *Ad Glauconem*. On this ensemble, and the *De podagra*, see 3.2.5 and 3.2.6.

[37] On the Arabic tradition of Alexander, see Puschmann, I, 92–5; Bloch, 537–8; Sezgin, 162–4; Ullmann, 85–6; Zipser, xviii–xix.

[38] A work on urine (mentioned by Zipser, xviii) may merit comparison with the pseudonymous work on the pulse and the urine discussed above. Cf. Puschmann, I, 93–4 n. 3, on the disease 'birsen', and Zipser, xviii n. 19.

[39] On the Hebrew excerpts, see Puschmann, I, 91; 96 (who also alludes to a possible translation of Alexander from Latin into Syriac), and Bloch, 538.

Much more significant, finally, are the excerpts from the Latin Alexander which appear, in Old English, in the medical compendium known as Bald's *Leechbook* (before A.D. 900; on which, see Cameron, 'Bald's *Leechbook*', and Adams and Deegan). Further description, and indeed collation and evaluation, of the Old English excerpts is a regrettable omission from the present work, and an important desideratum in further editorial work on the Latin text.

1.3. The Character and Reception of the *Therapeutica*

The *Therapeutica* sets out diagnosis and treatment of a large number of (mainly internal) diseases, ordered for the most part *a capite ad calcem*, from hair-loss to gout (see the summary in Table 2.1, pp. 15–16 below). The aim of the work throughout is thoroughly practical: it is to be a handbook of therapy for the practising doctor,[40] enabling the correct recognition of a disease and its treatment. While some parts of the *Therapeutica* are carefully composed and finished, others seem incomplete and resemble rather the notes and collected recipes of a busy doctor (Puschmann, I, 102; 104). The work is indeed based largely on the author's experience, and consequently — and appropriately enough in a therapeutic manual — relevant theory is, at most, mentioned in passing, and other areas of medicine — including anatomy, physiology, surgery, and gynaecology — are barely touched on.[41]

As for its medical background, the *Therapeutica* owes most to Hippocrates and Galen. Like all doctors of his time, Alexander belonged 'zu den galenischen Hippokratikern',[42] but gives perhaps a better picture than any later medical writer of the key principles that defined the Hippocratic doctor in the last centuries of antiquity.[43] Nevertheless, Alexander has been held to stand out from his contemporaries through a degree of eclecticism and originality, doctrinal independence reflecting his own experience, and the courage to speak his own mind. He cites by name numerous medical authorities in addition to those already mentioned, including Archigenes of Apamea, Asclepiades the Younger (ὁ φαρμακίων), Damocrates of Athens, Didymus of Alexandria, Dioscorides, Erasistratus, Philagrius, Rufus of Ephesus, and Xenocrates of Aphrodisias,[44] but he is anything but a mere compiler: his authorial persona (and personality) are ever present, he frequently recommends his own remedies,[45] and throughout his work the most important factor in his analyses and determinant of his prescriptions is his own personal experience, πεῖρα. As Duffy so aptly puts it, 'He chooses truth over authority, and the deciding factor is always experience'.[46]

[40] And ostensibly also for the interested layman — if, that is, we may take at face-value the final words of the preface (cf. n. 14 above).

[41] See Temkin, 'Hippokratismus', 39. On anatomy and physiology, see Puschmann, I, 108–11.

[42] Temkin, 'Hippokratismus', 36.

[43] See Temkin, *Galenism*, 118; 'Hippokratismus', 36, 39, including the remark that the absence of prognosis in Alexander is in striking contrast with the Hippocratic texts. Alexander praises Hippocrates and Galen together at the beginning of the book on fevers, I, 291, 6: τοῖς ἀρίστοις τῶν ἰατρῶν ἀποδέδεικται Γαληνῷ τε μάλιστα καὶ Ἱπποκράτει.

[44] For references, see Puschmann's index of personal names, II, 600; on Alexander's sources, see Puschmann, I, 85; on his place in the transmission of recipe-literature, see Sigerist, *Rezeptliteratur*, 186 (and Index, s.v. Alexander von Tralleis).

[45] See e.g. I, 547, 2: καὶ τοῖς ὑπ' ἐμοῦ κατασκευασθεῖσι καταποτίοις κεχρήσθωσαν, ὧν οὐδὲν εὗρον ἰσχυρότερον; cf. the similarly strong recommendation at e.g. II, 345, 6; 427, 5.

[46] Duffy, 25.

Alexander's professional and independent approach is most noticeable — and most remarked — in connection with Galen, who, although always quoted and referred to with the greatest of respect, is not infrequently criticized by Alexander, above all in the book on fevers.[47] At the start of this book, for example, he sets out expressly to follow as far as possible the teaching of Galen on quotidian fevers (I, 291, 2–3: τὴν τοῦ θειοτάτου Γαληνοῦ διδασκαλίαν, ὡς οἷόν τέ ἐστι, κἀνταῦθα μιμούμενοι). Within five pages, however, he has twice criticized Galen's mode of treatment (I, 297, 5ff.; 301, 12ff.). After the second occasion he adds an avowal that he does not mean to be contrary, but that the truth seemed to him to be so, and the truth was always to be honoured above all else.[48] The truth is emphatically assigned the same pre-eminent position after another extended criticism of Galen in which Alexander uses Galen's own words of criticism of Archigenes (*Comp. loc.* 2 = 12.535, 4–6 Kühn) (in the section on coughing, II, 155, 16–22, unfortunately not included in the Latin version): the truth must always be preferred, and moreover the doctor who has formed an opinion has a grave moral obligation to express it. Had he not thought silence to be a sin, and had the truth not given him courage, Alexander says here, he would not have dared to say such things about such a paragon of learning.[49] As Temkin observes,[50] Alexander does not find it easy to criticize Galen, and much prefers it when he can show that Galen was misunderstood.[51]

On the other hand, Alexander is not averse to criticizing the doctors of his own day (generally referred to as πολλοὶ, οἱ πολλοὶ, οἱ πολλοὶ τῶν ἰατρῶν): he takes them to task on dozens of occasions for applying — whether through ignorance, lack of concern, or both[52] — treatments that do more harm than good.[53] Alexander, although 'completely orthodox in theory',[54] is evidently aware that some of his treatments are out of line with current or even time-honoured practice. These include his preference for relying where appropriate on diet and exercise rather than on drugs,[55] and his avoidance of certain substances known to have potentially harmful side-effects.[56] Alexander's key criteria here, in advocating or rejecting a particular form of treatment, are the efficacy of

[47] In addition to the passages quoted in this paragraph, note e.g. I, 305, 11; 333, 6; 379, 19; 387, 14; 407, 22; 421, 4; II, 83, 15; 203, 23. Alexander's criticism of Galen is noted by among others Wellmann, 'Alex. Trall.', 1461; Kudlien in *DKP*, s.v. 'Alexandros' (23); Ullmann, 311, and idem, *Islamic Medicine*, 22, 107–8; Sezgin, 163 and n. 1 on Rhazes' frequent reference to Alexander's criticism of Galen.

[48] I, 301, 18–20: καὶ ταῦτα λέγω οὐδαμῶς εἰς ἀντιλογίαν ἀφορῶν, ἀλλ' ὅτι μοι τὸ ἀληθὲς οὕτως ἐφάνη ἔχον. δεῖ δὲ τὸ ἀληθὲς παντὸς προτιμᾶν ἀεί.

[49] II, 155, 16–18: καὶ ταῦτα δὲ λέγειν οὐκ ἄν ἐτόλμησα περὶ τηλικούτου ἀνδρὸς εἰς σοφίαν, εἰ μὴ τό τε ἀληθὲς αὐτὸ θαρρῆσαί με προετρέψατο καὶ τὸ σιωπῆσαι πάλιν ἀσεβὲς ἐνόμισα.

[50] Temkin, 'Hippokratismus', 36.

[51] As at I, 373, 30–2 (on tertian fever, where Alexander seeks to refute a misreading of a passage in a work of Galen (unidentified) Περὶ τροφῶν): ἔκαμον οὖν ἐγὼ οὐ μικρῶς, ἵνα δυνηθῶ πεῖσαι τοὺς παρακολουθεῖν δυναμένους, ὅτι οὐ χολὴν ἐνταῦθα λέγει τίκτειν αὐτοὺς, ἀλλὰ χολέραν ποιεῖν.

[52] Note e.g. I, 521, 22–3: πολλοὶ γὰρ ἀμελοῦσι καὶ οὐκ ἴσασιν, ὅσα δύναται βλάψαι καὶ ὠφελῆσαι ἡ δίαιτα τὸν κάμνοντα.

[53] Note e.g. I, 583, 2–3: πολλοὶ γὰρ ... οὕτω ποιοῦσιν οὐκ εἰδότες, ὅτι μᾶλλον ἄχρηστον αὐτὸ ἀπεργάζονται. For other criticisms of οἱ πολλοί, cf. e.g. I, 307, 6; 381, 22; 389, 8; 577, 3; II, 5, 2–4; 231, 13, 25; 397, 15, *et passim*.

[54] Duffy, 25.

[55] On diet, note e.g. I, 601, 10–11; II, 439, 3–8; on exercise, II, 457, 14–16. Note, however, that dietetics was about to enjoy a new wave of popularity in the West, witness Anthimus' (early sixth-century) treatise dedicated to Theoderic King of the Franks, and various dietetic compilations circulating already in ninth-century manuscripts, including one, the *Liber diaetarum* (3.2.4 below), excerpted mainly from the Latin Alexander. See MacKinney, *Medicine*, 42–5 and nn., esp. n. 75.

[56] Note e.g. I, 609, 22–7 against the use of white hellebore, notwithstanding time-honoured practice; II, 123, 19–21, against the use of the commonly-prescribed στρύχνος.

the therapy and above all the well-being of the patient. These criteria rely on his own practical clinical experience for their measurement and on his intellectual honesty and independence for their report.

These themes are also drawn together in another characteristic feature of Alexander's therapeutics, commented on in nearly all the handbooks,[57] namely the relatively significant role he assigns to magical remedies, including amulets and incantations. This has disappointed some of Alexander's admirers, although others excuse it as a superstition characteristic of the age.[58] In a refinement of the latter view, Nutton sees the prominence of φυσικά τε καὶ περίαπτα in Alexander's work as evidence of a new general feature of 'medicine in the Christian empire — the emergence into acceptability of remedies that had earlier been excluded',[59] and he cites the nice example of the remedy for epilepsy including gladiator's blood which was rejected by earlier medical writers as 'falling outside the profession of medicine', but which is given by Alexander as a well-proven remedy.[60] The remedies are certainly there, and it may well be that Christianity 'gave a sort of sanction to this white magic',[61] but, as Duffy shows,[62] to be fair to Alexander it is important to take account of what he says in his five or six discussions, some of them extensive, of the use of these so-called 'natural' remedies. It emerges clearly from Alexander's in places slightly defensive remarks that this is a delicate and controversial subject, and still far from central to standard medical practice. Because most people (doctors?) frown on those who use φυσικά, Alexander explains, he has avoided prescribing them incessantly, and favours instead the τεχνικὴ μέθοδος, which through diet and drugs yields excellent results (I, 573, 2–6). Nevertheless, in cases where a patient is unable to follow a diet or tolerate a particular drug, the doctor is obliged to use φυσικά (II, 579, 14), and indeed, in cases where all else has failed, it would be morally wrong (ἀσεβές) for him not to try every possible way of helping the patient (II, 319, 2ff.). These other remedies can be effective (I, 557, 16), as even Galen found (II, 319, 9f.; 475, 4ff.), and, as Alexander concludes in his first preamble on φυσικά (in the chapter on epilepsy), it is appropriate that they be set out for the interested doctor so that he has the full range of treatments available to him for helping his patient.[63] If some find this a weak justification for employing magic and superstition,[64] Alexander's defence of his approach provides further testimony to his own doctrinal independence, his intellectual courage in speaking out, and his emphasis on the well-being of the patient, and important evidence of on the one hand a more conservative medical establishment and on the other a greater openness to 'non-conventional medicine' among the upper classes than seems to be generally supposed.

[57] See e.g. Puschmann, I, 86–7, Strohmaier, 162f., and especially Thorndike, *History*, I, 579–82; the theme dominates Kudlien's short article in *DKP*, s.v. 'Alexandros' (23).

[58] See, for example, Meyer, II, 379–80; Wellmann, 'Alex. Trall.'; Neuburger, II, 110–11; Brunet, *Alexandre* I, 41–2.

[59] Nutton, 'Galen to Alexander', 8.

[60] Scrib. Larg. 17: 'extra medicinae professionem'; cf. Cels. 3.23.7; Plin., *Nat.* 28.4; Alex. Trall. I, 565, 7–10, ending δέδωκε δὲ πεῖραν πολλάκις ἐξαίρετον.

[61] Nutton, 'Galen to Alexander', 9.

[62] In his penetrating article on aspects of teaching and practice in sixth- and seventh-century Byzantine medicine, esp. p. 26, to which this paragraph is much indebted. Cf. also Brunet, *Alexandre* I, 42–4.

[63] I, 557, 17–18: ὥστε τὸν ἰατρὸν πανταχόθεν εὔπορον εἶναι εἰς τὸ βοηθεῖν δύνασθαι τοῖς κάμνουσιν. Cf. I, 573, 1: ἐγὼ δὲ φιλῶ πᾶσι κεχρῆσθαι.

[64] See, for example, Hunger, 298.

Although in Duffy's eyes 'a minute figure in the pageant of Greek Science' (contrast the selection of, say, Jacques Despars in the fifteenth century, below), Alexander wins high praise from the historian's point of view in that he 'deserves to be taken at face value' for being 'one of the very few Byzantine medical writers who bring us close to the physician in action'. Duffy's article is surely influential in the most recent evaluation of Alexander, that of Vivian Nutton in *DNP* (characteristically combining medical, philological, and medico-historical perspectives), which shows a new aspect to the appreciation of Alexander's work — viz. as a source of information on contemporary medical practice, in importance and reliability second only to the works of Galen.[65] In Alexander, given his practical and down-to-earth aims, his conscious effort to communicate, the candour and courage he displays in his remarks on magic (above), a long-unheeded voice is at long last heard and acknowledged as a trustworthy supplement, even replacement, for the one-sided evidence of papyri and hagiography, our only other sources for the little that we know of a doctor's life in the centuries just before and after the end of the Roman Empire in the West.[66]

This is not the only current view produced by the passing of the custody and criticism of texts in the history of medicine from doctors to historians and philologists. Other recent assessments of Alexander's significance are more sober, perhaps in reaction to the earlier exuberance of medical men. In particular, Alexander's originality is repeatedly called into question, notably by Gerhard Baader in the Dumbarton Oaks symposium volume,[67] and in the fifth edition of Meyer-Steineg and Sudhoff's textbook, which here may show the work of Fridolf Kudlien's revisor's hand:[68] at any rate, Kudlien's summing-up in his *DSB* article on Alexander is reserved almost to the point of grudgingness.[69]

Among his successors in the medical profession, however, Alexander has enjoyed consistently high renown, both as a doctor and as a medical writer. Daremberg's brief but elegant eulogy in *Histoire des sciences médicales* (I, 248) is notable for foregrounding the fact that Alexander practised in Italy: 'la Grèce reparaît un instant en Italie et non sans éclat'. To modern taste, perhaps, Puschmann and Neuburger wax rather lyrical on Alexander, Puschmann comparing him to fresh autumn shoots on the bare trees of a Byzantine scientific culture otherwise prepared for a long hibernation,[70]

[65] 'Seine Schriften vereinen beachtliche Kenntnis älterer Literatur mit Erfahrungsberichten aus seiner eigenen langjährigen Arztpraxis und vermitteln abgesehen von den Schriften Galens die besten Einblicke in den Arbeitsalltag eines antiken Arztes.'

[66] See Duffy, 25–7.

[67] Baader, 'Adaptations', 252: 'No Byzantine medical writings of significant originality were translated into Vulgar Latin, and these are the treatises which Temkin (*Double Face of Janus*, 202) has characterized as having a new combination of empiricism and tradition'.

[68] cf. Meyer-Steineg and Sudhoff, 102: 'heute in seiner Kompilatorenabhängigkeit erkannt, auch nicht frei vom Aberglauben seiner Zeit'.

[69] *DSB*, I, 121: 'In summary, one may state that Alexander was, as a representative of Byzantine medicine, rather refreshing, not uninteresting, and not, perhaps, altogether unimportant.' Kudlien regards Puschmann as 'perhaps biased in favor of his subject'.

[70] Puschmann, I, 74–5: 'Die byzantinische Culturperiode hat die Entwickelung der Wissenschaften nur wenig gefördert; aber ihr fiel die Aufgabe zu, die geistigen Errungenschaften der Vergangenheit zu erhalten und der Nachwelt zu übermitteln. Die Medicin begann den fast tausendjährigen Winterschlaf geistiger Erstarrung, aus dem sie erst durch die Glockentöne, welche mit dem Wiedererwachen der Wissenschaft die Freiheit des Forschens, das Morgenlicht der neuen Zeit verkündeten, zu neuer Thätigkeit erwachte. Aber gleich wie manchmal im Herbst die schon entlaubten Bäume noch einmal frische Blüthen treiben, so gebar diese Zeit einen Mann, der originell im Denken und Handeln, noch einmal den Glanz vergangener Pracht und Grösse entfaltete. Dieser Arzt, welchen Freind neben Hippokrates und Aretaeus stellt, ist: A l e x a n d e r v o n T r a l l e s.'

Neuburger invoking the image of an oasis in the desert of Byzantine literature,[71] but their verdicts and the virtues they single out for praise — Alexander's freshness, his originality, the high quality of his clinical observations — may be taken as representative of medieval and modern judgements down to the middle of the twentieth century. Lynn Thorndike writes of Alexander's originality, his resource and ingenuity, his medieval influence, and praises his 'concise and orderly method of presentation', which 'compares favorably with that of the classical medical writers',[72] while Félix Brunet in the long biographical introduction to his four-volume translation and commentary on the works of Alexander[73] is hardly less lyrical in his praise than Puschmann and Neuburger.[74] Paul Diepgen sees in the work of Aëtius, Alexander, and Paul of Aegina the acme of Byzantine medicine,[75] and for Loren MacKinney Alexander was simply 'the greatest Greek physician of the sixth century'.[76]

In the early modern period, Alexander became and remained a canonical author. He was, for example, one of only four Greek writers used by Jacques Despars in preparing (from 1432 to 1453) his commentary on the *Canon* of Avicenna (Ibn Sīnā; A.D. 980–1037).[77] His works were among the first ancient medical treatises to be printed, first in the ancient Latin version at Lyons in 1504 (**Plate VIII**), then in Humanist Latin versions, in Greek, and in bilingual editions (see Chapter 2), and he was included in Henricus Stephanus' collection of central ancient medical authors (1567).[78] He was set beside Hippocrates and Aretaeus by the great English doctor John Freind in his magnum opus, *The History of Physick*,[79] and retained in the same illustrious company in Albrecht von Haller's *Artis medicae principes*.[80] He was still a prescribed author in German medical faculties in the sixteenth and seventeenth centuries.[81]

The importance of Alexander's works for the medieval period is clear from the rich manuscript traditions of the *Therapeutica*, and from the extent to which Alexander is excerpted or used as a source by later medical writers and compilers. In the East, these

[71] Neuburger, II, 110–11: 'Dieses Werk bildet wahrhaft eine erfrischende Oase in der Wüste der byzantinischen Literatur, ja es erinnert stellenweise an die unbefangene Beobachtungskunst eines Hippokrates, an die lebendige, anschauliche Schilderung eines Aretaios ... Die Schriften des Alexandros übten sehr bedeutenden Einfluß auf die Entwicklung der Medizin; ...; durch sie blieb wenigstens ein nachahmungswürdiges Vorbild der echten ärztlichen Beobachtung und Kritik selbst in den dunkelsten Zeiten erhalten.'

[72] Thorndike, *History*, I, 575–84, here at 576.

[73] Brunet, *Alexandre*, I, 1–90.

[74] Brunet's work is subtitled *Le dernier auteur classique des grands médecins grecs de l'antiquité*. Cf. the assessment of Bariéty and Coury, 232, 'le plus grand sans doute de tous les médecins byzantins'.

[75] Diepgen, 167.

[76] MacKinney, *Medicine*, 48.

[77] Jacques Despars of Tournai (Jacobus de Partibus; 1380?–1458) worked directly from a corpus comprising the works of the five most famous Arabic medical writers (Avenzoar, Rhazes, Serapion, Mesue, and Averroes) and four Greeks, namely Hippocrates, Aristotle, Galen, and Alexander of Tralles. He tells us that he first corrected all the texts (except those of Rhazes), divided them into chapters, had them copied on parchment, and provided them each with a table of contents. Much of his work may be reflected in the ϕ recension of the Latin Alexander (4.5 below), which certainly contains many of his interlinear notes and glosses.

[78] In Winter's edition, on col. 133–346 of this monumental work, which contains 31 treatises in 1,940 pages. Cf. Wust, 82.

[79] John Freind (1675–1728) — chemist, doctor (from 1727 Court Physician), and politician — in the first section (on Alexander) of *The History of Physick; From the Time of Galen to the Beginning of the Sixteenth Century*, 2 vols (London 1725–1726; 5th edn 1758). Cf. the article on Freind by Marie Boas Hall in the *DSB*, V, 156f.

[80] In vols 6–7 of *Artis medicae principes*, recensuit praefatus est Albertus de Haller, 11 vols, (Lausanne, 1769–1774). I am grateful for this reference to Hubert Steinke. Cf. Wust, 82.

[81] Steudel, 396.

include Paul of Aegina,[82] Theophanes Chrysobalantes (formerly Nonnus),[83] Nicolaus Myrepsus,[84] and Johannes Actuarius.[85] And the same is true in the West, for — to return in conclusion to the main theme of this study — we do well to remember not only the influence that Alexander's works exerted in translation,[86] especially in Latin and Arabic, but also the esteem in which he and his writings were held, as attested by the very fact of their selection for the costly process of translation.[87] Writing of the West, and Anglo-Saxon medicine in particular, Cameron[88] includes (the Latin) Alexander with (the Latin) Oribasius and Cassius Felix as 'the three authors most influential in the transmission to later times of classical medicine in the tradition of Galen'. Some would disagree,[89] others might substitute or add one or more other names, or at least seek a definition of 'later times'. The fact remains that Alexander was chosen as one of remarkably few Greek medical authors for translating into Latin — probably the last so to be chosen at the end of antiquity.[90] That the translation was successful and important in the medieval West is seen not only in the strikingly large number of surviving complete manuscript copies, dating from about A.D. 800 (Par. lat. 9332) until the dawn of printing, but also in the extent to which the work was excerpted either piecemeal for later medical compilations or systematically to meet a particular demand for concise medical recommendations on specific subjects. Two sets of excerpts of the latter type (those on gout and the dietetic compilation known as the *Liber diaetarum*) came to constitute independent books, each came to form part of a larger, well-regarded standard medical work (the *Passionarius* of Gariopontus and the *Physica Plinii* corpus respectively), and each thus ensured its own rich manuscript tradition and its survival into the age of printing.

[82] Seventh century; Hunger, 302; for Sigerist, *Rezeptliteratur*, 15, the last great Greek doctor.

[83] Tenth century; Hunger, 305–6.

[84] Late thirteenth century; Hunger, 312.

[85] Fourteenth century; Hunger, 312–13.

[86] Rightly stressed by e.g. Neuburger, II, 111; Diepgen, 166.

[87] Alexander's name appears in a list (attributed to Alexander Neckam) from about 1190 of texts used for teaching in the Paris medical faculty (Seidler, 43–4; I owe this reference to Cloudy Fischer).

[88] Cameron, 67.

[89] Tempered by Baader, 'Adaptations', 252, who, while allowing that the influence of Alexander was stronger than that of Oribasius, seems to count the *Liber diaetarum* as more significant than the *Therapeutica* itself, and even here 'the influence of Alexander of Tralles was indirect, and dietetics was but a small portion of the transmitted material'.

[90] In wide circulation in the early Middle Ages were otherwise only Hippocrates (a few short works), Dioscorides, Galen (*Ad Glauconem* in two books, but otherwise only a few short works), and Oribasius. The first three are included in Cassiodorus' famous list (*Inst.* 1.31) of medical texts to be read in Latin collected in the library of the Vivarium at Ravenna.

CHAPTER 2. THE GREEK *THERAPEUTICA* AND THE LATIN VERSION

2.1. The Manuscript-Tradition of the Greek *Therapeutica*

In the context of editing the pseudonymous *De oculis* (p. 4 above), Barbara Zipser has recently considered the tradition of the *Therapeutica* as a whole, and has come to some important conclusions.[1] She lists eighteen manuscripts in which the Greek *Therapeutica* is transmitted in whole or in part.[2] On the basis of the collation of several passages, the arrangement of the *Therapeutica*, and the form and context of its transmission in all or most of the manuscripts, she establishes a stemma (*non vidi*) comprising four branches (her α, μ, π and L (= Laur. Plut. 74.10)), of which π and L constitute a sub-branch deriving from a complete copy intermediate between the acephalous μ and her archetype, the common ancestor of μ and the fragmentary α.[3] She shows that α, of which the Greek text is 'etwas eckig aber inhaltlich sehr gut', presents in numerous places superior readings (including *lectiones difficiliores*), and often agrees with the Latin Alexander against the rest of the Greek tradition.[4] Unfortunately, α contains of the Greek *Therapeutica* only Book 1 complete, together with extracts from Books 2 and 6. At the other extreme are π and L, which represent the results of at least one redaction, and present a text of which the Greek has been corrected and the content often trivialized. Regrettably, descendants of π, which according to Zipser came to constitute the *vulgata* version of the text, form the basis not only of the early printings of the *Therapeutica* but also of Puschmann's edition.

The consequences of these findings for the present work are essentially two-fold. On the one hand, by reconstructing part of the history of the Greek text, and by documenting the flawed principles of Puschmann's edition, Zipser has at last properly demonstrated the need for a new edition of the Greek *Therapeutica*; it follows that the authority of Puschmann's text is reduced, both in general and as a secondary witness for the text of the Latin Alexander. On the other hand, it is clear — and we may rejoice — that the Greek text used by the maker(s) of the Latin Alexander belonged to a superior branch of the Greek tradition. Especially given the fragmentary state of this branch among the surviving Greek manuscripts, this considerably increases the importance of the Latin Alexander as a witness for the Greek text.

2.2. Editions of the Greek *Therapeutica*

The first edition of the Greek *Therapeutica* was made by Jacques Goupyl (and printed by Robert Étienne) in Paris in 1548.[5] It was based on one (or more) of the

[1] I am very grateful to Barbara Zipser for letting me see some of her findings before their publication, and for several discussions of them in person with her. On the Greek manuscripts, see also Puschmann, I, 87–91.

[2] Zipser, xi–xii; she eliminates from the list of seventeen given by Diels, *Handschriften*, II, 11, the Par. Suppl. gr. 764, and adds Vat. gr. 1896 and Marc. gr. II 171.

[3] Zipser, xix–xxxvii; she seems to date her archetype to the tenth century, but if her α descends from her archetype and the Latin translator's copy from α (or even an ancestor of α), this needs to be brought forward by at least two centuries.

[4] Zipser, xxviii, xxxvii–xxxviii.

[5] *Alexandri Tralliani medici lib. XII. Rhazae de pestilentia libellus ex Syrorum lingua in Graecam translatus. Iacobi Gouphyli in eosdem castigationes.*

manuscripts deriving from Zipser's π (above),[6] and ignored the Latin tradition. (Like the common ancestor of Zipser's π and L, and the manuscripts deriving from it, it includes, beside Alexander, the Greek translation of Rhazes' work Περὶ λοιμικῆς.)

The second edition followed only eight years later, in 1556, the work of Johann Winter (or Winther — Ioannes Guint(h)erius) of Andernach, personal physician to the French king Francis I.[7] Winter added his own Latin translation (first published separately in 1549), which is praised by Puschmann (I, 98), but he also silently translated into Greek and included in his Greek text those parts of the Latin Alexander which are not in the Greek original, which makes his edition full of surprises![8]

Further editions were planned by Jac. Gronovius (1645–1702), Perizonius (1651–1715), both professors in Leiden, the Englishman Edward Milwards,[9] and Charles Daremberg. None was realized, with the result that Puschmann's was the first edition for more than three hundred years.[10]

Puschmann inspected, and presumably collated, virtually all the Greek manuscripts of Alexander then known (and a small number of the Latin as well[11]). He thus had access to all the branches of the family identified by Zipser, and his conclusions about the relations between the manuscripts match Zipser's closely: in a series of all-too-brief remarks (I, 89–91) he in effect establishes three branches, (in Zipser's terms) α, μ and L/π (he does not distinguish L and π); that α and μ, although very different, have a common ancestor; and that α (represented by Marc. gr. 295, his Mf) belongs especially closely with the Latin version. Then, however, apparently without considering the relations between his hyparchetypes, and without giving reasons for his decision,[12] Puschmann chose to base himself on the late recension represented by L/π (giving pride of place (I, 91) to the Laurentianus, Plut. 74.10, and Par. gr. 2201), using the other manuscripts only as sources of improvements to the text or of variants to report.

The extent to which Puschmann has rearranged the contents of π (here used in abbreviated reference to the common ancestor of Zipser's π and L) is immediately apparent from Table 2.1, which gives an overview of the contents of both Greek and Latin versions, including sections occurring only in the one or the other.[13] Possibly inspired by the Latin tradition (see II, 105 n. 5) Puschmann, like Winter before him, moved the chapters on parotis forward from between synanche and pleuritis to the end

[6] See Puschmann, I, 97–8; Zipser, xvii.

[7] *Alexandri Tralliani Medici libri duodecim, graece et latine, multo quam antea auctiores et integriores:* Johanne Guinterio Andernaco interprete et emendatore, etc. Henricus Petrus, Basel 1556. For a list of later editions, see Puschmann, I, 98–9, and Wust, 80–2.

[8] Most dramatically, Winter's edition gives the impression that we have large extracts from the lost authors Philumenus and Philagrius in Greek. Puschmann unmasks Winter, but defends and eulogizes him, *Nachträge*, v, 8–12. See also Masullo, 34–5, and n. 84.

[9] Milwards, 12, 189; Puschmann, I, 100.

[10] Meyer, II, 390; Puschmann, I, 101.

[11] Masullo, 36, thinks it improbable that Puschmann collated the Latin manuscripts personally, even for his edition (in the *Nachträge*) of the fragments of Philumenus and Philagrius, and states that the variant readings he reports in the Philagrius-chapters are frequently erroneous; Zipser (personal communication) reports the same for the chapters of the Greek text that she has collated.

[12] One might guess that he rejects μ because it 'macht den Eindruck der Interpolation' (I, 91), and α because it is fragmentary and so different from the rest of the Greek tradition.

[13] Zipser, xxxiv–xxxv, gives a useful overview of the arrangement of the contents of the Greek manuscripts, which goes well beyond what Puschmann offers in his notes.

Table 2.1: Overview of the contents of the Latin Alexander compared with the arrangement of Puschmann's edition and the Greek manuscripts (for the Greek sigla, see p. 13, for the Latin (P1, A, M), p. 38)

Book 1

chs in *ed.* (P1)	Subject	Puschmann	Pu.	Gk mss.
1–20 (1–19)	**Diseases of the hair and scalp**	I, 441–65	Bk 1	Bk 1 (all branches, incl. α)
21–33 (20–32)	**Headache: *cephalargia***	I, 465–483		
34–44 (33–43)	***cephalea***	I, 485–499		
45–51 (44–49)	***emigranium***	I, 499–509		
52–58 (50–56)	***Phrenesis***	I, 509–527		
59–60 (57–58)	***Lethargus***	I, 527–535		
61–74 (59–70)	**Epilepsy**	I, 535–567 +575		
not in the Latin	**further remedies**	I, 567–573		
75–84 (71–80)	***Melancholia***	I, 591–617		
85–107 (81–104)	**Eye-diseases**	II, 3–69	Bk 2	Bk 2 (all branches, incl. α [a frg. only])
108–130 (105–127)	**Ear-diseases,**	II, 71–105	Bk 3	Bk 3 π L Bk 2 μ
	incl. *parotis*	II, 105–25 Περὶ παρωτίδων		Bk 4 π L Bk 3 μ
131–135 (128–132)	**Nose, face and teeth**	**not in the Greek**		
136–142 (133–138)	***Synanche***	II, 125–145	Bk 4	Bk 4
143–149 (139–145)	***Pleuritis***	II, 229–243	Bk 6	Bk 6 π L Bk 5 μ

Book 2

chs in *ed.* (A)	Subject	Puschmann	Pu.	Gk mss.
1–13 (1–12)	**Coughing**	II, 147–167 + 185	Bk 5	Bk 5 π L Bk 4 μ
not in the Latin	further remedies for coughing	II, 169–183		
14–50 (13–47)	**Diseases of the digestive tract**	II, 245–313	Bk 7	Bk 7 π L Bk 6 μ and, frg. only, α
not in the Latin	Περὶ λυγμοῦ	II, 313–19		
51–56 (48–52)	***Cholera***	II, 321–335	Bk 8	
57–78 (53–69)	**Diseases of the liver**	II, 379–413	Bk 9	
79–103 (70–79)	**PHILUMENUS, on the stomach and intestines**	**not in the Greek**		
104–150 (80–99)	**PHILAGRIUS, on the spleen**			
151–157 (100–105)	**Dropsy**	II, 439–461	Bk 10	Bk 8 π L Bk 7 μ

Book 2: *Continued*

chs in *ed.* (A)	Subject	Puschmann	Pu.	Gk mss.
158–177 (106–114)	**Those spitting blood**	II, 187–209	Bk 5	Bk 7 π L Bk 6 μ
not in the Latin	Περὶ ἐμπυηματικῶν	II, 211–27		
178–203 (115–128)	**Diseases of the kidneys, bladder and genitals**	II, 463–501	Bk 11	Bk 8 π L Bk 7 μ
204–234 (129–133)	**Colic**	II, 335–377	Bk 8	Bk 9 π L Bk 8 μ
not in the Latin	Περὶ δυσεντερίας	II, 415–439	Bk 9	Bk 10
	Περὶ παρέσεως	II, 575–91	Bk 1	
235–271 (134–146)	**Gout**	II, 501–575	Bk 12	Bk 11 π L Bk 9 μ

Book 3

chs in *ed.* (M)	Subject	Puschmann	Pu.	Gk mss.
pr. (1)	Prologue, to Cosmas	I, 289		
1–9 (2–10)	***Ephemerae febres***	I, 291–311	sep. Bk, placed first	Bk 12 π L Bk 11 μ
10–20 (11–21)	**Fevers from corruption**	I, 311–27		
21–26 (22–27)	***Syncope* in fevers**	I, 329–37		
27–45 (28–46)	**Fainting**	I, 337–47		
46–66 (47–64)	***Hecticae febres***	I, 349–69		
not in the Latin	Περὶ τριταίου	I, 371–85		
	Περὶ ἀμφημερινοῦ	I, 385–407		
	Περὶ τεταρταίου	I, 407–39		

of the book on diseases of the ears.[14] Compared with π, then, Puschmann's Book 3 is relatively long, his Book 4 relatively short, and Puschmann similarly extended Book 5 by making it end with the chapters on αἱμοπτυϊκοί and ἐμπυηματικοί, which form the start of Book 7 in π. π's Book 7 is further shortened by the removal of cholera to Puschmann's Book 8 (mainly on colic, which is covered in Book 9 in π), and of liver-diseases to Puschmann's Book 9 (which also contains dysentery, the first part of Book 10 in the manuscripts, the other part of which, on paresis, Puschmann moved to between epilepsy and melancholy, at the end of his Book 1!). Puschmann divided Book 8 of π

[14] All the Greek manuscripts have *parotis* after *synanche*; Puschmann's arrangement here agrees with the Latin.

into two parts, namely his Book 10 on dropsy and his Book 11 on kidneys, bladder, and genitals, and finished with his Book 12 on gout (= Book 11 in π), having thus made twelve books out of eleven in π (and only ten in μ[15]). (For a much more detailed survey of the Latin Alexander, see the Appendix to this book.)

The most dramatic aspect of Puschmann's rearrangement, however, concerns the book on fevers, together with the preface to Cosmas. As already noted, in the Greek (as in the Latin) manuscripts, these come at the end and together constitute the last book of the *Therapeutica* (Book 12 in π, Book 11 in μ, Book 3 in the Latin version). Puschmann brought them both right to the front, and printed the book on fevers (preceded by the preface to Cosmas) as a separate work before Book 1 of the *Therapeutica*.

2.3. General Comparison of the Latin Version with the Greek

2.3.1. Content and Arrangement

With regard to the order of the material, the Latin version agrees with the Greek tradition most importantly in broad terms in the sequence of major components: diseases from head to toe — preface to Cosmas — fevers. The book on fevers (Book 3 of the Latin Alexander) stops abruptly at the end of the section on hectic fevers, and we have no trace of a Latin translation of Alexander on tertian, quotidian, and quartan fevers. The Latin preface to Cosmas is hardly more than a brief summary of the Greek, as we shall see in detail below (p. 32).

Book 1 of the Latin Alexander — all but the last seven chapters (1.143–9 on pleuritis: see below) — corresponds closely to Books 1–4 of the Greek tradition, covering, broadly speaking, diseases of the head. Both traditions treat almost the same material: there are some minor omissions of Greek material from the Latin, and the more significant addition of five chapters (1.131–5) on diseases of the nose, face, and teeth (see below, p. 25), which are placed appropriately between ears and throat. Diseases are dealt with in the same order in Greek and Latin, with two exceptions: (a) parotis comes at the end of ears in the Latin (as in Paul. Aeg. 3.23.13) but after synanche in the Greek tradition; and (b) in the Latin version, pleuritis (the Greek Book 6) comes before rather than after coughing (the Greek Book 5, the start of the Latin Book 2) — here Paul agrees with the Greek Alexander, treating coughing (3.28) before pleuritis (3.33).

The remainder of the Latin Book 2 (2.14ff.) corresponds to Books 7–11 of the Greek tradition. Again there are important omissions: seven pages of further remedies against coughing (part of the Greek Book 5), the chapters on hiccoughing and suppurations in the lung (both from Book 7), and those on dysentery and on paralysis (the whole of the Greek Book 10); but again, there are equally important additions, in the extensive extracts from Philumenus on dysentery (replacing Alexander on dysentery) and diseases of the intestine, and those from Philagrius on diseases of the spleen. This supplementary material from Philumenus and Philagrius is placed,

[15] According to Zipser, xxxvi, xxxviii, the shift of books in μ (and, she believes, α) — leading to μ (and, in Book 6, α) being a book behind π/L in the numeration — was caused by the interpolation without the marking of book-divisions of two books *De oculis* between Alexander on the eyes and Alexander on the ears.

appropriately enough, between diseases of the liver and dropsy. This leaves colic (treated next to dysentery in the Greek Alexander, Paul. Aeg. 3.42–3) rather isolated between genitals and gout, but this is a consequence of the treatment in the Greek of diseases of the genitals immediately after those of the bladder and the kidneys: in Paul. Aeg. we have all the internal organs dealt with together (3.37–46: in the sequence stomach — intestines — kidneys and bladder — liver) followed closely by dropsy (3.48) and much later by diseases of the genitals (3.54–9). The only significant departure from the Greek in the order of the diseases in the Latin version is that the chapter on those spitting blood comes oddly between dropsy and diseases of the kidneys, much later than in the Greek Alexander, where (as in Paul. Aeg. 3.31) haemoptysis is treated among the diseases of the thorax and immediately precedes suppurations in the lung. Whether the omission of the latter from the Latin version is related to the misplacement of haemoptysis, we may only speculate. With these few exceptions, then, the Latin Alexander presents in Books 1 and 2 a largely sensible *a capite ad calcem* ordering.

2.3.2. Length

It is important to stress that the Latin Alexander is not so much shorter than the Greek as is often stated or implied.[16] The Greek text occupies in Puschmann's edition 457 pages. By my calculations, which at this stage necessarily involve some estimation, the Latin Alexander as a whole is only about 7 per cent shorter than the Greek, and even if one disallows the extensive excerpts from Philumenus and Philagrius, and other additions, notably the chapters on the nose, face, and teeth (1.131–5), the Latin still accounts for about 80 per cent of the Greek Alexander.[17]

2.3.3. The Division into Books

With one single exception, all of the mainstream Latin manuscripts, from Paris, lat. 9332 (around A.D. 800) to London, Harley 4914 (after 1500), transmit the Latin Alexander in three books (1: hair-loss to pleuritis; 2: coughing to gout; 3: fevers); the end of the third book is explicitly noted also by the scribe of one of the oldest excerpting manuscripts, Vat. regin. lat. 1143 (below, p. 97). On the origin of this division we can only speculate. The book on fevers is self-contained and requires no further comment, but there is no natural break between Books 1 and 2, unless we imagine an earlier version with pleuritis in Book 2, which would allow us to characterize Book 1 as diseases of the head.

At some point before 1200, the Latin Alexander was rearranged into seven books — perhaps more than once. A redivision into seven books is physically exemplified in only one surviving manuscript, Paris lat. 6882 (my P3). Book 1 is divided in two

[16] I have found this acknowledged only in Thorndike, *History*, I, 577 n. 8 ('not as abbreviated as one might infer from Rose').

[17] Translated into Latin are about 364 of the 457 pages of Puschmann; the excerpts from Philumenus and Philagrius occupy 57 Puschmann pages (in the *Nachträge*), the chapters on the nose, face and teeth, a further 6, yielding a total of 427 Puschmann pages for the Latin Alexander as a whole.

(1.1–84, diseases of the head and nervous diseases; 1.85–149, diseases of the eyes, ears, nose, face and teeth, synanche, and pleuritis); Book 2 is divided into four books (2.1–78, coughing to diseases of the liver; 2.79–157, Philumenus, Philagrius, and dropsy; 2.158–234, those spitting blood to colic; 2.235–71, gout); Book 3 is left untouched as Book 7. The contents are unaffected by this redivision. If the intention was to produce more thematically-coherent books, this was achieved only for new Book 6 (on gout; and perhaps for new Book 1, on the head and nervous diseases). The effect of the redivision was simply to produce a series of books of more uniform and manageable size. The choice of the number seven may be in direct imitation of earlier medical classics, in particular the encyclopaedia of Paul of Aegina, the early medieval Galenic and pseudo-Galenic ensemble, and Gariopontus' *Passionarius* (see 3.2.6, below).

The name of Gariopontus occurs in an apparent reference to a second rearrangement of the material of the Latin Alexander contained in the first four folios of another manuscript copy (also now in Paris) of the three-book Latin version (Par. lat. 6881, my P2). The content and import of this 'preface' remain to be elucidated: they are beyond my competence, even now that a fresh autopsy has solved the problems posed by the poor legibility of the microfilm of these four folios. I now incline to think that the work in seven books referred to here ('Diuiditur autem h<o>c opus in VII libros') is not simply a version of Alexander but a compilation, otherwise unknown, made from several works including that of Alexander ('Opus istud compilatum est ex diuersorum au<c>torum operibus.s.g.(?) Pauli Alexandri Theodosii prsc(?) (Prisciani?) et Democriti'); this would be in spite of the prominence accorded Alexander in the opening sentence of this 'preface',[18] and in spite of the fact that these folios stand before a roughly-contemporary manuscript copy of Alexander alone. It is thinkable that the author of this 'preface' regarded the Latin Alexander as a compilation, but the content of each of the seven books is then summarized in such a way that one wonders whether this really can be the Latin Alexander of the rest of the tradition.[19] There are similarities (e.g. Book 2 beginning with coughing; the incorporation of a book of Philumenus), but some important differences, too (e.g. the removal of the book on diseases of the eyes;

[18] Par. lat. 6881, f. 1ra: 'Cum post tempora Ypocratis plurimi auctores tam ueteres quam moderni in phisica facultate studuisse inueniantur, secundus post Galienum excellentiorem locum obtinuisse creditur Ale[n]xander, qui, rogatus a discipulis suis Cosma et Damiano, paucarum egritudinum sed earum plenissime causas et significationes exposuit <et> curas, subitiens eas qui(dem?) nn (?) quas uel ipse probauerat uel ab amicis probatas acceperat.'

[19] Par. lat. 6881, f. 1vb: 'Continet iamque primus liber tractatum passionum capitis et parcium capiti adiacentium ut aurium dentium uue faucium atque genarum. Liber autem oculorum depertus (decerptus?) est ex hoc libro et per se inuenitur. Secundus continet passiones cordis pulmonis eparis stomachi diafragmatis atque costarum. Tercius uero splenis intestinorum renum uesice et uirge. Quartus a(utem?) scie(ntiam) genuum articulorum manuum et pedum et partium tractatus particularium. Quintus continet tractatum omnium et uniuersalium nisi febrium et cardiace passionis. Huic et alligatus liber est Filomini(?) (flonu *or* flomi?). Sextus autem est scientia febrium et criticorum dierum et cardia[r]ce. Septimus uero de sinthomatibus febrium?et sig(nis??) (*or* dig(erit), *or* ag(it)?). Sed quia in hoc libro ... [*numerous further medical definitions and notes*] ... f. 2va ... Variis et c(?) ostenso de passionibus capitis et parcium cerebri transiturus ad passiones parcium capitis adiacentium repetit de dolore capitis ... Postquam eg(it) de passionibus capitis, ag(it) de c(ausis) parcium capitis adiacentium dicens. *Aurium* et c(ausa?) ex reumatismo.i. ex fluxu ... Hic fuit appositus tractatus oculorum sed fuit subtractus a quodam medico Sequitur tractatus dentium ... [*more notes and definitions*] ... f. 2vb Secundus incipit. Tussis est motus spiritalis uirtutis ad expellendam s(upe)r fluitatem insp(irit)ualibus habundantem uel comprimentem ... f. 3ra ... Tertius. typus a figura. *Vulneratio corporis* in cruribus et tibiis *nascitur*. In hoc tractatu splenis ferrum ponitur pro qualibe (chalybe?) ... f. 3va ... Quartus. *Seri(um?)*.i. carum (??) *Psialgia* ... *Podagrica*(?) ... [*I cannot find* Quintus!] f. 4rb ... SEXTVS. dieticos. dicte congrue interfontes (sontes, *or* inidentes??) ... f. 4va ... Septimus. In hoc libro tractat de febribus uel? sinthomatibus in est quod inducit de dol(ore) capitis et si similiter uideatur ...'

the apparent division of fevers between Books 6 and 7; the inclusion of *cardiaci* with fevers in Book 6). At all events, it is hard to imagine that this is a summary of the seven-book version copied by the original maker of P3 (above), so that — even granted the possibility that the 'preface' to P2 is describing a version of the Latin Alexander[20] — we should have to reckon, as noted, with more than one redivision into seven books. In view of the puzzling order of the transmitted parts of both Greek and Latin Alexanders (*a capite ad calcem* — preface — fevers), it is interesting to note the reference in P2's 'preface' to an earlier version of the work commented on in which, as in Puschmann's edition of the Greek Alexander, the treatment of fevers was placed first. It is stated explicitly that the order of the work discussed has been subject to change ('Ordo uero alius est secundum modernos alius fuit secundum antiquos'): while 'Priscianus' put the treatment of diseases affecting the whole body (i.e. mainly fevers) before those affecting particular parts ('Priscianus etenim, qui[bus] operis institutor extitit, tractatum uniuersalium passionum praemisit particularibus'), Gariopontus of Salerno reversed the order ('Garipontus uero Salernitanus transmutauit ordinem et praemisit tractatum particularium'). Further research is needed on the background and the implications of the first four folios of Par. lat. 6881.

Apart from P3 (and possibly P2), however, there is no evidence of a Latin version of Alexander in other than the standard three-book arrangement.[21]

2.4. Other Discrepancies Between the Latin Version and the Greek

Discrepancies between the Latin Alexander and the Greek original are broadly speaking of three sorts: either the Latin version has material not in the Greek; or the Greek original has material not in the Latin; or corresponding passages of the 'same' text differ in the two versions. It will be part of the job of the full edition of the Latin Alexander to indicate all such differences. For present purposes, I content myself with brief description and illustration of the ways in which the Latin version departs from the Greek. I begin with departures in corresponding passages of the 'same' text, as this type of discrepancy illustrates also the first two types in miniature and, more significantly, raises an important uncertainty which must be kept in mind when we consider major instances of Latin or Greek material apparently unmatched in the other version.

2.4.1. Differences Between Latin and Greek Versions of the 'Same' Text

Much of the Latin Alexander looks like a word-for-word translation of the Greek. Often, however, there are differences between the two versions, ranging in scope from a single word (even a single grammatical feature, e.g. singular vs. plural or present vs. future) to a passage of several sentences. The possible reasons for the Latin version on a given occasion saying something different from what the Greek says at the same point are essentially three: either the makers of the Latin version misunderstood

[20] As far as I can see, although P2 contains only this 'preface' and the three-book Latin Alexander, the preface makes no mention of a version in three books.

[21] The reference in the chapters of the Latin Alexander from Philagrius to 'the fourth book on gout' (2.122: 'in quarto libro de podagricis'; cf. also 2.112: 'sicut dictum est in podagrica cura'), while consistent with the book-division of the work described in the preface to P2, is most probably original to Philagrius on the spleen, rather than added by the maker of the Latin Alexander. We are fortunate enough to know that Philagrius wrote a work on gout in at least five books. Cf. Orib., *Syn.* 9.59 (p. 312, 1 Raeder) = Philagrius, frg. 8 Masullo. Masullo, 75–124 collects the fragments on gout.

the Greek; or they had before them a version of the Greek text different from that edited by Puschmann; or they or later redactors revised the Latin text. Let us look straightaway at an example, from early in Book 1 of the Latin version (= Book 1 Greek).

1.4 *ad fin.* and 1.5 *ad init.* (text of Angers 457 [A])	Puschmann's Greek text I, 445, 7–447, 7
1. Stercus autem catti cum aceto illitum bene operatur. +–I, 445, 8–9 (also Mf) –+	**1**. Ἄλλο. Κόπρον αἰλούρου μετ' ὄξους κατάχριε· καλόν ἐστι +– καὶ πάνυ φυσικὴν ἀντιπάθειαν ἔχει πρὸς τὸ πάθος.–+
2. Nucibus integris ustis et cum oleo tritis inunge; ante radens ipsa loca. +– Et euforbium tritum cum oleo et illitum frequenter multis sanauit.–+ **3**. (1.5. t.) De compositis medicamentis +– ad tineam capitis–+ **4**. +– Operatiua enim sunt et compositis medicamenta quae ab antiquis dicta sunt, multa sunt ex simplicibus confecta; sed omnia scribere superfluum est. Sed ea tantum tradimus quae experimentata habemus uel probata a certis amicis qui nobis ea tradiderunt medicis.	**3**. Περὶ συνθέτων βοηθημάτων. **6**. Χαλκοῦ κεκαυμένου δραχ. β′ θείου ἀπύρου δραχ. β′ ἀσφοδέλου δραχ. β′ λειάνας σὺν κρόκῳ ᾠῶν καὶ ἀνατρίψας τὸν τόπον χρίε. **2**. Ἄλλο· Κάρυα βασιλικὰ καύσας ὁλόκληρα λείου μετ' ἐλαίου καὶ κατάχριε προξυρήσας τὸν τόπον.+– –+ +– **4**. –+
5. Recipit autem unum ex his haec. –+ Adipe ursino ÷ I. adarcis ÷ I. fimo murium ÷ III. pice liquida ÷ III. oleo usto ex lucerna ÷ IS. teres; et omnia miscens lines. Sed antea rades capitis loca; et sic perunges ipsa loca; +– et miraberis quomodo curabit tineam capitis. etiam si antiquissima sit. –+	**5**. +– –+Ἄλλο· Στέατος ἀρκτείου οὐγγ. β′ ἀδάρκης οὐγγ. γ′ μυοχόδων οὐγγ. γ′ πίσσης ὑγρᾶς οὐγγ. γ′ λυχνελαίου ἀπὸ καύματος δραχ. α′s" ἀναλαμβάνων τὸν τόπον προξυρῶν χρίε.+– –+
6. Item aliud. Calcu cicaumeno ÷ II. sulphure uiuo ÷ II. asfodillo <radicibus> II. teres cum uitellis ouorum et fricando caput uteris.	
7. Item aliud Aceto acro ÷ I. allio ÷ I. oleo roseo ÷ I. fricabis locum cum panno laneo; et sic linens +– mirabiliter faciet.–+	**7**. Ἄλλο· Ὄξους δριμέος οὐγ. α′ σκορόδων οὐγ. α′ ῥοδίνου ἐλαίου οὐγ. α′ τρίψας τὸν τόπον ῥάκει ἐρίου κατάχριε.+– –+
8. Item aliud +– ualde mirabile –+ Ranarum +– ustarum cinere –+ ÷ III. murium fimo ÷ I. pice liquida ÷ I. cedria quod sufficit. +– –+ +– hoc enim etiam si diuturnae sint sanat alopicias.–+	**8**. Ἄλλο· Βατράχων+– –+οὐγγ. γ′ μυοχόδων οὐγ. α′ καλάμου φλοιοῦ τέφρας οὐγ. α: πίσσης ὑγρᾶς οὐγ. α′ πράσου σπέρματος οὐγ. α′. κεδρέα ἀναλάμβανε +–καὶ οὕτω περίχριε.–+ +– –+

The differences between Puschmann's Greek text and the Latin version affect virtually every sentence of this short passage, and exemplify the various types of divergence to be encountered in systematic comparison of the two texts. The passage also illustrates the special position of Greek manuscript Mf (Marc.gr.295), which, while sometimes agreeing with the rest of the Greek tradition against the Latin, more often agrees with the Latin against Puschmann's edition of the Greek version.

In the passage quoted above, Mf agrees with the rest of the Greek tradition (numbers refer to sections of the chapter):

(a) **1**, in having a second sentence in the recommendation which is not in the Latin;

(b) **2**, in the designation κάρυα βασιλικά (the Latin has just *nucibus*);

(c) **2**, in the omission of the second recipe in **2** ('Et euforbium ...');

(d) **6**, in making **6** follow **1** (although in the placement of the title **3**, Mf agrees with the Latin version);

(e) **8**, in having ἀναλάμβανε after κεδρέα (contrast Latin 'cedria quod sufficit').

On the other hand, Mf agrees with the Latin version against the other Greek manuscripts:

(a) **3**, in making the title follow **2**;

(b) **4** and **5**, in containing text corresponding to **4** and the first sentence of **5** in the Latin;

(c) **5**, in prescribing one ounce of ἀδάρκη, rather than three;

(d) **5**, in having the recommendation at the end of **5**, as in the Latin;

(e) **6**, in having ῥιζῶν, κρόκοις, χρῶ: cf. Latin *radicibus*, *uitellis*, *uteris*;

(f) **7**, in having a recommendation at the end of **7** (θαυμάσεις) similar to that in the Latin ('mirabiliter faciet');

(g) **8**, in having two words[22] after ἄλλο almost certainly corresponding to Latin 'ualde mirabile';

(h) **8**, in having κεκαυμένων after βατράχων:[23] cf. Latin 'ranarum ustarum';

(i) **8**, in concluding this recipe with a sentence corresponding to the Latin version, and not the Greek.

Reading on through the next few chapters of Book 1, we see that these findings are repeated, and for longer stretches of text. So, for example, on the one hand, the Latin chapters 1.7 and 1.8 are absent from all the Greek manuscripts, including (as far as I can see) Greek manuscript Mf. On the other hand, Mf alone has text to match the following passage towards the end of 1.6 of the Latin version (what would be between lines 6 and 7 of I, 451 Puschmann):

> 1.6 Haec scientes, dicere oportet ad unamquamque passionem expedientia adiutoria. Diuersa enim et quam plurima sunt scripta ad fluxus capillorum. Quae ergo noscimus esse probabilia et experimentata, uel a nobilissimis et caris amicis didicimus, haec etiam uobis fideliter tradimus cum quibusdam unctionibus prouisis composita medicamenta. Quod laudauit Galienus fieri ad rarefactos poros uel condensatam cutem de ladano medicamento confectum, quod hoc modo fit.

And likewise Mf alone has text corresponding to 1.9 of the Latin version (what would be before line 1 of I, 453 Puschmann):

> 1.9 (entire) Cogimur saepius ab amicis ut nigros faciamus capillos, et maxime a potentibus aut regibus, interdum etiam aut flauos uel albos. Necesse est ergo ut ex his aliqua dicamus. Suadeo tamen non satis eos qui habent caput naturaliter frigidum frequenter ex his ungui. Stiptica sunt enim haec omnia talia et austera et densatiuam habentia uirtutem. Propter quod utilissimum est aliqua quae subtiliant et paulatim calefaciunt in his quae tingere possunt admisceri quia descendunt in profundum, et magis ea quae innigrant capillos. Et ideo si addantur quae leniter calefaciant, minus laedere possunt. Conuenit autem per dies quattuor aut quinque adhiberi medicamen. Nam si per singulos dies adhibeatur, multo magis periculum incurrunt, ita ut maxime catarrizent, et peripneumonici *aut* epylemptici aut apoplectici fiant et exinde moriantur. Melius est ergo ut non in his causis incidant malis. Remouenda est enim frequens inunctio.

[22] The first is λίαν; the second I cannot read from the photocopy of Mf.
[23] A conjecturable correction, perhaps, as Puschmann reports this also for C (a daughter of Zipser's π).

On a smaller scale again, the Latin Alexander at 1.11: 'et tunc lauari iubebis' appears to overtranslate the Greek at I, 455, 4 καὶ ἀπόνιπτε, until, that is, one reads the Greek manuscript Mf at this point, which has καὶ τότε ἀπονίψασθαι κέλευε. And two lines later in 1.11 the Latin version agrees with Mf in omitting two commands present in the rest of the Greek tradition at I, 455, 6–7: κυπέρου φύλλα βρέξον χυλῷ στρουθίου καὶ χρῶ τῷ ἀποβρέγματι (having them instead a dozen lines later, just before 1.13 (= I, 455, 17ff.), the Latin being 'cyperi folia infundes in suco strucii et uteris illa infusione').

These findings naturally prompt even greater caution when it comes to characterizing independent work on the part of the maker(s) of the Latin Alexander in those books — the large majority — not transmitted by Mf, for it is only when the Greek tradition is unanimously against the Latin version that we can think in terms of interventions on the part of the Latin translator(s)/redactor(s) — and even then of course only provisionally. In passages for which we do not have Mf, such as the two examples below, chosen at random from Book 2 of the Latin Alexander, this is a standing and important caveat. The departures of the Latin version from the Greek in the form and detail of the instructions to the drinker of the remedy (at the start of the first example, from 2.67), and in the list of ingredients for the remedy διὰ βακάνου, are just like the sort of discrepancies we saw illustrated above between Mf and the rest of the Greek tradition. The divergences between the Latin and Greek introductions to simple remedies for diseases of the liver which follow in 2.67 are much more radical (apart from the difference in length, note the naming of Oribasius in the Latin, presumably for ὁ σοφὸς γέρων in the Greek), but, in the absence of a systematic comparison of Mf with Puschmann's text, we must reserve judgement on the question whether they reflect recension of the Greek tradition, or of the Latin, or of both.

2.67 *med.* iaceat +–qui biberit–+ in latere dextro +–manu dextra sub capite posita et extensus hora media–+.	II,395,4–18 +–κέλευε–+ δὲ εἰς τὸ δεξιὸν ἀνακεῖσθαι πλευρόν.+– –+
Item aliud diabacanum Bacano ÷ i. costo ÷ i. folio .2 viii. Pipere +–albo–+ .2 vi. +–spica nardi .2 vi.–+ melle quod sufficit. Dabis autem cotidie lib() i. cum condito in balneo. Et hoc enim experimentatum est. Maxime autem haec potio facit ad eos quibus de spisso et pingui humore fit infraxis.	Ἄλλο τὸ διὰ βακάνου Κόστου οὐγ. α′ βακάνου οὐγ. α′ φύλλου γρ. η′ πεπέρεως γρ. ς′ μέλιτος τὸ ἀρκοῦν. δίδου κοχλ. μετὰ κράσεως κονδίτου ἐν λουτρῷ. καὶ τοῦτο διὰ πείρας μάλιστα πρὸς τὰς ὑπὸ γλίσχρων καὶ παχέων γενομένας ἐμφράξεις.
Item ponimus simplicia adiutoria **Uribasii** auctoris uel a diuersis nobilibus uiris probata adiutoria ad epar.	ὅπως δέ ἐστι και δυνατὸν συντιθέναι φάρμακον, οἷον βούλεται, ἁρμόζειν δυνάμενον πρὸς τὴν ὑποκειμένην διάθεσιν καὶ πρὸς τὴν τοῦ κάμνοντος δύναμιν καὶ κρᾶσιν καὶ ἡλικίαν καὶ πρὸς ἕκαστον τῶν ἄλλων ἀποβλέπων, εἰς ὅσα καὶ **ὁ σοφὸς γέρων** ἐδίδαξεν ἀποβλέπειν, ἐξεθέμην ἁπλᾶ βοηθήματα, ὡς καὶ αὐτῶν εὐπορεῖν συντόμως καὶ ἄλλα δὲ συντιθέναι ἐξ αὐτῶν, ὡς ἂν ἕλοιτό τις εὐχενρῶς δύνασθαι. Ὅσα πρὸς ἧπαρ ἁπλᾶ βοηθήματα.

(Note that, in 2.67, while the Latin resumes agreement with the Greek for some lines after the end of the comparison above, the final 130 words of the chapter in the Latin version are not in Puschmann's text of the Greek; these additional words are quoted on p. 27 below.)

Equally, in the second example below, an extract from 2.217, while the relative fullness and clarity of the Latin version could plausibly be taken as the work of the translator (or his editor), unless and until we can identify Latin linguistic features characteristic of — ideally, peculiar to — such expansions, we must leave open the possibility that they are faithful translations of a lost Greek recension.

2.217 Haec enim omnia extenuant et digerunt omnem corporis superfluitatem et confortant totam habitudinem corporis ut ea quae molestantur iam non possint +–laedere nec–+ frigidum congregare humorem. Sed neque his qui ex alio fluit loco in eum qui laesus fuit supercurrit quia non recipitur ab eo qui fortior effectus est loco.	II, 361, 14-17 ταῦτα γὰρ πάντα λεπτύνει καὶ διαφορεῖ καὶ τὸ πᾶν ἀπέριττον διατίθησιν ἀναρρωννύντα τὴν ὅλην ἕξιν, ὡς τοῦ λοιποῦ μηκέτι τὰ πεπονθότα δύνασθαι ψυχρὸν ἀθροίζειν χυμὸν, ἀλλὰ μηδὲ τὸν ἐξ ἑτέρου ἐπιρρέοντα ἑτοίμως ἐπιδέχεσθαι πρὸς ἑαυτά.

2.4.2. Latin Material Not in the Greek Original

We saw in the last section some instances of apparently additional material in the Latin Alexander, whether a few words or whole chapters, sometimes matched by part of the Greek tradition and sometimes not. My main concern in this section is to highlight the fact that the Latin Alexander is to a significant degree a compilation: that is to say, the earliest version that we can reconstruct contains material demonstrably from other sources which has been deliberately worked into the Latin text at more or less appropriate places. This is seen on a small scale at the very beginning of Book 1 in the definition of *alopecia* and *ofiasis*, which is more elaborate than that offered at the opening of the Greek text, and is drawn from the start of the seventh chapter of the first book of Theodorus Priscianus,[24] as is clear from the comparison below:

1.1 *init.* (text of A) +–I, 441, 1–6–+	Theod. Prisc., *Eup. faen.* 16, p. 16, 14ff. Rose	I, 441,1–6 +– Ἡ ἀλωπεκία πάθος ἐστὶ τριχῶν μάδισις, οὐκ ἐκ μιᾶς δὲ αἰτίας, ἀλλ' ἐκ διαφόρων καὶ ποικίλων ἔχει τὴν γένεσιν· –+

[24] Theodorus is named as the source of a remedy for epilepsy in both Greek and Latin versions, and may be the source of several others in the same chapter: 1.72: 'In LVIII titulo Theodorus. Epylemptico autem cadente, si de maioribus digitis pedum eius sanguinem tollas et linias labia eius et frontem, mox surgit' = I, 559, 18–561, 1: Περὶ θεραπείας ἐκ τοῦ δευτέρου Θεοδώρου. 'Επιληπτικοῦ δὲ καταπεσόντος ἀπὸ τῶν μεγάλων δακτύλων τῶν ποδῶν αὐτοῦ αἷμα ἀποξύσας χρῖσον αὐτοῦ τὰ χείλη καὶ τὸ μέτωπον καὶ παρ' αὐτὰ ἀναστήσεται; cf. Theod. Prisc., *Physica* 6, p. 254, 9–11 Rose: 'in ipsis uero commotionibus, si sanguinem de eius pedem digitis elicias quoquo pacto, et eius frontem ex eo tangas et labia, continuo exsurget', and see Rose's apparatus here for other places where Theodorus may have been used by Alexander.

+– Contingit haec duplex passio cadentibus capillis, ut aliquando defectu quodam cadant et nudando partes capitis turpent. (2) Fit uero ophyasis, quae, uelut serpentinis squamulis superficiem cutis mentiatur. (3) Alia uero uulneribus horridis plerunque uisibus occurrit, cuius foeditas uulpinis uulneribus exhibet similitudinem, quam alopiciam uocant.–+	Contingit haec in capite duplex passio cadentium capillorum, ut aliquando defectu quodam cadant et nudando partes capitis turpent, (cf. 3) aliquotiens ut eorum uulnerum horridus plerumque uisus occurrat. ergo defectus, ut prius diximus, cum contigerit caluitium facit. foeditas illa uero uulpini uulneris exhibet similitudinem, (cf. 2) ut etiam serpentis aliquando squamosi superficiem mentiatur.	+—+
(4) Fit autem passio ...		γίνεται γὰρ ...

A much longer supplement to the Greek text is inserted by the makers of the Latin Alexander at 1.131–5, between the end of *parotides* and the start of *synanche*. These chapters are composed very largely of miscellaneous extracts from Books 3 and 5 of Galen, Περὶ συνθέσεως φαρμάκων τῶν κατὰ τόπους,[25] interspersed with some other recipes apparently from other sources,[26] and some editorial intervention, including perhaps the particle *quippe* (prec. n.) and a mildly ridiculous summing up at the end of 1.131.[27]

The longest supplements by far are the extracts in the middle of Book 2 from Philumenus on the stomach and intestines (2.79–103≈6.5 per cent of the Latin Alexander) and Philagrius on the spleen (2.104–50≈6.5 per cent of the Latin Alexander). These hardly require illustration, as they have attracted interest as the sole or principal fragments of two otherwise lost Greek doctors: both excerpts have been edited together twice, by Puschmann (in his *Nachträge*) and Mihăileanu respectively, and Philagrius separately by Masullo. In the absence of the Greek originals of the texts from which these extracts were drawn, comparisons may be made at most with surviving fragments of other works. With regard to the making of the Latin Alexander, an important question — which applies also to the Galen excerpts mentioned above — is whether our translator(s) excerpted a ready-made Latin translation or turned Greek excerpts into Latin as they worked. I am as yet unable to give anything like a definitive answer to this

[25] 12.678–9, 688–95, 807, 812, 816, 848–9, 853–61, 869, 882, 880, 877, 883–6 Kühn. There are some divergences between the Latin Alexander and Kühn's text of Galen, e.g. between 1.134 and Gal. 12.849, 15–17. Note that Book 3 of Galen's κατὰ τόπους is referred to also by the Greek Alexander, at II, 81, 24 = 1.114 Latin (12.603–4 Kühn); cf. II, 163, 18 = 2.13 Latin (Book 7, 13.43 K.), II, 293, 18 = 2.44 Latin (Book 8, 13.118 K.).

[26] For example, the prescriptions eight lines into 1.131 beginning (text of A): 'ad roborandum igitur caput hoc modo uteris. deraso quippe capiti imponendum est emplastrum diaiteon aut barbara ...': compare the pseudo-Galenic Εὐπόριστα (14.336 Kühn), Theod. Prisc. 1.42 p. 43, 15–44, 4: '... post rasuram uero emplastrum dia iteon aut barbaram imponendo'; Cass. Fel. 31.1 Fraisse (pp. 62, 16–63, 2 Rose): 'medicamentis desiccatoriis capiti praeraso impositis curabis, ut est dia iteon emplastrum aut barbara'.

[27] 'Manifestum est autem in his passionibus ut considerata uniuscuiusque corporis natura si nihil impediat sanguis detrahatur. Etiam et catarticum dandum est et diaeta obseruanda est et caput radendum est et medicamentis desiccandum est et apoflegmatismi sunt adhibendi' (text of A). Cf. the misleading summary of Gal. 12.853, 17–854, 13K at the end of 1.134: 'alia igitur medicamenta aut stiptica sunt adhibenda quae reprimant aut certe quae digerant'.

question. My general impression is that in terms of their Latinity these excerpts have enough in common with each other and with parts at least (the stylistically higher parts) of the Latin Alexander to make it likely that the several translations belong closely together. In Chapters 4 and 5 below, I offer some particular comparisons and contrasts, but regretfully postpone a systematic study of the Latin Philumenus, the Latin Galen, and the Latin Philagrius transmitted with the Latin Alexander.

Here and there in the Latin Alexander are sizeable chunks of Latin material apparently additional to the Greek text but of unidentified origin. By way of illustration, I reproduce below two examples (constituting complete, if small chapters) from that part of Book 1 devoted to diseases of the eyes.

1.92 (text of A; just before II, 29, 6 Puschmann) +– Signa infraxis in oculis factae
Infraxin autem humorum in oculis factam hoc modo cognosces. Cum tumore enim eleuantur fortiter, et sine uenarum sanguine plenae sunt existentiae, sed et tensionem sentiunt in ipsis oculis. Haec ergo signa ostendunt satis pinguissimos humores infraxin fecisse in oculis.–+

1.95 (text of A; just before II, 31, 17 Puschmann) +– Signa qui flebotomari opus habent uel qui catartico purgari
Ex sanguinis autem abundantia si fiat flegmon, siquidem absque tensura est repletus qui inflammatus est locus cum tumore magno plus a natura rubro colore. Multa autem fit cognitio. Lacrimatur enim et lippes facit. Fit enim tensio intolerabilis in profundo oculorum, ut simul exprimi et rumpi uideantur. et cum pulsu interdum subleuantur palpebrae et euertuntur; et uix mouentur et album oculi altius nigro fit. Hos autem tales mox flebotomabis. Si autem flegmaticus aut colericus aut melancholicus fuerit, his catharticum dandum est. Quorum signa sunt haec. Si flegmaticus sanguini mixtus sunt haec. Album colorem et rubrum permixtum habent simul. et media natura flegmati mixtus est sanguis; et magis in uespera accessiones fiunt per singulos dies. Colericus autem humor si fuerit, calor sentitur multus. Mordens autem quam plurime est et lacrimae subrubro colore et subflauae; et tertia die fit accessio. Quodsi melancholicus fuerit sanguis, accessiones quarto die magis consurgunt. Quomodo autem debeant agnosci, in podagricis passionibus dixi.–+

In the absence of direct or indirect evidence of an independent source, we cannot exclude the possibility that these passages, and others like them, were in the translator's copy of the Greek Alexander; indeed, the last four words of 1.95 (underlined above) constitute a plausible reference to the chapters on gout at the end of Book 2. Naturally, as in the reference to Theodorus in both Greek and Latin traditions quoted in n. 24 above, an explicit reference to another book may have been taken over by the translator from his Greek original. Again, we cannot exclude this for cases such as the alternative version of a recipe, not in Puschmann's text, in the middle of 1.84, which begins: '+– In duobus autem libris nouiter scriptis, haec confectio ita habetur . . .–+'. Our best hope in such cases is to identify either a source that Alexander cannot have known or features of the content or the language that set them apart from the rest of the Latin Alexander, or both. I conclude this paragraph by quoting in full two further examples, this time from Book 2, of substantial pieces of unidentified additional material in the Latin Alexander, in order to increase the probability of the source, if extant, being identified.

2. 67[28] *ad fin.* (a continuation of the Greek chapter ending II, 397, 4 Puschmann; text of A) +–Itemque purgant simam epatis popondion herba mercurialis cum mite lateride cum oximelle camelea cum absintio et ydromelle potata, brasicae sucus datus, nitrum cum mulsa potatum, cyclamidis radix, lupinorum apozima, oleum, mel, nitrum, lactis serum galliae tusti ius, ciceris ius. Adiuuant haec diuturnas flegmonas quae fiunt in sima epatis. Et quae purgant cirtam epatis: nardus Celtica potata, amonii apozima, squinoantum, acori radix, agaricum cum uino et melle potatum, gentiana cum aqua potata, picci albi folia cum mulsa, lauri radicis cortice cum uino oboli tres potati, reoponticum, gliciricae sucus cum sapa, quinquefolii sucus de radicibus, agni sperma, daucus, apii semen, petrosilinum, bacani folia, cardamomum centaurea glicidis quae et pionia semen, anisus pefrigmenus, absintium, costum, opobalsamum, smirnis, fu, asarum, meu. Haec diuturnas aegritudines epatis, siue cum tumore aliquo fuerint, siue distemperantia sit, et dolores ex epate sanant.–+

2. 187 *ad fin.*–188 (a continuation of the Greek chapter ending II, 485, 19 Puschmann; text of A) +– ne pus coaguletur intus ad flegmonem uesicae et renium: lini seminis puluere .L ii. amilo .L i. dabis in aqua coclearium unum bibendum. Trociscus ad renium et uesicae ulcera et antidotum ad ulcera et uulnera et dolores in ipsis locis consistentes, quod mox subuenit, recipiens haec: pipere albo .L xx. iusquiamo .L xx. opio .L i. croco .L iii. peretro .L i. euforbio .L i. Haec quidem confectio Philonii antidotum est, cui addantur in confectione: cucumeris domestici semine .L vi. apii semine .L vi. conii semine .L iii. lappatii semine .L iii. amigdalis amaris .L iii. feniculi semine .L iii. melle quod sufficit. Dabis autem sicut Philonium antidotum.

2. 188 +– De trociscis et antidotis ad renum et uesicae ulcera

Item dia fisallidon trociscus, qui facit ad nefreticos et ad ulcera in renibus et uesica: cucumeris domestici semine .L xii. feniculi semine .L vi. lappatii semine .L iii. nucleis pineis pefrigmenis .L iii. croco .L vi. opio .L iii. iusquiami albi semine .L iii. amigdalis amaris pefrigmenis .L iii. fisallidon (quam Latini uesicaginem uocant) grana numero uiginti quinque, conii (id est cicute) semine .L iiii. Cum sapa autem facies trociscos dragmeos, et dabis cum uino dulci, qui non febriunt aut sapa, qui autem febriunt, cum aqua tepida. Facit ergo hic trociscus ad renium et uesicae passions, quibus pus cum urina redditur aut sanguis aut muccis simile aut sablonis cum urina iactant ex multo calore. Qui autem in uesica aut in uritra ulcera aut uulnus habent, inities per uritram (id est uirgam) cum lacte asinino aut muliebri aut cum sapa.–+

A second type of demonstrable Latin addition to the content of the Greek Alexander that merits a brief word here is the glossing, or more elaborate explication, of technical terms and concepts which are employed, usually without explanation,[29] in the Greek original. An extended example is seen in the explanation of the three types of blood-loss at 2.158 (for the Greek and Latin texts, see 4.10.5 below), but there are at least a dozen such instances in Book 2 alone. Usually, these involve either simply highlighting that the word is Greek, as e.g. at 2.181: 'quod Graeci pentafilon uocant' (cf. II, 465, 21: τῆς πενταφύλλου βοτάνης),[30] or providing a Latin gloss or terminological equivalent, as e.g. at 1.143 (text of A): 'in epyzogoto membrano, id est in omento uel cingulo quo circumdantur latera' (cf. II, 229, 4: τοῦ τὰς πλευρὰς

[28] Other divergences between the Latin and Greek versions of this chapter are set out on p. 23 above.

[29] Note, however, e.g. 2.258: 'ad eos (*scil.* neruos) quos Graeci ankilas uocant' (beside II, 539, 32: τὰς καλουμένας ἀγκυλώσεις); 2. 266: 'cerota de opio confecta quae et ciliogrisa Graeci uocant' (beside II, 561, 18: ἃς οἱ παλαιοὶ καὶ χιλιοχρύσους καλεῖν ἀξιοῦσιν).

[30] At 1.144, the Latin Alexander provides a second Greek synonym that is absent from Puschmann's text at least: (text of A) 'peganisa +–quam quidam diapegason appellant–+ ... potest ... digerere' (cf. II, 233, 27: ἡ πηγανερὰ καλουμένη ... διαφορεῖν δύναται).

ὑπεζωκότος ὑμένος), again usually with an explicit reference to Greek terminology, as e.g. at 2.197: 'Cognosces igitur uesicam scabram esse quod Graeci propriasin uocant ...' (cf. II, 491, 12: Διαγίνωσκε τὴν ψωρίασιν τῆς κύστεως ...); 2.204: 'multi eorum flegmaticum et quem Graeci yalodem, id est similem uitro, flegmatis secessum faciunt' (cf. II, 337, 29–30: πλεῖστοι δ' αὐτῶν τὸν φλεγματώδη καὶ τὸν ὑαλώδη μᾶλλον ἐκκρίνουσι χυμόν); 2.269: 'potiones ad podagras quae sine dolore faciunt quas Graeci anodinas uocant' (cf. II, 569, 2: πρὸς τὰς ποδαγρικὰς ἀνωδυνίας ποτά). A more elaborate case is seen in the treatment of Greek ὀρ(ρ)ώδης, which receives a rudimentary etymology at 2.42 (below), and occurs twice more at 2.249.[31]

II, 289, 29–30 +––+ Εἴπερ ὀρρῶδες εἴη καὶ λεπτὸν καὶ μὴ ἄγαν ἐμπεπηγὸς ἐν τῇ γαστρὶ, οὐ χρὴ πολυπραγμονεῖν	2.42 +– Orus dicitur serus, id est ab humore pingui si tenuis decurrat; sic et liquidus humor a pingui defluens a Graecis orodis appellatur.–+ Quodsi orodis fuerit, id est tenuis a pingui fluens humore in uentrem non oportet remorari

In a third, straightforward but welcome and useful sort of case, the 'extra' material was not added to the Latin version but lost from the Greek. In fortunate circumstances, the Latin version makes it probable or certain that the translator's Greek text contained words lost through a mechanical copying error in an ancestor of the surviving Greek manuscripts. A clear example of this is the absence of the Greek words corresponding to the end of 1.145 and the very start of 1.146 (see the comparison below) caused by a *saut du même au même* from σύμπτωμα (Latin *simptoma*) to σύμπτωμα (Latin *accidentia*).

1.145 *ad fin.* Sic ergo oportet pleureticis si non aliud aliquid adsit simptoma +– quod prohibeat praedicto ordine fieri adiutoria.	II, 239, 14–17 οὕτως οὖν διαιτᾶν δεῖ τοὺς πλευριτικοὺς, εἰ μηδὲν ἄλλο τι παρείη σύμπτωμα +–
1.146 De uentris fluxu pleuresis Quodsi ut saepius contingere solet e contrario agat accidentia,–+ tunc oportet et adhuc insistere, quale est si cum dolore flegmone laterum non secundum naturam uenter excernat sed inordinate	 –+καὶ τότε δεῖ καὶ πρὸς ἐκεῖνο ἐνίστασθαι, οἷον, εἰ συμβῇ μετὰ τοῦ ὀδύνην εἶναι καὶ φλεγμονὴν περὶ τὸ πλευρὸν, μὴ κατὰ φύσιν ἐκκρίνειν τὴν γαστέρα, ἀλλ' ἀτάκτως,

[31] At 2.249, first it is glossed with Latin *aquosus*, then in the very next sentence it recurs in a *quod Graeci uocant* formula, where Puschmann's text has not ὀρρώδης but λεπτός: 2.249: 'dandum est catarticum quod possit educere pingue et spissum flegma et non orode id est aquosum et tenue urinae simile, quemadmodum multi faciunt dantes lacterides et opos titimali et cnidium coccum admiscentes et sic euacuant tenuiores humores quos Graeci orodes uocant' (II, 521, 5–7: τὸ δυνάμενον ἑλκῦσαι παχὺ φλέγμα καὶ ὀρρῶδες, ὥσπερ ποιοῦσι πολλοὶ λαθυρίδας τε καὶ ὀπὸν τιθυμάλλου καὶ Κνίδιον κόκκον παρέχοντες αὐτοῖς, οἳ τὰ λεπτὰ κενοῦντες ῥεύματα).

2.4.3. Material in the Greek Original Missing from the Latin Version

The converse of the glossing of Greek terms, touched on in the last paragraph, is seen in the translator's removal (sensible enough) of the Greek apology for the use of a Latin term. So, for example, 'barley-water' referred to by the Latin term at II, 191, 21: τῷ παρὰ Ῥωμαίοις καλουμένῳ φαριχύλῳ, appears in the Latin version simply as *sucus farris* (2.168: 'Non autem praesenti tisan<a> suco uteris farris'). Other minor omissions of Greek material we have already seen illustrated (e.g. on pp. 21–2 above). In this section, I wish to draw attention to three types of omission on a larger scale, and in particular the reduction of material devoted to theory and to magic, respectively.

Some substantial cuts amount to the omission of whole discussions of particular diseases. This is true of internal abscesses and hiccoughs (both originally in Book 7 of the Greek), of dysentery and paralysis (which constitute Book 10 in the Greek manuscripts), of tertian, quotidian, and quartan fever (about the last 40 per cent of the book on fevers), and, on a smaller scale, of ἄνθρακες of the eye (II, 59, 1–65, 28, between 1.104 and 1.105). These chapters were either absent from the translator's text, or omitted by editorial decision, whether because they were thought to be insufficiently important, or because other treatises on these subjects were available and preferred. The latter was probably the reason for the omission of Alexander on dysentery, as this disease is covered in the extracts from Philumenus on the stomach and intestines.

Other large omissions occur in lists of remedies in the Greek text which (presumably) seemed excessively long. In Puschmann's edition no fewer than fifteen pages are occupied by treatments for epilepsy, conventional (I, 545–57) and magical (I, 557–75), of which the Latin version lacks most of the second half of the latter (I, 567, 18–573, 14), resuming about a page from home and then translating to the end. A similar pattern is seen in remedies against coughing, which also claim fifteen pages of the Greek text (II, 157–85). Of these pages the Latin version translates the first five (II, 157, 1–167, 2), and then cuts almost ten pages of Greek, retaining only the very last two recipes in this very long chapter (II, 185, 26–34).

It is important to note that, while the remedies against epilepsy are mixed, conventional and magical, none of the treatments prescribed by Alexander for coughing are labelled as φυσικά, 'natural', medico-magical remedies: in this case at least, the abbreviation of the Greek text was not prompted by the desire to eliminate unconventional therapies from the Latin version. Thorndike observes correctly (*History*, I, 584) that the Latin Alexander omits 'many, although not all, of the chapters devoted to physical ligatures', but overstates her case in concluding that 'the early medieval translator and adapter, instead of retaining and emphasizing the superstition of the past, has largely purged his text of it'. It is true that the majority of the Greek medico-magical passages discussed by Thorndike (*History*, I, 579–84) do not appear in the Latin version,[32] but enough magic survives in the Latin to throw serious doubt on the very

[32] Note for example the substantial portions of Greek text absent from the Latin Alexander at 1.73 (I, 567, 18–573, 14) and 2.184 (II, 473, 28–475, 24).

idea of a deliberate purging. This is illustrated not only by the chapters on epilepsy outlined above (1.71–2) but also in the last three chapters on the treatment of colic (2.232–4), which open, also in the Latin version, with an acknowledgement of the need to say something about magical remedies. I reproduce both versions side by side below.

II, 375, 11 Puschmann	2.232 (text of A)
	t. De fisicis [et] ligaturis et potionibus et caracteribus ad colum
Cf. 1. ἀλλ' ἐπειδὴ τῶν περιοδευομένων πολλοὶ καὶ μάλιστα τῶν πλουσίων οὔτε πίνειν ὅλως θέλουσι φάρμακον οὔτε κλύσμασι θεραπεύειν τὴν γαστέρα, **διὰ δὲ περιάπτων φυσικῶν ἀναγκάζουσιν ἡμᾶς ἀποπαύειν αὐτῶν τὴν ὀδύνην**, ἐσπούδασα καὶ περὶ τούτων ἐκθέσθαι ὑμῖν, ὧν τε αὐτὸς ἔσχον πεῖραν καὶ ὅσα παρὰ φίλων ἀληθινῶν ἔγνων ὠφελεῖν δύνασθαι.	**1**. Quoniam multi qui colum patiuntur et maxime diuites neque ex toto aliquid bibere uolunt neque iniectionem sibi consentiunt fieri, propterea **necesse est nobis de fisicis ligaturis aut caracteribus aliqua dicere**. Quae si fiant mox relaxari solent uel amputari dolores et ideo ea quae ab antiquis uel postea a nobis probata sunt scribere non omittam et quae resistunt et patientibus colum praebent remedium.
+–καὶ τοὺς ἀρίστους δὲ τῶν παλαιῶν εὕρομεν μαρτυρήσαντας, ὅπως μηδὲ ἡ τέχνη ἄπειρος εἶναι νομισθῇ καὶ ἀσυμπαθὴς μήτε οἱ περιοδεύοντες ἀφιλόκαλοί τε καὶ ἀσυμπαθεῖς εἶναι δόξωσιν, ὡς ἀγνοοῦντες τὰ τῆς φύσεως ἀσυμπαθῆ τε καὶ συμπαθῆ.–+	+– II, 375, 16–22 –+
Cf. t. Περίαπτα φυσικὰ πρὸς τοὺς κωλικὴν ἔχοντας διάθεσιν +– Περίαπτον ἀδιάπτωτον, οὗ καὶ ἡμεῖς ἔσχομεν πεῖραν καὶ πάντες δὲ ὀλίγου δεῖν ἄριστοι τῶν ἰατρῶν εὐδοκίμησαν. –+	
Cf. 2. λαβὼν ἀφόδευμα λύκου, εἰ δυνατὸν, ἔχον ὀστάρια κατάκλεισον εἰς σωληνάριον καὶ δὸς φορεῖν περὶ τὸν δεξιὸν βραχίονα ἢ μηρὸν ἢ ὀσφὺν ἐν τῷ παροξυσμῷ κατὰ τοῦ ἀλγοῦντος μέρους φυλαττόμενος, ὡς μήτε τῆς γῆς μήτε λουτροῦ θίγειν.	**2**. In primis ergo accipiens fimum lupi — et si possibile est ex eo qui ossa comedit — claudes in testeo uase et ligabis in dextro brachio aut in humero id est collo aut ad coxas suspendes in ipsa commotione doloris. Obseruabis autem ut neque terram tangat neque in balneum secum ferat. **3**. Item aliud.[33] Et hoc experimentatum est. Corallium habens incendes et teres et quantum sunt coclearia duo aut tria ieiuno potum dabis per dies tres aut quattuor. Facit enim bene ad colicas passiones.
Cf. 4. Ἄλλο καὶ αὐτὸ διὰ πείρας. Κορυδαλὸς ἐσθιόμενος τὸ αὐτὸ ποιεῖ καλῶς. οἱ δὲ Θρᾷκες ἔτι ζῶντος τοῦ κορυδαλοῦ ἐξαιροῦντες τὴν καρδίαν περίαπτον ποιοῦσιν ἐν τῷ μηρῷ τῷ ἀριστερῷ περιθέντες αὐτό.	**4**. Item aliud.[34] Hoc ipsum corallium acceptum in cibo sanat. Item aliud. Qui autem scindunt eum et cor eius sublatum appendunt in coxa sinistra carent coli dolore

[33] The following is recipe 2/4 in 2.233.
[34] The following are recipes 3/4 and 4/4 in 2.233.

+–Ἄλλο φυσικὸν δεδοκιμασμένον. Χοίρου λαβὼν ἐκ τοῦ τυφλοῦ ἐντέρου τὸ μασθοειδὲς, σμυρνιάσας και ἐνδύσας δέρματι λυκίῳ ἢ κυνίῳ δίδου φορεῖν ἐν ἀποκρούσει σελήνης καὶ θαυμάσεις.–+	+– Gk II, 377, 1–4 –+
Cf. 5. Ἄλλο περίαπτον. Εἰς λίθον Μηδικὸν γλύψον Ἡρακλέα ὀρθὸν πνίγοντα λέοντα καὶ ἐγκλείσας εἰς δακτυλίδιον χρυσοῦν δίδου φορεῖν.	(*ed.* 2.234 De lapide medicon) **5**. Item aliud. De lapide medicon sculpens in eo Heraclea[m] rect*um* suffocantem leonem includes in anulo aureo et dabis ad utendum in digito et sanus erit
Cf. 3. Τὸ αὐτὸ πάλιν. Κορυδαλὸς καιόμενος καὶ λειούμενος καὶ διδόμενος, ὅσον κοχλιάρια β′ ἢ γ′, προποτιζόμενος ἐφ' ἡμέρας γ′ ἢ δ′ ποιεῖ πάνυ πρὸς κωλικὰς διαθέσεις.	**6**. Item aliud.[35] Physicum faciens ad colum experimentatum est ualde. Lupi fimum terens in subtilissimum puluerem cernes et dabis patienti in aqua calida coclearium in mesum.
Cf. 7. Ἄλλο λίαν δραστικόν. Παιδίου ὀλίγον ἐκτμηθέντος ὀμφαλοῦ εἰς ἀργυροῦν ἢ χρυσοῦν ἔγκλεισον μεθ' ἁλὸς ὀλίγου. ὁ φορῶν τὸ περίαπτον τοῦτο ἄπονος ἔσται εἰς τὸ παντελές.	(*ed.* 2.233 De caracteribus) **7**. Item aliud ualde bonum.[36] Accipiens nascente infante modicum de inciso umbilico eius includes in argento aut aureo metallo. Hoc enim secum portans sine dolore erit semper.
Cf. 8. Ἄλλο· Αἴγειον ἧπαρ καύσας λείωσον καὶ δὸς πιεῖν μετ' οἴνου· πάνυ βοηθεῖ αὐτοῖς.	**8**. Item aliud (Gk II, 377, 16).[37] Caprae epar ustulans teres et dabis bibendum cum uino. Satis enim iuuat hoc +–et amputat coli dolorem.[38] –+
+–Δακτύλιος πρὸς τὸ αὐτό. Λαβὼν δακτύλιον σιδηροῦν ποίησον γενέσθαι τὸ κρικέλλιον αὐτοῦ ὀκτάγωνον καὶ οὕτως ἐπίγραφε εἰς τὸ ὀκτάγωνον ... ... γινέσθω δὲ ὁ προϋποτυπωθεὶς δακτύλιος ιζ′ τῆς σηλήνης ἢ κα′.–+	+– Gk II, 377, 18–28 –+
Cf. 6. Ἄλλο φυσικὸν ποιοῦν πρὸς κῶλον διὰ πείρας. Λαβὼν λύκου ἀφόδευμα τρίψας χνοωδέστατον πάνυ καὶ σήσας δίδου τῷ κάμνοντι εἰς ὕδωρ θερμὸν κοχλιαρίου τὸ s″.	

This longish comparison not only illustrates the survival of magic in the Latin version, but also offers another extended example of how different the Latin may be from the Greek,[39] in terms both of arrangement and of content: notice especially the content of Section 1.[40]

Another possible criterion for the shortening of the Greek original — whether by a Greek redactor or by the maker of the Latin Alexander — may have been a prejudice in

[35] The following is recipe 2/3 in 2.234.
[36] The first four words not in *ed.*; the following is recipe 1/4 in 2.233.
[37] The following is recipe 3/3 in 2.234.
[38] Here *ed.* repeats from end 2.232: 'Obseruabis autem ut neque terram tangat neque in balneum secum ferat'.
[39] To say nothing of divergences within the Latin tradition: see preceding nn.
[40] The numbering of sections here is to be regarded for the moment as purely ad hoc.

favour of purely factual and practical medicine matched by a consistent lack of concern for medical theory or debate. Such leanings are implied quite generally by the nature and form of those medical texts selected for translation and copying in the medieval West. Writing of the High Middle Ages, Danielle Jacquart observes[41] that '[l]a principale carence des textes véhiculés au Haut Moyen Age réside dans la quasi-absence d'un propos théorique'. She cites Alexander as an example, and characterizes the Latin translations of his *Therapeutica* and of the *Euporista* and *Synopsis* of Oribasius as 'compendia à usage pratique'. The observation gains in force when one notes that frequently even those limited passages on theory in the original do not appear in the Latin version. In view of the importance of the Latin Alexander as a witness for the Greek text, this is regrettable — regardless of one's taste concerning what constitutes more and less interesting medical prose — as the missing material includes quotations from, allusions to, and discussions of doctrines of important medical predecessors of Alexander, as well as personal reflections on his approach to healing and anecdotes from his own practice. There is an important example in the chapters on coughing (edited in Chapter 5 below), where, while the Latin version contains the case of the man who coughed up a stone,[42] it omits twenty lines of Greek containing Alexander's famous criticism of Galen using Galen's own words of criticism of Archigenes, and Alexander's assertion, quoting Aristotle, of the overriding importance of truth over authority (II, 155, 2–22 Puschmann). At 1.58, on diet in the treatment of *phrenitis*, the Latin version has the opening sentence criticizing the ignorance of many doctors in this regard ('Multi enim ignorantes cibos ministrant, et nesciunt utrum potius laedant aut sanent'), but then jumps directly to Alexander's first prescription ('Mox ergo a primordio ptisanae sucus ministrandus est bene coctus'), omitting the fairly rhetorical tirade against contemporary doctors, which includes a reference to Galen and an appeal to personal experience (I, 521, 23–523, 7 Puschmann).

A particularly good example of severe compression of the Greek text at the expense of discursive, personal anecdotal material, so as to leave a bare minimum of functional statements, is the Preface to Cosmas at the start of Book 3 of the Latin Alexander (Book 12 of the Greek manuscripts). Much of what the Latin tradition presents as the Preface is in fact the first section on ephemeral fevers (I, 291 Puschmann). In fact, the interesting and colourful Greek preface, which contains important information about Alexander's practice and the circumstances and intended style of composition of the promised work, is reduced to barely a quarter of its length in the Latin. See the comparison below.

The Greek dedication to Cosmas	The Latin dedication to Cosmas
I, 289 Puschmann Αἰτήσαντί σοι, Κοσμᾶ φίλτατε,+– τὰς ἐκ πείρας ἡμῖν πολλάκις ἀνυσθείσας –+ ἐπὶ διαφόρων νοσημάτων +– –+	3. pr. (text of *ed.*) Petisti a me, carissime Cosma, ut +––+ de diuersis passionibus +–membrorum et

[41] Jacquart, 'Transmission', 253.

[42] Albeit with a disastrous mistranslation, 2.11.5 'ita defunctus est' for II, 155, 1 ἂν ἀπώλετο.

ἐκθέσθαι θεραπείας ἑτοίμως ὑπήκουσα χάριτας ἀμφοτέροις εἰκότως ὁμολογῶν σοί +–τε καὶ τῷ σῷ πατρὶ τῆς εἰς ἐμὲ παρ' ὑμῶν φιλοφρόνως ἑκάστοτε γενομένης εὐνοίας· ὁ μὲν γὰρ ἐξ ἀρχῆς εὐθὺς οὐ μόνον ἐν τοῖς ἔργοις τῆς τέχνης, ἀλλὰ καὶ τῶν κατὰ βίον πραγμάτων ἁπάντων δεξιὸς ὑπουργὸς ἐγένετο· σὺ δὲ μετὰ βαρβάρων τὴν ἀναστροφὴν μὲν ποιούμενος διὰ τὴν τῶν βιασαμένων ἡμᾶς πραγμάτων περίστασιν παριδεῖν οὐκ ἐκαρτέρησας· διὸ καὶ γέρων λοιπὸν πειθαρχῶ καὶ κάμνειν οὐκέτι δυνάμενος τοῦτο τὸ βιβλίον ἔγραψα συντάξας τὰς μετὰ πολλῆς τριβῆς ἐν ταῖς τῶν ἀνθρώπων νόσοις καταληφθείσας πείρας, τέρψει δὲ πολλοὺς εὖ οἶδα τῶν εἰς φθόνον μὴ θελόντων βλέπειν τό τε εὐμέθοδον τῶν θεωρημάτων καὶ τὸ σύντομον ἅμα καὶ σαφὲς τῆς λέξεως. ἐσπούδασα γὰρ, ὡς ἐνδέχεται, κοιναῖς καὶ μᾶλλον εὐδήλοις χρήσασθαι λέξεσιν, ἵνα καὶ τοῖς τυχοῦσιν ἐκ τῆς φράσεως εὔλυτον εἴη τὸ σύνταγμα.	febrium generalibus tibi signa–+ et curationes breuiter exponerem. Obediens ergo petitioni tuae in utroque me parare confiteor +–et inceptum possibile est de febrium diuersitatibus signa et curationes breui stilo scribam.

This is not so much a translation as a bare-bones summary. It is interesting to note the addition of *signa* (twice, in the clumsily-repeated *signa et curationes*) and even more so the introduction of fevers (also repeated). The repeated mention of fevers here suggests that the maker of the Latin Preface was trying to make sense of the placement of the Greek Preface in his exemplar towards the end of the work and immediately before the book on fevers; the Greek Preface, on the other hand, makes no mention of fevers and implies that it is introducing a medical work of much broader scope (note especially I, 289, 1–2: +– τὰς ἐκ πείρας ἡμῖν πολλάκις ἀνυσθείσας –+ ἐπὶ διαφόρων νοσημάτων +– –+ ἐκθέσθαι θεραπείας, and 9–10: τοῦτο τὸ βιβλίον ἔγραψα συντάξας τὰς μετὰ πολλῆς τριβῆς ἐν ταῖς τῶν ἀνθρώπων νόσοις καταληφθείσας πείρας); on the implications of this for the original arrangement of the work, see above (p. 17). With regard to the apparent elimination of original Greek material, we can be thankful that not every passage as engaging and personal as this appears so reduced in the Latin version!

If excisions of this sort make sense in a recension aimed at distilling the practical at the expense of the theoretical or discursive, on other occasions the Latin version lacks material which ought to have commended itself for out-and-out practical purposes, including differential diagnosis and lessons to be learned from case-histories. So, for example, at 1.54, the Latin version lacks the section on how to distinguish phrenitis from delirium (οἱ παραφρονοῦντες), on the one hand, and madness (οἱ μαινόμενοι), on the other. The Latin implies that there is a condition that resembles but is not phrenitis, but gives a (flawed) translation of only the last sentence of the Greek chapter headed Πῶς χρὴ διορίζειν τοὺς παραφρονοῦντας ἀπὸ τῶν φρενιτικῶν; (I, 511, 21), as in the comparison below.

I, 513, 4 Puschmann +–… ταῦτα μέν ἐστι τὰ σημειᾶ τῶν κυρίως φρενιτικῶν, ἐφ' ὧν καὶ ξανθὴ χολὴ μόνη στηριχθεῖσα ἄνευ ἄλλης ὕλης τὴν διάθεσιν εἰργάσατο, –+ ὥσπερ εἰ μιχθείη τῇ ξανθῇ χολῇ φλέγμα, νόθη φρενῖτις ἡ τοιαύτη καλεῖται καὶ τὸ καλούμενον ἐργάζεται ἄγρυπνον κῶμα.	1.54 *ad fin.* (text of A) +– … –+ Quodsi mixta fuerint rubea colera flegmati, et haec uocatur frenesis, quia exinde insomnietas fit corporis, sed non est uera frenesis.

Again, at 1.83, on the treatment of melancholia, although we have in Latin the case of the woman who believed she had swallowed a snake, we lack the famous case[43] (preceding in the Greek, I, 605, 26–607, 5) attributed to the great Hellenistic doctor Phylotimus[44] of the curing of the man who thought he had been beheaded for being a tyrant.

Broadly-characterized recommendations or prescriptions for treatment couched in general terms, although of obvious practical value in the right hands, may have been perceived as quasi-theoretical, or at least insufficiently specific, and are on occasion omitted from the Latin version. So, for example, at 1.44 the Latin Alexander is innocent of the elegant last four lines, beginning καθ' ὅλου εἰπεῖν, on general principles to be observed in the treatment of chronic headache (I, 499, 1–4 Puschmann). Similarly, at 2.202 the Latin Alexander lacks the last twelve lines on the treatment of 'gonorrhoea' (II, 497, 24–499, 10 Puschmann), which also begin καθόλου (was this a signal to the translator to switch off?) and speak almost entirely of classes of foods and medicaments (those which cool, those which dry, etc.).

Surely of no less practical value from the point of view of the user/reader are programmatic statements about diseases to be discussed in coming chapters, such as the long list of eye-diseases at II, 31, 12–16. If these were in the original Greek text, they are absent from the end of 1.94 of the Latin version, on the treatment of constriction of the 'pores' of the eye (πύκνωσις).

Occasionally, one wonders whether the content of some missing material was the reason for its omission. At 1.139, for example, there is no trace of the twenty-eight lines of Greek (II, 137, 17–139, 14) on the preparation and use of human faeces as an ingredient in remedies for the treatment of angina. A few lines earlier, Alexander actually anticipates patients' (and perhaps doctors') refusal to use this ingredient: II, 137, 11–13: εἰ δέ τινες διὰ τὸ βδελυρὸν παραιτοῦνται χρῆσθαι τῇ ἀνθρωπείᾳ κόπρῳ, ἀρκοῦσι καὶ τὰ δύο μόνα, καὶ τὸ ἐλατήριον καὶ ἡ κυνεία κόπρος διαχριομένη. Alexander's assurance that the prepared juice of the squirting-cucumber and canine faeces suffice on their own might have suggested this excision to a squeamish redactor. Equally, at 2.203, the chapter on priapism, one wonders whether the sexual content of the missing lines (II, 499, 18–24, including references to pornography and to a case of a posthumous priapic erection) may account for their omission. The aversion to more theoretical statements may explain the absence of the last five lines of this chapter (II, 501, 2–6, from πάνυ γάρ), the redactor perhaps overlooking the specific physiotherapy recommended at the very end.

[43] It is reported also by Galen (19, 701) and Aëtius (6.9).

[44] More often written 'Philotimus', also by Puschmann. On the spelling, see von Staden, *Herophilus*, 48 n. 32.

Finally, we have to reckon in certain instances with purely accidental loss of original material, at whatever stage of the tradition. At 1.83, for example, the chapter on the treatment of melancholia (mentioned above for omission of another sort), the case-history of the second woman, rendered melancholic by her husband's long absence, is cut abruptly short: in the Latin Alexander, between the phrases 'Quam ego hac ratione curaui' and 'In primis scilicet catharticum dedi', we have lost the equivalent of about a page of Puschmann's text (I, 607, 12–609, 11), detailing the sudden cure of the woman thanks to the sudden reappearance of the husband,[45] and containing also the start of a new chapter, on chronic cases of melancholy. However the mistake was made in the first place, it was not apparent to superficial scrutiny — the reader was expecting some form of treatment for the melancholic woman — and hence the slip was allowed to stand until it was irrecoverable. A second example of apparently accidental loss is seen at 2.204 (on colic). A comparable amount of Greek text — just over a page of Puschmann — appears to have been lost. Latin manuscript A (closely matched by *ed.*) has:

Fit (*scil.* colica passio) et per alia multa, et non solum +– (Gk II, 335, 19–337, 25) –+ flegmate imposito in intestino grauitas esse sentitur.

This time, the result — with the abrupt jump from causes to symptoms — is more obviously nonsensical in the Latin version, and so more probably the consequence of an accident within the Latin tradition.

It is probably fair to conclude that material was lost from the Greek Alexander in the processes of recension (in Greek and/or Latin) and translation (into Latin) sometimes by accident and sometimes as a result of deliberate excision. Some deliberate omissions were probably in some degree principled. Their main effects have been to shorten excessively long lists of remedies and to reduce the numbers of generalities, of theoretical and other discursive comments, and of magical remedies surviving in the Latin Alexander. If these were also deliberate policies, none has been carried through systematically. It bears to be stressed again that it is normally unclear — and in many cases probably unknowable — whether a given excision occurred among the ancestors of the Greek exemplar used by the maker(s) of the Latin Alexander, or in the preparation of that text for translation, or in subsequent editing of the first Latin version.

2.5. The Date and Place of Origin of the Latin Version

There is to my knowledge no external evidence as to where the Latin Alexander was made, or by whom. As to the question when, the only hard and fast *terminus ante quem* is the date of the earliest Latin manuscript copy, Par. lat. 9332 (my P1), around A.D. 800. Nevertheless, many scholars have pronounced more or less tentatively on these questions — presumably on the basis of probability and circumstantial evidence, for no arguments are produced — and a fairly firm consensus appears to have

[45] Note that the Greek Alexander, unlike the Latin (with 'ego curaui'), takes no credit for the cure.

emerged that the Latin Alexander was made soon after the Greek original (whenever that was!),[46] and in Ravenna or Rome.[47]

This is certainly plausible enough a priori, given what we know of the production of medical literature in Latin in the sixth and seventh centuries A.D. Hard evidence for the medical establishment in this period is slight in the extreme, but from the few hints that we do have 'there can be no doubt that in the history of early mediaeval medicine Ravenna in the 6th century played a very important part', as important as 'a Western Roman Alexandria'.[48] One or two other known centres of medical learning and activity (such as Monte Cassino) may offer themselves as possible alternatives, but as MacKinney stresses,[49] it was 'Ravenna and other *non*-monastic [emphasis implicit in the original] centres that took the lead in the translation of Greek medical texts and their transmission to the Latin West'. The connection of the Latin Oribasius with Ravenna was posited by Mørland (Oribasius, 191–2) on the strength of direct and indirect references to Ravenna in the text. This connection is now widely accepted, and more recently other late Latin medical texts have also been attributed to the putative output of the Ravenna redactors and translators, notably the Latin Galen.[50] If, as may be the case, we can establish close linguistic links between the Latin Alexander and the Latin Oribasius, we may perhaps suppose that they were made close together in time and space. However, in the absence of external evidence as to when and where the Latin Alexander at least was made, the best — really the only — way forward is through close linguistic study, and comparisons with other texts, on the basis of a sound text.

[46] Relative datings are offered by e.g. Rose, *Anecdota*, II, 108 ('an alter dem griechischen original fast gleich'); Sigerist, *Rezeptliteratur*, 15 ('schon zu Lebzeiten'); Ieraci Bio, 'Interferenze', 285 ('quasi coeva all'autore') — all three begging the question of Alexander's own dates. Absolute datings range only from the sixth to the seventh century A.D.: cf. e.g. Wellmann, 'Alex. Trall.', 1461 ('wohl noch im 6. Jhdt.'); Ieraci Bio, 'Trasmissione', 195 (sixth century), eadem, 'Interferenze', 285, and 'Centri', 28 (sixth–seventh century); Sudhoff, 'Unterricht', 32 (after A.D. 600); Seidler, 45 ('im 7. Jahrhundert'). To the best of my knowledge, the earliest dating is that implied by Rose's comparison (*Anecdota*, II, 45) of the language of the Latin Alexander with that of the early sixth-century treatise on dietetics by the exiled Byzantine doctor Anthimus (the *De obseruatione ciborum*, prefaced with a letter to Theoderic, king of the Franks (r. A.D. 474–526); further references in Langslow, *Medical Latin*, 67).

[47] Mørland, 'Nachträge', 92, 93, (followed by Beccaria, 'Sulle tracce', II, 59) associates the excerpts from Philagrius and Philumenus with the 'Ravenna-Kreis', and this association is made for the Latin Alexander as a whole by MacKinney, *Medicine*, 218; Mazzini, 'secoli V e VI', 435 n. 10; Ieraci Bio, 'Trasmissione', 195, and 'Interferenze', 285 (in the latter article with the qualification 'o comunque all'asse Roma-Ravenna'); and more cautiously by Cavallo, 'Cultura Scritta', 99 ('non si può escludere che, come per quella di Oribasio (e di Dioscuride?), ne sia stata sede la stessa Ravenna'). Rome is favoured as the place of origin of the Latin Alexander by Sudhoff, 'Unterricht', 32; Riché, 185; and Vázquez-Buján, 670.

[48] Sigerist, 'Latin med. lit.', 135.

[49] MacKinney, *Medicine*, 52.

[50] See Mazzini and Palmieri, 286–7, 294–6.

CHAPTER 3. THE MANUSCRIPT TRADITION OF THE LATIN VERSION

This chapter describes, and offers a preliminary evaluation of, the manuscript tradition of the Latin Alexander. This tradition is one of the richest, if not the richest, known for such an early medieval Latin medical text as the Latin Alexander must be, in particular for such a long text.[1] To date we know of twenty-one complete copies of the text,[2] dating from the ninth to the sixteenth century, even if only four of these are from before 1100. On the other hand, the text was evidently subject to excerpting from a very early date, being used as a source for various compilations, at least three of which are transmitted by three or more manuscripts. It is noteworthy that the manuscripts so far identified as containing excerpts are by and large significantly older than the mainstream tradition; this is a well-known phenomenon which applies both to other medical texts (such as Cassius Felix, who indeed is represented in the same collections as Alexander Trallianus) and more generally.[3] I embarked with some trepidation on an account of the secondary tradition, as it is so very complex, and it seemed that, whenever I spent time with it, the material grew — further witnesses were identified — and the questions multiplied. My hope is that, although I fail to specify closely the origins of the various branches of the secondary tradition, it will have been worthwhile to include my findings so far, as in most cases it has seemed possible to give a clear preliminary assessment (with examples) of their potential value for the editing of the Latin Alexander as a whole, and several of them are clearly going to be important.

The present chapter, then, comprises three parts. The first (3.1) gives a conspectus of the manuscripts so far identified which transmit the text of the Latin Alexander as a whole. They are listed below in chronological order, but for ease of reference their descriptions are ordered alphabetically by siglum. For each manuscript, I offer a bibliography; a physical description; a summary of the contents; and details of the Latin Alexander material transmitted (some notes on the form of the Latin in each manuscript, and the extent and nature of any secondary material or other interventions in the text, may be found in 4.9, 4.10.1 and the Appendix).

The second part (3.2) offers an account of the more important strands of the secondary tradition of the Latin Alexander, including sample comparisons between the excerpting and the mainstream manuscripts. It begins with an overview, partly in tabular form, of all the excerpts from the Latin Alexander so far collected, and then considers in turn several important sets of excerpts, each of which has its own, more or less separate manuscript tradition, namely the *Liber passionalis*, the so-called *Tereoperica* (*Therapeutica*) ascribed to Petroncellus of Salerno, the *Liber diaetarum diuersorum medicorum*, the *De podagra* often ascribed to Galen (drawn from the chapters on gout at the end of Book 2 of the Latin Alexander and appearing also in Book 4 of the *Passionarius* of Gariopontus of Salerno), and the so-called *Bamberg Surgery*.

[1] Leaving aside short tracts such as Vindic., *Ad Pentad.* and the Ps. Hippocratic letters (both late antique rather than early medieval).

[2] I include Chartres 342 and Metz 278, both destroyed in World War 2, and Vatican, BAV, Pal. lat. 1209 and Oxford, Bodleian Library, Bodl. 524 (twelfth century), which I have not yet seen.

[3] This is true of, e.g., Gargilius Martialis, the *Medicina Plinii* (see Fischer, '*Lib. Byz.*', 291 n. 49) and indeed of Pliny's *Natural History* as a whole.

Finally (3.3), the principal manuscripts containing these several parts of the secondary tradition — at least, those that I have examined and worked with — are described as in the first part of the conspectus, again in alphabetical order by siglum.

In order to give an initial impression of the extent and spread of the tradition known to date, both mainstream and secondary, I list below in chronological order: (1) the complete copies so far identified; (2) the excerpting manuscripts and the secondary tradition, first those manuscripts containing miscellaneous excerpts only, and then works which have used Alexander as a source (listing for these last at most only those manuscripts which I have used).

(1) Complete Copies[4]

P1	Paris, BN, lat. 9332 (early 9th cent.)
M	Montecassino, Archivio della Badia 97 (early 10th cent.)
A	Angers, Bibl. mun. 457 (11th cent.)
O	Orléans, Bibl. mun. 283 (end 11th cent.)
	[Oxford, Bodleian Library, Bodl. 524 (12th cent.) — *nondum uidi*]
(Ch	Chartres, Bibl. mun. 342 (12th cent.) (surviving only in a few photographs))
D	Durham Cathedral, C. 4. 11 (end 12th cent.)
G1	Glasgow, University Library, Hunter 435 (12th–13th cent.)
Mu	Munich, Bayerische Staatsbibliothek, clm 344 (12th–13th cent.)
Ox	Oxford, Pembroke College 8 (12th–13th cent.)
C	Cambridge, Gonville & Caius College 400 (early 13th cent.)
Ge	Geneva, Bibl. publ. et univ. 78 (13th cent.)
Ma	Madrid, BN, 1049 (13th cent.)
P2	Paris, BN, lat. 6881 (13th cent.)
P3	Paris, BN, lat. 6882 (13th cent.)
L2	London, British Library, Royal 12. B. XVI (late 13th cent.)
	[Vatican City, Bibl. apostolica vaticana, Pal. lat. 1209 (13th cent.) — *nondum uidi*]
B	Brussels, KBR 10869 (14th cent.)
G2	Glasgow, University Library, General 1228 (second half 15th cent.)
L1	London, British Library, Harley 4914 (16th cent.)

(2) Excerpting Manuscripts and the Secondary Tradition

(2.1) Miscellaneous excerpts

vat1	Città del Vaticano, Bibl. apostolica vaticana, regin. lat. 1143 (first half 9th cent.)
u	Uppsala, Universitetsbibliotek, C 664 (9th or 10th/11th cent.)
v1	Vendôme, Bibl. mun. 109 (11th cent.)

[4] cf. the lists in Puschmann I, 91–2; Diels, *Handschriften*, 11–12; Thorndike, *History*, I, 566–7, 576–7; Thorndike and Kibre, 259, no. 13.

v2 Vendôme, Bibl. mun. 172 (11th cent.)
v3 Vendôme, Bibl. mun. 175 (11th cent.)

(2.2) *Liber passionalis*

be Berlin, Deutsche Staatsbibliothek Preußischer Kulturbesitz, Phillipps lat. 1790 (second–fourth quarter 9th cent.)
s Sankt Gallen, Stiftsbibliothek 752 (10th cent.)

(2.3) *Tereoperica* [=*Therapeutica*], a compilation ascribed to Petroncellus of Salerno, part of it transmitted already in Paris, BN, lat. 11219 (early 9th cent.), etc.

(2.4) *Liber diaetarum diuersorum medicorum*

s Sankt Gallen, Stiftsbibliothek 752 (second half 9th cent.)
co Copenhagen, Koninglike Bibliotek, Gamle Koninglike Samling 1653 (11th cent.)
v1 Vendôme, Bibl. mun. 109 (11th cent.)
l2 London, British Library, Royal 12. E. XX (12th cent.)

(2.5) *De podagra*

po Poitiers, Bibl. mun. 184 (11th cent.)
vat2 Città del Vaticano, Bibl. apostolica vaticana, Barb. lat. 160 (11th cent.)
vat3 Città del Vaticano, Bibl. apostolica vaticana, lat. 4417 (11th cent.)
vat4 Città del Vaticano, Bibl. apostolica vaticana, lat. 4418 (11th cent.)
[**v1** Vendôme, Bibl. mun. 109 (11th cent.)[5]]
l2 London, British Library, Royal 12. E. XX (12th cent.)

(2.6) *Passionarius* (*Galeni* or *Garioponti*) of Gariopontus of Salerno, an important eleventh-century synthetic redaction, transmitted in over fifty manuscripts, and including the Latin Alexander, *De podagra.*

(2.7) '*Bamberg Surgery*', an anonymous, early twelfth-century(?) compilation on surgery, transmitted in Bamberg, Staatsbibliothek, med. 3 (L. III. 11) (mid-12th cent.), etc.

[5] Included here because Vendôme 109 also contains the chapters on gout, but evidently directly from the mainstream tradition.

3.1. Conspectus of the 'Mainstream' Latin Manuscripts

3.1.1. Complete Copies

A Angers, Bibliothèque municipale 457 (442) (autopsy April 1999) **Plate III** (Beccaria, *Codici*, 125f.; Bischoff, *Katalog*, 21; *Cat. gén. Dép.*, XXXI, 345; Mihăileanu, 94f. [in Rum.]; Puschmann I, 91; Stoffregen, 25f.; Vezin, 98, 106 n. 43, 160; Wickersheimer, *Manuscrits*, 15f.)

Eleventh century (Wickersheimer, Bischoff).[6] Of local manufacture,[7] at some point 'Ex libris monasterii S. Albini Andegavensis Congregationis S. Mauri'.[8] Vellum, 325×254mm, ff. 142. Large and clear and beautiful minuscule, in two columns of about 33 lines, chapter-numbers and chapter-initial capitals in red, titles (including sub-titles, such as *Item aliud*) in red lower case, or in black lower case underlined or boxed in red, or in black capitals each highlighted in red (with or without red underline), *capitula* numerals in red, initial capitals highlighted in red. The whole is carefully and clearly corrected.

Contents: two erased folios used as fly-leaves
2r–139v Alex. Trall.
140r–142v Alexander, *De pulsibus et urinis*: in a similar but smaller hand (at least 45 lines in a column, 2 columns)

Alex. Trall.: Book 1: 144 *capitula* numbered, 2ra–3rb, numerals always on outer edge of column; 144 chapters exactly fill 3v–51v. There is confusion in the copying of 1.6–12.[9]
Book 2: 146 *capitula* numbered, 52ra–53vb, numerals to left of column 52rv but on outer edge of column 53rv; 146 chapters 53vb–129va.
Book 3: 65 *capitula* numbered,[10] 129va–130ra, numerals to left of column; 34 chapters, 130rb–139vb, the text breaking off abruptly in 3.34, line 4 (XXXV) with 'Si autem non facile uomit calefieri oportet'.

B Brussels, Bibliothèque Royale, 10866–10869 (autopsy January 2000) (Calcoen, 40–1; Durling, *Guide*[1], 342; Kristeller III, 100; Puschmann I, 91; Silvestre)

Ff. 1–4 twelfth century, the rest fourteenth century (Calcoen). Liège, S. Laurent.[11]

[6] The ninth-century dating offered by *Cat. gén. Dép.* and Beccaria is rejected by Bischoff, *Katalog*, 21 (a reference I owe to Professor David Ganz).

[7] So Bischoff (*apud* Beccaria) and Vezin.

[8] These words are in the lower margin of 1r in seventeenth-century letters. The ms. is not, however, listed in a twelfth-century inventory of this library.

[9] **A** at first omits 1.6–12, save the first recipe of 1.7. **A** 4rb after 1.5: 'Deest una sententia [i.e. chapter!]. VII. Vt furfures non nascantur. Calicanto absintio arceutido ana ÷ vi. [1.7 in **A** has the first recipe in *ed.* but *ed.* omits the first ingredient and adds 'adianntos [*sic*] mirte nigre galle asiane ana ÷ vi' before *trita*.] Trita hec infundes in oleo diebus vi colabis et uteris. *Hic desunt vi sententie omnino superflue*. XIIII. Ad pitiriaseos. ...' At 6ra, however, **A** has second thoughts, and the missing chapters appear as 6ra–8va, including the start of 1.7 for the second time: **A** 7ra 'VII Ad capillos cadentes et caluos. Vt non cadant capilli et ne furfures nascantur' — then the first recipe exactly as before (see above); the rest of 8v and all of 9r are blank. The tradition of this group of chapters is confused also in the Greek Alexander: see 2.4.1 above.

[10] Ending 'LXIIII. Lyxoperita epitimata et embroce febrientibus Marturii medici. LXV. Epitimata Galieni quibus usus est ad humectandum diuersas febres': cf. **Mu** and **O** below.

[11] cf. 5r, before the *capitula*, in another, much larger hand, '.P. (?) Sa(ncti) Lauren(tii) in Leodip.'; and 142r, after 'explicit', in the same hand, '.P.(?) Sa(ncti) Lauren(tii) in Leod.'.

Parchment, ff. 203, octavo (ff. 74–144 are *c.* 5mm smaller than the others), in single columns of 40–41 lines. Alex. Trall. chapter-titles (in large lower case) and initial capitals in red (presignalled in brown in the margin). Many marginal notes[12] and corrections appended in the same hand(?). A number of folios were damaged before being used, holes or unusable areas being written around.

Contents: 1r of medical content, in the same hand as 1v–4v
1v–4v *Speculum medicorum*
5rv a paragraph on weights and measures, then the *capitula* to Constantinus
6r–72r Constantinus Africanus' Latin translation of Ibn al-Jazzar, *Viaticum*
72v–73v obscure
74r–114v Matthaeus Platearius, *De simplicibus medicinis*
115r app. of medical content
116r–142r Johannes Platearius, *Practica*
143r–200v Alex. Trall.

Alex. Trall.: Book 1: unnumbered *capitula* in 3 columns 143r, 1 column 143v; chapters 143vb–166r.
Book 2: unnumbered *capitula* in 3 columns 166r–167r; chapters 167r–200r. Note that ff. 169–180 (2.97–206) have changed places with ff. 181–191 (2.22–97).
Book 3: unnumbered *capitula* in 3 columns 200r, 2 columns 200v (ending with the title of 3.66), and then, 200v (just less than half a page of the start of Book 3): (3. Pr.) 'P etisti [*sic*] a me Cosma ... Inprimis ergo de effimeris simplicibus febribus q(ue) etiam frequenter solent p(ro)uenire hominibus. (3.1) E ffimere [*sic*] febres. Q(ue) tantum in sp(irit)u qui est in corde consistunt. n(ihil?) a(utem?) in se habent manifestius.'

C Cambridge, Gonville & Caius College 400 (729) (autopsy October 2002) (James II, 464–5 and *Suppl.*, xxiii; Puschmann I, 92)

Early thirteenth century (James). Made in England (James, *Suppl.*). Vellum, 232×172mm, ff. iii + 90 + ii. Well and clearly written in a small hand, for the most part in single columns of 38 lines (ff. 84–93, in 2 columns of 37 lines), with lovely illuminated book initials, ornate chapter-initials in red, blue, green, and yellow, and foliation in red.

Contents: 3 fly-leaves+2 at the end (all with thirteenth-century writing)
4r blank
4v–83v Alex. Trall.
84ra–90va *Liber cyrurgie* (i.e. the *Bamberg Surgery*, 3.2.7 below)
90va–93ra *Liber flebotomie*
93ra–93vb *De theriaca* (in another, slightly later hand)

[12] Above all, these draw attention to remedies attributed to Alexander himself: e.g. 152r (1.70) beside three remedies is, respectively, 'nota opus Alexandri', 'nota', and 'nota dignum'. Note also 157r (1.99) about a third of the way down, in the first hand, 'totus iste uersus corruptus est'.

Alex. Trall.: Book 1: 147 unnumbered *capitula*, 4v (3 columns) and 5r (2 columns), with initials alternately red and blue; the sections on the eyes, ears, and nose each have an additional title underlined in black; 5v–34v text of Book 1.
Book 2: only 75 (*sic*) unnumbered *capitula*,[13] 34v–35r (in 2 columns); 35r–75v text of Book 2.
Book 3: 62 unnumbered *capitula*, 75v (3 columns) and 76r (2 columns), ending with the title of 3.66; 76r–83v text of Book 3, including all but the very last recipe of 3.66.

D Durham Cathedral Priory, ms. C. IV. 11

End twelfth century, made in Italy.[14] Parchment, ff. 139, written in 2 columns of about 32 lines, with decorated initials at ff. 51 and 123. Some of the chapters are numbered.

Contents: 1r '1. Liber alexandri yatros sophiste [fourteenth century] De medicinis'
1v a list concerning the colours of urine
f. 2 apparently cut in half vertically; 2r is blank
2v–137va Alex. Trall.
137vb–139v a short text on the seven branches of learning in a later (fifteenth-century?) hand

Alex. Trall.: Book 1: (the *capitula*, 1.1–5 and the first three lines of 1.6 are missing); 2v–49va text of 1.6 line 4 to end of Book 1.
Book 2: 49va–51ra 148 unnumbered *capitula*, the start of each on a new line; 51ra–122vb text of Book 2.
Book 3: 122vb–123rb about 64 unnumbered *capitula* written continuously, ending with the title of 3.66; 123rb–137va text of Book 3, to end of 3.65 followed by 'EXPLICIT ALEXANDER YATROS SOPHOS'.

Ge Geneva, Bibliothèque publique et universitaire, ms. lat. 78 (Petau)
(Aubert, *Notices ... Genève*, 41–4)

Two manuscripts (of which the second (ff. 145–315) contains Alex. Trall.), thirteenth/fourteenth century (ff. 1–144) and thirteenth century (ff. 145–315), respectively. Parchment, ff. 317 (several ff. having been lost), 230×165mm; the second manuscript beautifully written in single columns of about 32 lines, with chapter-titles in red, chapter-initials alternately in red and blue (in the lists of *capitula*, in red), and originally with very elaborate, lovely book-initials in gold and various colours (the f. containing the initial to Book 1 is lost). No chapter numbers. Annotated throughout in a much later, minute hand.

[13] Not all '*capitula*-titles' are in the text (e.g. after (2.29) *De siti*, the title (2.30) *Ad eos qui habent ardorem* ... is not in the text, 38v). On the other hand, in the '*capitula*-titles' for Book 2 there are only three entries between (2.68) *De athonia epatis* (text 45r) and (2.235) *De podagra* (text 69r), and in general there are more titles in the text than in the *capitula*.

[14] I am very grateful to Alan Piper, Archives and Special Collections, Durham University Library, for information about the manuscript. He informs me: 'it contains [1r] a Durham letter-mark (L) and note of content in a hand of the later fourteenth century. Subsequently it is entered in the 1392 catalogue of the books kept in the Spendement, the strong-room adjoining the cloister.' The Hill Monastic Manuscript Library catalogue entry, reproduced at the front of the microfilm, gives as the date of the ms. thirteenth century.

Contents:[15] 1–126 Rhazes, *Liber uocatus Almanzor* (alias *El-Mansour*) or *Verba Albubecri*, Latin translation from the Arabic by Gerard of Cremona
126–144v an anonymous treatise on fevers (by Johannicius? Johannes Ferrarius?)
145–289v Alex. Trall. (145 is blank, being the original end-paper)
290v two hexameter quatrains in a fourteenth-century hand
291–314 blank
315r a summary table of contents to Alex. Trall.

Alex. Trall.: Book 1: (one f. missing, containing the *capitula*, 1.1–4 and most of 1.5); 146r–197r text of Book 1, from 1.5 line 9.
Book 2: 197r–198v 141 unnumbered *capitula* in 2 columns; 198v–274v text of Book 2 to the end of 2.271.[16]
Book 3: 275r the *capitula* of 3.64, 65, 66 in 2 columns at the top; 275r–289v text of 3.1–65. There follows, 315r (in a later hand, fourteenth or fifteenth century), a table of contents summarizing all three books in a column and a half (with the entry *De ethica* after (3.65.t.) *De marasmode*!).

G1 Glasgow, University Library, Hunter 435 (autopsy January 2006) **Plate V** (Puschmann I, 92; Schenkl, 32; Young and Aitken, 358 [I quote their description below, with a few modifications prompted by autopsy])[17]

Twelfth/thirteenth century, made in France(?) (Young and Aitken; end twelfth-century, Schenkl). Vellum, 242 × 165mm, ff. vii+132+ii (of which iii + ii are recent; foliated in 1961), originally ff. 138; beautifully written (?in France), in single columns (with a few exceptions) of 30 lines, each 165 × 89mm, ruled and margined with plummet. No signatures or foliation, probably cropped, catchwords, chapter-titles (and subheadings) in red, chapter-initials alternately red decorated with blue and blue decorated with red, the three book-initials in red, blue and green (2r; 45r; 111v), small red and blue initials (alternately) in lists of chapters preceding the three books, careful marginal and interlinear notes throughout in more than one hand. Vellum defective in places and sewn, square place-finding tabs cut in 5, 5 and 15, 8, much cropped, otherwise well preserved and clean.

Contents: iv verso in twelfth/thirteenth-century uncials 'ALEXANDER AD COSMAM ET DAMIANVM'[18]
v recto–verso *Pharmacopoeia*
vi recto–vii verso *Ponderum et mensurarum explicatio*
1r–124r Alex. Trall.
124v–126v *Nominum medicorum explicatio*
127r–132r Anonymus, *De passionibus mulierum*[19]
132v Constantinus Africanus, *Viaticum*, excerpts on epilepsy and menstruation.[19a]

[15] Note that the manuscript has been refoliated since Aubert.

[16] *Pace* Aubert, we have not lost the end of Book 2, merely the explicit and the first (approximately) 63 *capitula* of Book 3. It is surprising that the latter should have occupied a whole folio.

[17] For assistance and information relating to both of the Glasgow manuscripts, **G1** and **G2**, I am grateful to David Weston, Keeper of Special Collections, Glasgow University Library.

[18] For this pair of names, cf. the 'foreword' to **P2** (below).

[19] In the same hand as the Alex. Trall., it begins 'Incipit Genecia Prisciani', and is version B in the terms of Green, '*De genecia*'.

[19a] I am grateful to Monica Green for this information.

Alex. Trall.: Book 1: 1r–2r 139 unnumbered *capitula* written continuously in 2 columns; 2r–43v text of Book 1.
Book 2: 43v–45r 135 unnumbered *capitula* written continuously in 2 columns; 45r–110v text of Book 2.
Book 3: 110v–111v 69(!) unnumbered *capitula* written continuously in 2 columns;[20] 111v–124r text of Book 3, including all but the very last recipe in 3.66 (no Explicit).

G2 Glasgow, University Library, General 1228 (autopsy January 2006)
(Durling, *Guide*², 348; Ker, II, 926; Kristeller, IV, 31a; Schenkl, 34)

Second half fifteenth century, probably made in France (Ker, Kristeller; fifteenth century, Schenkl). Vellum, 305×215mm (the written area 190×110mm), ff. ii+413+ii (ff. 1 and 415 being medieval parchment fly-leaves). Large size, Northern hand (Kristeller), 'a large ugly set hybrida' (Ker), in single columns of 25 lines. Three-line red chaper-initials, a few of them illuminated (e.g. 63r, the face of a man in the 'N' of 'Non una est …', the start of 1.75 *De Melancholia*), red chapter-titles and section-initials throughout. Neat marginalia and interlinear notes in several hands throughout.

Contents: only Alex. Trall.

Alex. Trall.: Book 1: 2r–4va 149 numbered *capitula* in 2 columns; 5r–147r 149 chapters.
Book 2: 147v–153v 271 numbered *capitula* in 1 column; 154r–368v 271 chapters.
Book 3: 368v–370v 66 numbered *capitula* in 1 column; 370v–413r 66 chapters.

L1 London, British Library, Harley 4914 (autopsy January 2003)
(*Cat. Harley*, III, 220; Durling, *Guide*², 348; Kristeller, IV, 181b; Puschmann I, 92)

Sixteenth century, written in France. Paper, ff. 316 (+4 prepared but unused), paginated. Clearly written in single columns of 26 lines. Lined in red throughout, and with chapter-numbers, titles, initials, and paragraph markers in red throughout.

Contents: only Alex. Trall.

Alex. Trall.: Book 1: 1r–4v 147 unnumbered *capitula*; 5r–112r 149 numbered chapters.
Book 2: 112v–118v 271 numbered *capitula*; 118v–281v 271 numbered chapters.
Book 3: 282r–283v 66 numbered *capitula*; 283v–316v 66 numbered chapters.

L2 London, British Library, Royal 12. B. XVI
(Warner and Gilson, II, 15)

Late thirteenth century. Formerly belonged to Athelney Abbey, Somerset (f. 2v 'Athelnay pertinet'). Vellum, ff. 113, 216×152mm. Clearly written in two columns of 35 lines (save the *capitula* of Book 1, in 3 columns). Elaborate book-initials, and chapter-initials throughout (save in the *capitula* to Book 3). Chapter-titles written into the gaps only on the first side of the first folio of Book 1 (4r). Damage to the outside central section of ff. 42 and 43 affects mainly the *capitula* of Book 2.

[20] Ending: 'De lixoperitis pannis et embrocis. <A>liud ad idem. De epithimate. | De epihimate ad febrem. De catarticis. Antidotum' — i.e. subdividing 3.66, as in the text of **G1**.

Contents: only Alex. Trall.[21]

Alex. Trall.: Book 1: 3rv unnumbered *capitula*, initials alternately in ?red and blue?; 4ra–42vb unnumbered chapters.

Book 2: 42vb–43vb unnumbered *capitula* written continuously (and hard to read); 44ra–102vb unnumbered chapters.

Book 3: 102rb–vb unnumbered *capitula* without initials, ending with (3.61) *De uino*; 102vb–113vb unnumbered chapters ending with the end of 3.65.

Ma Madrid, Biblioteca Nacional ms. 1049 (L. 115)
(Domínguez Bordona I, 255, no. 520; Durling, *Guide*², 349; Gallardo, 163; *Inventario* III, 274; Kristeller IV, 521a)

Thirteenth century (Kristeller; *Inventario*). From the Primitiva Biblioteca Real. ff. 162+2. Vellum, 243×150mm. Written in single columns (the *capitula* in double columns) of 30 or 31 lines, 140×90mm. No numbers, and no chapter-titles in running text: gaps were left for titles; some were sketched in, but none were written in. Elaborate chapter-initials; each book begins with a wonderful illuminated initial. Numerous corrections and marginalia throughout. f. 143 was evidently accepted for use lacking its bottom third: no text is lost.

Contents: **1–161 Alex. Trall.**
162rv an alphabetical medical glossary, mainly Greek-Latin, A–T

Alex. Trall.: Book 1: 1r–2r 142 unnumbered *capitula* in 2 columns; 2v–56v text of Book 1.

Book 2: 57r–58v 269 unnumbered *capitula* (the last being that of 2.269); 58v–144r text of Book 2.

Book 3: 144r–145r 66 unnumbered *capitula*, ending with the title of 3.66; 145r–161v text of 3.1–65, followed by Explicit.

M Montecassino, Archivio della Badia, V. 97 **Plate II**
(Beccaria, *Codici*, 297–303; Beccaria, 'Sulle tracce', II, 27; *Cat. Casin.*, 96ff.; Glaze, *'Passionarius'*; Howald and Sigerist, v–vi; Loew, *Beneventan Script*, *passim*; Loew, *Scriptura Beneventana*, tab. xxxvi, p. 543; MacKinney, *Medicine*, 163, n. 77, 168, n. 97; MacKinney, 'Ethics', 8, 24 n. 39 (no. 4); Mihăileanu, 97f. [in Rum.]; Orofino, 58–72; Puschmann I, 91; Stoffregen, 41–2)

Early tenth century (Loew; Beccaria), less probably ninth century (Howald and Sigerist), probably made in the Abbey in Montecassino. Vellum, 414×300mm, pp. 552, some folios having been lost (including one of Alex. Trall.). Beneventan minuscule, perhaps by a single hand (Beccaria), in 2 columns of 40 lines, with titles and numbers in red, and chapter-initials generally decorated and coloured. Occasional marginal and interlinear glosses, corrections and additions in contemporary, sometimes slightly later, ordinary minuscule.

Contents: 1a–1b *Sapientia artis medicinae*; 1b–3a pseudo-Hippocratic and other anonymous prognostic texts 3a–4a *Incipiunt indicia ualitudinum Yppogratis*; 4a *Quomodo uisitare debes infirmum*; 4a–4b *Cura febrientibus*

[21] On f. 2v is the false title 'Constantini monachi viaticum' (in a sixteenth-century hand).

4b–6a Vindicianus, *Epistula ad Pentadium*
6a–8a Vindicianus, *Gynaecia*
8a–10a *Incipit epistula Yppogratis de fleubothomia*; 10a–10b *De mensura tollendo sanguinem in magnitudine aegritudinis et fortitudo uirtutis*; 10b–12b Pseudo-Aristotle, *Problemata*; 12b–13b *De passionibus unde eueniunt*
13b–20b Isidore, *Etymologiae* 4.1–12
20b–23b Hippocrates, *Epistula ad Antiochum regem*; 23a–24a *Item alia aepistula*; 24a *Item alia aepistula*; 24a *Alia*; 24a–26a *Epistula de ratione uentris uel uiscerum*; 26a–26b *Item alia aepistula de pulsis et urinis*
26b–33a *De pulsibus et urinis*
33a–199b the pre-Gariopontean ensemble minus *De podagra*:
 33a–89a Galen, *Ad Glauconem de medendi methodo* 1–2
 89a–108b *Liber tertius*
 109a Theod. Prisc., end of Book 2
 109a–131a *Liber Aurelii*
 131a–199b *Liber Esculapii*
199b–282a Commentary (Lat. A) on Hippocrates, *Aphorisms*, 1–7
282a–466a Alex. Trall.
466a–474b Galen, *Alphabetum ad Paternum*
477a–522b Apuleius Platonicus, *Herbarius*; 475b–476a *De herbis*
476a–476b, 523a–532b Dioscorides, *Liber medicinae ex herbis femininis*
532b–545a *Incipit de quadrupedibus*: 532b–533a *De taxone liber*; 533a–545a Sextus Placitus, *Liber medicinae ex animalibus*
545a–552b Galen, *Alphabetum ad Paternum*

Alex. Trall.: Book 1: 282a–284a 145 numbered *capitula*; 284a–346a text of Book 1. Book 2: 346a–349b 262 numbered *capitula*; 349b–442b text of Book 2, but missing a folio between pp. 394 and 395 containing the text of 2.137 (here CXVIIII) line 9–2.144 (here CXXV) line 3; the last chapter is numbered 264.
Book 3: 442b–443a 64 numbered *capitula* (the numbers XXXIIIff. are invisible because of the binding);[22] 443a–466a text of Book 3 ending with the penultimate recipe of 3.66 (minus the last three words); the last chapter, numbered LXV (*Lyxiperitus et inbrocas Galieni ad febres*), begins at 3.66 line 9.

Mu Munich, Bayerische Staatsbibliothek clm 344 (autopsy January 2001) (*Cat. Monac.*, I, 90; Mihăileanu, 97 [in Rum.])

Twelfth/thirteenth century, written in Italy (*Cat. Monac.*). Vellum, ff. 81 (but f. 61 twice), written in 2 columns of 52 lines. Highlighting in red: chapter-titles and numbers and a few chapter-initial capitals ff. 1–28r (the initial C of 1.1 is in blue); then again 44r–45r but with some titles missing and others very faint 44v–45r. Then only isolated initial capitals 45v–50v, 54va, 59rv, 60r. The text of Alex. Trall. has been corrected and annotated throughout, in places (e.g. 2.235–6) several times and by a different hand. ff. 1–61 (=Alex. Trall.) have been rebound and recut, f. 44 carelessly so that the text

[22] Ending with: 'Lyxiperitus et embrocas febrientibus. Lyxiperitus et inbrocas Galieni ad febres.'

leans into the binding, and part of a marginal note (44rb) is lost. The left margin of the lower half of f. 51ra is difficult to read because of the binding. There are some empty or barely-used sides: 37va (last few lines), 37vb contains only 'CVRATIO VENTOSITATIS' at the bottom; 43va (most of it), vb empty; 51rb uses only a few lines; 51va uses only a few lines (a recipe: 'Ad ictericiam. Apium cum modico aceto ... per urinam fel deducit'), 51vb is empty, and 51v contains a faint sketch of a man's bearded face. There is quite a bit of staining, smudging, and rubbing throughout. Particularly bad are 1rv top, 2r top, 24v top, 25r top, 26v top, 27r top, 44v, 45r, 55ra (part of the prologue to Book 3), 58v top–61r top. These parts would have been top outside corners in the original binding.

Contents: **1–61ra Alex. Trall.**
61bis–80va a commentary on Alex. Trall. Book 1 and part of Book 2 (to about 2.22)[23]
81 43 hexameters on matters grammatical

Alex. Trall.: Book 1: 1ra numbered *capitula* for C–CXLV only; 1ra–22vb text of Book 1.
Book 2: 22vb–23va 146 numbered *capitula*; 23va–54va text of Book 2: a folio is lost between ff. 40 and 41, so that we jump from 2.147 line 10 to 2.161 (CIX) line 4.
Book 3: 54vb 65 numbered *capitula*[24] divided by a wiggly line into two columns in order to fit all the *capitula* into 54vb; 55ra–61ra text of Book 3 to the very end of 3.66 (EXPLICIT LIBER ALEXANDRI).[25]

O Orléans, Bibliothèque municipale 283 (237) (autopsy April 1999) **Plate IV**
(Pellegrin, 'Fragments', 351; Septier, 136–7; Wickersheimer, *Manuscrits*, 191–2)

A small book, with covers of wood more than 10mm thick, containing two fragmentary manuscripts, of which the first (pp. 1–77) contains the Latin Alexander. Second half eleventh century (Septier, Wickersheimer),[26] *c.* 1100 (Ganz, pers. comm.); earlier belonged to the Abbey of Saint-Benoît-sur-Loire, Fleury. Vellum, pp. 77. Written in a minute hand (8 pt or smaller), 'a very informal, scholarly hand' (Ganz, pers. comm.), with many abbreviations, in single columns of about 59 lines. Chapter- and section-titles and chapter-initial capitals are highlighted in red (which makes the titles appear as if they have been crossed out!). This highlighting is also used to pick out other items judged significant, including personal names (e.g. 35b 'Iacobus') and statements in the first person (e.g. 35a 'Ego autem'[27]). There is some, mainly interlinear, glossing, and a

[23] In red, on a folio pasted to the inside of the front cover: 'Libri Celeberrimi medici | Alexandri Atrosophiste | tetrapeuticum. Et sunt | libri tres. Deinde | commentum et expositio Doctoris Hartmanni | Schedel de Nurenberga | .413. | Alexander Lythos hoc est medicus | cognomento sophista per hoc tempus | ob ingenii magnitudinem medicorum | princeps habitus; totius medicine | disciplinam tribus libris explanauit | et alia quedam composuit.' The reference is to Hartmann Schedel, the humanist and doctor (b. Nürnberg 1440, d. Nürnberg 1514), who was brought up by his older cousin, the humanist and doctor Hermann Schedel (Nürnberg 1410–1485). (On Hartmann Schedel's books, see Stauber.)

[24] The last two (LXIIII and LXV) are exactly as in **A** (n. 10 above), except that LXIIII lacks the word *febrientibus*.

[25] 61rb contains a recipe for a 'Medicam(en) pro locutione ammissa'.

[26] The second manuscript (pp. 78–109) is in Beneventan script, probably of early twelfth-century date (Wickersheimer, *Manuscrits*).

[27] This highlighting may be an error: it immediately follows the unhighlighted section-title (2.11) *De lapide sputato*.

few marginal notes picking out points judged important (e.g. 11a 'fuge frigidam aquam'!). The pages are in varying condition: some were clearly accepted for use in a damaged or misshapen condition (e.g. 7–8, 19–20, 20–1, each of which is very short with a sharply curved bottom edge); many show signs of heavy wear and the text has been rubbed completely away at numerous points. The tiny hand and frequent abbreviations have as a consequence that a small area of damage or severe wear renders a large stretch of text illegible. For no apparent reason, the lower half of 42a (end of 2.52) and all but the very bottom of 42b (start of 2.53, without title) are blank.

Contents: p. 1 Hippocrates, *Indicia ualetudinum*
pp. 2–77 Alex. Trall.[28]
pp. 78–109 Dioscorides, *De materia medica* (the alphabetically-ordered recension)

Alex. Trall.: Book 1: 2a–3a 145 numbered *capitula*; 3a–33a text.
Book 2: 33a–34a 146 numbered *capitula*; 34b–74b text.
Book 3: 74b–75a 58 *capitula*[29] (not numbered and with initial capitals in column and set off from the second letter in each line); 75a–77b text, breaking off abruptly after (3.13 *ad fin.*) 'Et magis si egrotantem uideris aquam desiderare frigidam adtendere autem si'.

Ox Oxford, Pembroke College 8 (autopsy June 2003)[30]
(Durling, *Guide*^{2}, 349; Ker III, p. 678; Kristeller IV, 267a)

Twelfth/thirteenth century, perhaps written in France (Kristeller). Parchment, ff. i + 121 + i, 240 × 135mm, ff. not numbered (but see below). Well written in single columns of 34 lines, with wide margins to the sides and below and interlinear and marginal notes in various hands, above all in a minute fourteenth-century(?) hand giving numerous explanatory notes between vertical lines ruled in the very wide margins; there are also marginal addenda, of material originally omitted, added in the first hand(?), often in the form of a triangle or diamond and surrounded by a red line; with a fine initial in blue, gold, red, and white at the beginning of each book (excised from Book 1[31]), chapter-titles in red, the first two or three words of each book in alternating red and blue capitals (not done for Book 2[32]), and chapter-initials[33] alternately in red decorated in blue and blue decorated in red. There is a large Roman numeral decorated in red at the bottom of the verso of every eighth f., the last being XIV at the bottom of f. 111v, but only the following ff. have modern numbering: 9, 17, 25, 33, 41, 49, 57, 65, 73, 81, 89, 97, 105, 112, 121. Both foliations ignore the fact that what was originally f. 110 has been cut out (see on Book 3 below).

[28] Note the ascription to Theod. Prisc. in the incipit (in a different hand) on p. 2b 'Passionalis liber Theodori Prisciani sophiste de diuersis morbis et curis eorum incipit'.

[29] The last two are exactly as in **Mu** (n. 24 above).

[30] I am very grateful to Mrs Naomi van Loo, Deputy Librarian of the McGowie Library, Pembroke College, Oxford, for information relating to this manuscript, and for supplying me with a copy of an extract from typescript notes by Miss A. Anderson entitled 'Some medical manuscripts' and describing Pembroke College mss. 8, 10–13, 15 and 21, which are listed in the Appendix to the Sixth Report to the Historical Manuscripts Commission, but which (*pace* Masullo, 31) do not appear in Coxe.

[31] There is consequent loss on f. 1v of a square of text *c.* 35 × 35mm from (1.4) *De simplicibus medicamentis*. The blade used to remove the illuminated C at the start of Book 1 cut through as far as f. 11, but without causing further damage to the text.

[32] Of the opening words 'Tussis quidem accidentia', only the 'T' (illuminated) is present.

[33] Only very rarely omitted, e.g. 2.3.1 '<T>ussiunt'.

Contents: only Alex. Trall.

Alex. Trall.: Book 1: incipit 1r, expl. 43r (with damage to the text of 1.4: see n. 31).
Book 2: incipit 43r, expl. 108r.
Book 3: incipit 108r, expl. 119r (end of 3.65), but lacking, because of the loss of f. 110, from 3.6 v. 23 ('ipsas solas micas de ...') to 3.9 v. 20 ('... et maxime eos quibus pinguis superfluitas').
The *capitula* to all three books are at the end (119v–121v), in 3 columns save on the last side (121v) in 2 columns, the last title in Book 3 being (3.65) *De marasmode perfectius existente*.

P1 Paris, Bibliothèque Nationale, lat. 9332 (autopsy April 1999, June 2000, and August 2004) **Plate I and Cover**
(Beccaria, *Codici*, 157–9; Bischoff, *Studien*, II, 291; III, 16–17; Delisle, 28; Dubief, 48f., pl. 8 (=f. 140r); Homburger, *Bern*, 34, 40–1, 44, 47; Lowe, *CLA*, VI, xix; Lowe, '*Membra disiecta*'; MacKinney, *Medicine*, 111–14, 196 n. 213, 197 n. 218, pl. III (=f. 140r); MacKinney, *Illustrations*, 169; Mihăileanu, 95f. [in Rum.]; Molinier, *Oeuvres* VI, xviii (frontispiece=f. 30); Mostert, 226; Wickersheimer, *Manuscrits*, 89–93 (with illus. of ff. 182v, 223r, 226v))

Late eighth century (MacKinney, *Medicine*, 111), *c.* 800 (MacKinney, *Illustrations*, 169), or early ninth century (Beccaria, Bischoff, Mostert, Wickersheimer), made at or in the region of Fleury (Beccaria; Bischoff; Lowe, *CLA*; MacKinney, *Medicine*; Mostert),[34] formerly belonged to the Chapter of the Cathedral of Chartres.[35] Vellum, 392×270mm, ff. 321, written in minuscule in various hands,[36] in 2 columns of 36 lines; titles and numbers in red or green, and with frequent elaborate illuminated initials, sometimes in one colour, sometimes in several (all now much faded), although chapter-titles are occasionally not written in Book 1 (as early as 1.13) and are frequently left undone from early in Book 2. f. 140r is filled by a picture of a double arch with Alexander seated under the left arch holding a medicine case or book (MacKinney, *Illustrations*) and under the right arch a cross with a prayer for salvation beginning, 'scancta crux psalua nos' (see Bischoff, *Studien*, II, 291). Many ff. are in places worn, spotted, or stained to the point where even the original is impossible to read. Some ff. were accepted for use in a damaged state (with holes or with a corner missing). One f. has been torn out between ff. 184 and 185; its stub is still bound in. Six ff. are missing after f. 242, the end of Alex. Trall. and the start of Dioscorides.

Contents: 1va–138va Oribasius, *Synopsis ad Eustathium filium* 1–9 (including an added recipe, 69rb)
138vb–242vb Alex. Trall. (including an added spell and recipes, 233vab)
243ra–321va Dioscorides, *De materia medica*: the start is lost — it begins XXXIII. *De balanino* (including *Epistula de uulture*, 251va–vb, and an added recipe, 321va)

[34] Less probably in Italy (Molinier). Lowe, '*Membra disiecta*', argues for an Insular exemplar.

[35] Bern, Bürgerbibliothek, A. 91, frg. 7 (2 ff. containing the start of the Latin Dioscorides) once belonged to this manuscript (see Beccaria, *Codici*, 352f., Homburger, *Bern*, and Lowe, *CLA*, who associates **P1**+Bern with a group of Fleury manuscripts from around A.D. 800).

[36] The hands appear to change sometimes for as little as part of a single column: e.g. there is a change to a much cruder hand for the lower two thirds of 167rb, but we are back to 'normal' at the top of 167va; a cruder hand appears again for just the last 2 vv and a word of 168ra and the top 7 vv of 168rb, and for exactly one column at 170rb, 172va.

Alex. Trall.: Book 1: 138vb–139vb 143 numbered *capitula*, with one number repeated (in an eleventh-century hand (Beccaria)); 140vb–179va text of Book 1. There is some confusion in the copying of 1.16–17.[37]
Book 2: 179vb–180vb 145 numbered *capitula*, with 5 numbers repeated; 180vb–233va the text of Book 2 (missing one folio, the stub of which can still be seen, between ff. 184 and 185 containing 2.26 v. 11–2.32 v. 3).
Book 3: 234ra–rb 64 numbered *capitula*;[38] 234rb–242vb the text of Book 3, breaking off at 3.63 (LXI): 'De testicolis qui para<s>tatas uocantur. Testiculus uero gallorum dare semper oportit hicticis'.

P2 Paris, Bibliothèque Nationale, lat. 6881 (autopsy April 1999, June 2000, and August 2004) **Plate VI**
(Mihăileanu, 96 [in Rum.]; Puschmann I, 91)

Thirteenth century. Vellum, ff. 121, the folios edged in gold, beautifully written in single columns (save in *capitula* and in text completing a page containing *capitula*, where there are 2 columns) of 33–5 lines. Lovely ornate book-initials, chapter-titles in red, initials of *capitula* in red; chapter numeration is sporadic, chapter-initial capitals in running text are missing throughout (although the letters to be supplied by the rubricator are written very small on the left of the left-hand margin). The text has been carefully corrected, not only with an eye to accuracy in matters of detail but also more substantially, apparently against another exemplar (in places where we can guess at it, the original seems to have been closer to the text of **A**; see 4.7.1 below[39]). There are numerous marginal glosses in a third hand, and frequent occurrences of the word 'Nota' or a picture of an arm with the index-finger pointing at a section of text.

Contents: 1–4va apparently an essay, in a thirteenth-century(?) hand, on a medical work in seven books which, while probably not the Latin Alexander, at least draws significantly on it; the 'essay' is interspersed with — indeed, dominated by — numerous medical glosses, notes, and etymologies; it contains references to Theodosius (presumably for Theodorus) Priscianus, Paul (of Aegina?), Democritus, and 'Garipontus Salernitanus', who is said to have reordered the material of the seven books, which used to begin with fevers (see 2.3.3 above).
4vab medical glosses
5ra–121v Alex. Trall.

Alex. Trall.: Book 1: 5ra–6rb 137 *capitula*; 6rb–45v text of Book 1.
Book 2: 45va–47ra 136 *capitula*; 47ra–110ra text of Book 2.
Book 3: 110ra–110va 59 *capitula*, ending with the title of 3.66; 110va–121v text of Book 3, ending with 3.65.

[37] Immediately after 1.15 (numbered 14), **P1** has (a) 1.17 (numbered 15) as far as 'impetiginosas', then (b) most of the recipe omitted by *ed.* ('Item aliut ad ea que in capite scauias sunt ... oliue folia'), followed by a repetition of the end of 1.15 ('ad autem humidioris pitiriasis ... experimentatum multum abeo'), then (c) 1.16 (numbered 16), then (d) a new chapter numbered 17 but without a title ('Ad psidracia et ad ea que in capite scauias sunt ...'), with the whole of the recipe just mentioned (ending 'cum mel catapl()'), and the last recipe in 1.17. There are marks indicating that (b) should follow (d).

[38] The last is 'LXIIII. Lixoperito et inbrocas Galine ad febris'. Note also 'LXIII. De pomis modis febris' (a blend of 3.64 *De pomis* and 3.65 *De marasmode*).

[39] At 2.236.6 (4.10.6 below), the corrector's version of the definition of *duplicata distemperantia*, which is written over four erased lines of the original is almost identical with that of ϕ.

P3 Paris, Bibliothèque Nationale, lat. 6882 (autopsy April 1999, June 2000, and August 2004) **Plate VII**
(Avril and Załuska, I, 26 (no. 48), pl. XIV (f. 102v); Dubief, 50f., pl. 10 (f. 74v); Mihăileanu, 96f. [in Rum.]; Puschmann I, 91)

Last quarter twelfth century, or twelfth/thirteenth century, made in central (south-central?[40]) Italy (Avril and Załuska). Vellum, ff. i+114, 280×190mm, beautifully and clearly written, in single columns of 38 or 39 lines; chapter-titles in red, with chapter-initial capitals alternately in red and blue, both in the *capitula* and in the running text; wonderful illuminated initials at the start of each of the *seven* books of this edition (cf. the description of **P2** above),[41] each of which also has its own *capitula* (see below). There are numerous corrections, additions, and marginal notes on nearly every page, many of them extensive, in three separate hands.[42]

Contents: only Alex. Trall.

Alex. Trall.: Book 1: f. 0rv 79 unnumbered *capitula* in a single column, the first 1.1, the last 1.84; text of 1.1–84; 19r 'Incipiunt capitula **libri secundi** ad oculorum passiones' (my emphasis): 19rv 59 unnumbered *capitula* in 2 columns (of 'Book 2'), the first 1.85, the last 1.149; text of 1.85–149.
Book 2: f. 37v 76 unnumbered *capitula* in 2 columns (of 'Book 3'), the first 2.1, the last 2.78; text of 2.1–78; 54v–55r 86 unnumbered *capitula* in 2 columns (of 'Book 4'), the first 2.79, the last 2.157; text of 2.79–157; 74rv 84 unnumbered *capitula* in 2 columns (of 'Book 5'), the first 2.158, the last 2.232/233 (but 2.234 is in the text); text of 2.158–234; 90v 36 unnumbered *capitula* in 2 columns (of 'Book 6'), the first 2.235, the last 2.269 (but 2.270–271 are in the text[43]); text of 2.235–271.
Book 3: ff. 101v–102r 71 unnumbered *capitula* in a single column (of 'Book 7'), the first 3.1, the last 3.66;[44] ff. 102v–114v the text of Book 3, breaking off without an Explicit after only 8 lines of 3.66 (just before *Emplastrum Galieni*).

3.1.2. Lost Copies

Ch Chartres, Bibliothèque municipale 342 (383)
(*Cat. gén. Dép.*, XI, 165; Dronke, 125; MacKinney, *Medicine*, 211 n. 282; Puschmann I, 91)

Twelfth century (*Cat. gén. Dép.*). Chapitre de la Cathédrale de Notre Dame. Parchment, 250×163mm, ff. 140. Minuscule, in single columns of about 40 lines (but 140r has 65 lines!). This manuscript was destroyed in May 1944. The University of North

[40] Avril and Załuska include it in their chapter on 'l'aire bénéventaine et du royaume normand'.

[41] i.e. there are book-initials at the start of 1.1 (1r), 1.85 (19v), 2.1 (38r), 2.79 (55v), 2.158 (74v), 2.235 (90v), and 3.1 (102v). According to Avril and Załuska, while the first, second, and fifth show 'rapports avec le style géométrique tardif d'Italie centrale', the others do not, and are presumably the work of a second artist.

[42] 1. The original is fine dark brown, quite angular. 2. The first corrector is rounder, thicker and lighter brown; occasionally he adds or corrects chapter-titles using red ink. 3. The corrector of both 1. and 2. is fine black. He also makes some additions. 4. The latest is fine, very dark brown. He glosses heavily and provides a sort of running header vertically down the outer edges of the folios.

[43] However, the middle of 2.269 and the second half of 2.270 were added in a different hand (m2?) at the bottom of 101r and in the margin of 101v, respectively.

[44] The form of the last — *De lixoperitis pannis et embrocis* — is identical with the last *capitulum* in **G1** (n. 20 above).

Carolina at Chapel Hill has photographs made by L. C. MacKinney of seven sides (see below).[45] MacKinney thought that this manuscript 'appears to have been copied from the former Chartres ms., now Paris B. N. 9332' (**P1** above), but my collations do not bear this out.

Contents: the entry in the *Catalogue général* is very brief, but it is clear that the manuscript contained only Alex. Trall., and all three books. The Chapel Hill photographs depict the following:

3r[46] 'Incipiunt capitula Primi libri Alexandri yatros' | chapter-titles I–XXVII (=1.1–28)

68rv 1.145 (CXLI), v. 7 'coques'–149 (CXLV) end '... Incipiunt capitula libri secundi Alexandri. | I De tusse. | II De tussis cognitione que de calida distemperantia generatur'

127v–128r 2.268, v. 4 'aloe'–2.271 '... Incipiunt capitula libri tercii'

140r vv. 1–32: 3.66 complete[47]

vv. 33–45: 'Cordapsus id est dolor ylii ... Ventrem procurabis ex lacte decocto in quo q(ui?)s facies uel dissolui aut aloe aut scamonee'

vv. 46–55: 'Debilitatur uox aut p(er) clamorem aut p(er) frigorem aut p(er) estum nimium ... et antidotum becicum aut catapodias ad hanc causam confectas'

vv. 56–65: 'Arteriaci sunt quibus fauces reumatizant ... aut purum (parum?) oleum infundendum est secundum qualitatem temporis sicut sepe docuimus'

140v last side: 'lib(er) medicinal(is) Alexandri yatros'

Metz, Bibliothèque de la Ville, ms. 278
(*Cat. gén. Dép.*, V, 118; Diels, *Handschriften*)

Early thirteenth century (*Cat. gén. Dép.*). This manuscript was destroyed in September 1944; no reproductions of, or studies bearing on it, are known.[48] The entry in the *Catalogue général* makes clear that the manuscript ('petit in-folio sur vélin') contained only Alex. Trall. lat. It describes the contents as 'Alexandri Iatrosophistae de morbis dignoscendis et sanandis libri III', and gives the Incipit ('dempta praefatione') as 'Incipit ejusdem de allopicia. Contingit hec dupliciter passio', and the Explicit as 'Explicit liber

[45] I am very grateful to Christiane Pollin of the Bibliothèques de Chartres for information about the manuscript, and to Michael McVaugh for his kind assistance in the matter of acquiring reproductions of the Chapel Hill photographs. There is, however, no mention of this manuscript in Bischoff, *Nachlaß*, nor in the papers of Loren C. MacKinney at the University of North Carolina at Chapel Hill (I am indebted to Eliza Glaze for this information), nor in the Handschriftenscheden of the *CMG/CML* in the Berlin-Brandenburgische Akademie der Wissenschaften (I am indebted to Diethard Nickel for this information). For a complete list of the Chartres material preserved, see Behrends. (A BBC News Online article of 4 July 2003 reports the possibility of using multispectral imaging to render some of the Chartres material legible.)

[46] Behrends wrongly reports 1r.

[47] The *Catalogue général* quotes '... ferens inchoantem marasmon. Explicit liber tertius Alexandri'. This, the end of 3.65, was presumably on f. 139v. Why was the Explicit placed here, rather than after line 32 on f. 140r? The *Catalogue général* reports f. 140 as containing 'recettes médicales', apparently not recognizing the first as Alex. Trall. 3.66.

[48] I am grateful to Dr Philippe Hoch, the Conservateur en chef of the Bibliothèque de la Ville de Metz, for this information. There is no mention of this manuscript in Bischoff, *Nachlaß*, nor in the papers of Loren C. MacKinney at the University of North Carolina at Chapel Hill (I am indebted to Eliza Glaze for this information), nor in the Handschriftenscheden of the *CMG/CML* in the Berlin-Brandenburgische Akademie der Wissenschaften (I am indebted to Diethard Nickel for this information).

Alexandri medici Iatrosophistae, translatus a Johanne episcopo, cui benedicat Deus', without in the latter case quoting the last sentence of the translation.

3.1.3. Unconfirmed

Oxford, Bodleian Library, Bodl. 524
(Madan and Craster, no. 2586; incorrectly given as 'Digby 524' by Thorndike and Kibre, 259, no. 13)

Twelfth century (Madan and Craster, Thorndike and Kibre), written in Italy (Madan and Craster). Parchment, iii+277 pp., in two hands (a slightly later one beginning on p. 222), with some illuminated initials, etc., in a thirteenth-century English binding.

Contents: apparently only Alex. Trall., in three books each with a list of chapters, plus an additional Latin recipe on p. 277

Vatican, Città del Vaticano, Bibl. apostolica vaticana, Pal. lat. 1209
(Kristeller VI, 358b; Schuba, 198)

Thirteenth century. Parchment, ff. vi (a–f)+92+vi (93–8, blank), 180 × 130mm, written in early Gothic minuscule in several hands, in single columns (the *capitula* in 2 columns) of 35 lines, with interlinear and marginal glosses of thirteenth/fourteenth century.[49]

Contents: only Alex. Trall.

Alex. Trall.: 2r the start of Book 1.
37r the start of Book 2.
81v–92r Book 3, ending with the end of 3.66, 'cum oleo roseo ungito et uteris'.

3.1.4. Corrigendum

Paris, Bibliothèque de l'Arsenal, ms. 867 (end thirteenth century, Glaze,[50] ff. ii+265+ii) does not (*pace* Diels, *Handschriften*, II, 12) contain the Latin Alexander. Its principal contents are:

1r–72v Johannes Platearius, *Practica*;
73r–170v Gariopontus, *Passionarius* (with the prologue beginning 'Iste liber ex diuersis auctoribus' (=Glaze's Prologue B, *Medical Books*, 309ff.);
171r–235v *Liber Constantini* (*de febribus*), beginning 'Quoniam te karissime fili Iohannes lacrimas mesto cordis dolore';
236r–239v Constantine, *Liber pauperum*;
240r–249v the Latin Hippocratic *Aphorisms*;
249v–256r the Latin Hippocratic *Prognostics*;
256r–258r *De pulsibus*, ascribed to Philaretus;
258r–263v *De urinis*, incomplete, ascribed to Theophilus.

[49] The index on f. c and notes on ff. 1–6 are in the hand of the (fifteenth-century) Heidelberg doctor Martinus Rentz.

[50] See Glaze, *Medical Books*, 183 n. 41, 312; eadem, '*Passionarius*'. Cf. also *Cat. gén. Arsenal*, II, 142–3.

3.2. The Secondary Tradition

In the following paragraphs, I give a brief introduction to, first, miscellaneous excerpts (which include for editorial purposes some of the most important of the excerpts), and then, in a plausible chronological order,[51] each of the late antique or medieval Latin compendia which have used the Latin Alexander directly or indirectly as a source, and which have independent manuscript traditions of their own (the *Liber passionalis*, the *Tereoperica* ascribed to Petroncellus, the *Liber diaetarum*, the *De podagra*, the *Passionarius* of Gariopontus, and the so-called 'Bamberg Surgery').[52] Time has not permitted systematic collations of these secondary traditions with the mainstream, but I offer for each a sample portion of text, for which I have collated at least some of the manuscripts, with the purpose of giving a flavour at least of each work, of illustrating how each has made use of the Latin Alexander, and of showing (if possible) how the source of each is related to the mainstream tradition and what value, if any, each has as a potential witness for the reconstruction of the mainstream text. There follow (3.3), in alphabetical order by sigla, descriptions of some of the manuscripts of the secondary tradition that I have inspected and worked with.

Table 3.1 offers an overview of many of the excerpts from the Latin Alexander known to date,[53] and of all those noted in the present work.

Table 3.1: An overview of the secondary traditions of the Latin Alexander
(*for a more detailed conspectus of* Lib. pass., Lib. diaet. *and* De podagra, *see Tables 3.2, 3.5 and 3.7*)

Book 1 **Alex. Trall. lat. *ed.***	***Lib. pass.***	***Lib. diaet.***	***Ter.***	**v1**	**Misc.**
1.1 De allopitia et ophiasi	83 (84)		*Ter.* 1.3-4		
1.2 Signa ex quo humore allopitia generata sit					
1.3 Cura ad tineam capitis					
1.4 De simplicibus medicamentis					
1.5 De compositis medicamentis ad tineam capitis					
1.6 De capillis cadentibus		1			
1.13 Ad capillos auro similes faciendos	83 (84) cont.				
1.14 Ad capillos albos faciendos					
1.17 Ad psidracia et exantimata in capite facta	84 (85)		*Ter.* 1.12		
1.19 De acore signis	85 (86)		*Ter.* 1.13		
1.20 Curatio achorarum					

[51] The order I have chosen reflects the age of the oldest manuscript in each case, but also deliberately juxtaposes two pairs of texts which it is desirable to compare, *Liber passionalis* and *Tereoperica*, and *De podagra* and Gariopontus' *Passionarius*.

[52] None of these exists in a reliable modern edition, although all but the *Tereoperica* and the *Passionarius* are of a very manageable size, and the *Liber diaetarum* and the *De podagra* in particular would make excellent PhD projects.

[53] There are almost certainly more to be found: two, very different, sources which will probably merit systematic study are, on the one hand, the Latin Oribasius and, on the other, the material referred to in Sigerist, *Rezeptliteratur*.

Table 3.1: Continued

1.25 Si de nimio epatis calore caput dolet		2			
1.32 (1.31bis) Curatio si ex uino caput doleat	80 (84)	3			
1.33 (1.32) Si ex percussura caput doleat		4			
1.58 De cibis in frenesi		5			
1.59 De litargico .i. obliuioso	23 (24)		*Ter.* 2.5		
1. 60 Curatio litargicorum		6			
1.63 Cura epileptie		7			
1.64-67 De apozimis et cathaputiis dandis; De catarticis; De apoflegmatismis; De uomitu	(80–83) (**be** only)				
1.81 De cibo dando menomenis uel melancolicis		8			
1.91 Curatio hiis qui de colerico et acro humore laborant		9			
1.100 Ad nictilopas .i. eos qui post transmutatum solem non uident			*Ter.* 1.21		
1.103 De mulsa				**v1**, 1r	**v2**, 1r **v3**, 2rv
1.107 Ad egylop<a>s	78 (79)		*Ter.* 1.20		
1.108-123 De passionibus aurium – (123) Ad aures surdas				**v1**, 59v -63r	
1.119 Si in aure fuerit aliquid ingressum					*'Bamberg Surgery'*
1.124-128 De parotidis – (128) Curatio si ex colerico humore fiant parotide	76 (77)				
1.130 De dieta (*scil.* in parotidis)		10			
1.131-133 De narium passione; Ad sanguinis fluxum de naribus; De liuore in facie				**v1**, 63v -65r	
1.131 De narium passione	77 (78)				
1.134-135 De dentium causis id est passionibus; De dentium dolore cura				**v1**, 65r -66r	
1.136 De squinance uel sinance					Cf. **v3**, 49r
1.140 De flobothomia et catartico ac uentosis sinancis					Cf. **v3**, 49r
1.142 De dieta sinanticorum		11			
1.145 De cibis dandis sinanticis		13			

(*continued*)

Table 3.1: Continued

Book 2 **Alex. Trall. lat. *ed.***	***Lib. pass.***	***Lib. diaet.***	***De podagra***	***Ter.***	**v1**	**Misc.**
2.18 Curatio si ex frigido contingat cynorodoxeos		14 (15)				
2.21 Curatio si ex frigore imbecillis fiat cateltica uirtus						
2.22 Curatio si ex calore nimio fuerit imbecilla cateltica uirtus		15 (16)				
2.26 Si de spissis et glutinosis humoribus fastidium fiat		16 (17)				
2.27 Si de calida distemperantia facta fuerit absque humore de solo calore anorexia		17 (18)				
2.36 De cardiaca passione					**v1**, 59r	**u**, pp. 320-2
2.37 Curatio cardiace		18 (19)				
2.40 Si melancolicus aut colericus humor uomitum excitet		19 (20)				
2.50 De hiis qui satis <spuunt> et humidum habent stomachum	20 (21)			*Ter.* 1.47		
2.55 Curatio (*scil.* ad colericam pass.)		20 (21)				
2.61 Curatio de flegmone epatis		23 (24)				
2.62 De potionibus et apozimatibus						
2.73 Curatio calide distemperantie epatis		24 (25)				
2.74 Curatio epatice dissinterie de frigida epatis distemperantia		(26)				
2.79 De reumate uentris Filominis					**v1**, 68v-70v	
2.86 De cibo dissintericorum		(27)				
2.94 De pomis						
2.108 Curatio frigide et humide distemperantie splenis		(28)				
2.109 Curatio calide et humide distemperantie		(29)				
2.135 De cibo						
2.156 De dieta ydropicorum		(30)				
2.164 De dieta emoptoicorum		(31)				
2.180–184 Curatio nefreticorum – (184) Curatio de flegmone cum inflammatione facto in renibus					**v1**, 71r-73r	
2.184 Curatio de flegmone cum inflammatione facto in renibus		(32)				
2.187 De hiis qui pus per urinam faciunt		(33) **co** only				
2.200 Curatio dyabetis		(34)				

Table 3.1: Continued

2.205 De dieta (*scil.* colicae passionis)		(35)				
2.222 Curatio si de colerico humore colica fuerit passio generata		(36)				
2.235–270 De podagra – (270) De antidotoalio podagricis dando per totum annum					**v1**, 75v-86v	
2.235 De podagra			1			
2. 236 De podagre causis						
2.237 Signa si de colerico humore podagra fuerit generata			6			
2.238 Curatio podagre calide de coleribus adhibenda			7			**v3**, 93rv
2.239 Podagricis que sunt extrinsecus adhibenda			8			
2.240 De embrocis			9			
2.241 De dieta		(37)	10–18			
2.242 De balneis			(22)			
2.248 Curatio flegmatice podagre			19			
2.249 De catarticis			19bis			
2.250 Oximel Iuliani catarticum			20			
2.251 De cathaputiis dandis			21			
2.261 Curatio podagre ex sanguine generate			2			
2.262 De localibus curis			3			
2.263 Ad porros hoc est si in nodis tumores fuerint et lapides			4			
2.264 De antidotis						
2.265, 267, 270 Ad porros; Catarticum de hermodactilis; De antidoto alio podagricis dando per totum annum			5			
2.267 Catarticum de hermodactilis						**v3**, 93v

Book 3			
Alex. Trall. lat. ***ed.***	***Lib. pass.***	***Ter.***	**Miscellaneous excerpts**
3.46–47 De ethicis febribus; De marosmode	72 (73)	*Ter.* 2.17.2(?) (**l3**, f. 113rv)	
3.66 (part) Lixoperita epithimata et embroce et emplastra febrientibus Martyrii medici			**vat1**, 87v-88v

Perhaps the most striking feature revealed by Table 3.1 is the almost complete lack of excerpts from the third book of the Latin Alexander, on fevers. Apart from 3.66, which is not in the Greek Alexander as we have it, and which could be an addition to the original version of the Latin Alexander, I know of only one passage drawn from Book 3, namely chs 46–7 (*De icticis febribus* and *De marasmode*), which incidentally (like several other chapters) appear both in the *Liber passionalis* (3.2.2 below) and in the *Tereoperica* (3.2.3 below). The excerpting of Books 1 and 2 is the work predominantly of the makers of the *Liber passionalis*, the *Liber diaetarum* (3.2.4 below), the *De podagra* (3.2.5 below), and of Vendôme ms. 109, the most important of the manuscripts containing 'miscellaneous excerpts', with which I begin.

3.2.1. Miscellaneous Excerpts

The Vendôme medical manuscripts are described in detail in a long article by Henry Sigerist,[54] which includes a considerable amount of transcribed material and photographs of several folios, which I will not repeat and to which I refer for further detail. Three Vendôme manuscripts contain excerpts from the Latin Alexander, namely mss. 109 (=**v1**), 172 (=**v2**), and 175 (=**v3**), all of the eleventh century. Of these three, **v1** is for present purposes far and away the most important, in that it contains very substantial extracts (a total of 65 chapters: 22 from Book 1, 43 from Book 2) faithfully copied without editorial intervention from a complete copy of at least Books 1 and 2 of the Latin Alexander. The faithfulness of the copying extends to the (for the purposes of **v1**, pointless) reproduction of some of the chapter-numbers of the original. These match the numeration of **M** and **P1**, and given numerous errors in common with these two mainstream manuscripts, it is clear that at least one of the copies used by the maker of **v1** was closely related to γ, and probably a descendant of β (see 4.2 below). I say 'at least one of the copies' because the maker of **v1** evidently had two versions of part of 1.114, the second (presumably discovered only after the first act of copying was complete) being written in-between the lines of the first version (f. 61v), and neither of these versions is close to γ (though the interlinear text is almost identical with that of **A**: see pp. 100–1 below). It is equally clear that – again, presumably at different times – two versions of the *Liber diaetarum* were used (see 3.2.4 below). Whether it is by chance that there is virtually no overlap (just a few lines in 2.79) between the *Liber diaetarum* and the other Alexander extracts in **v1**, or whether the maker of **v1** knew that he was about to copy the *Liber diaetarum* and, aware of its contents, avoided duplicating them, one can only speculate. The excerpts in **v1** from the mainstream Alexander are all in their original order, save 1.103 *De mulsa* and 2.36 *De cardiaca passione*. The latter chapter, also in **u** (p. 96), immediately precedes the big run through Books 1 and 2, which dominates **v1** ff. 59v–86v (although interspersed with material from other sources). The former, the *Mulsa Alexandri* for treatment of the eyes, is in fact the earliest chapter of Book 1 to be reproduced by **v1** (the next being 1.108), but it is put at the front of the codex and functions practically as a frontispiece not only in **v1** (f. 1r) but in **v2** (f. 1r) and **v3** (f. 2rv) as well. This is surely not coincidental, but must reflect a scriptorium decision to reproduce such a highly-recommended remedy[55] over and over again right at the front of

[54] Sigerist, 'Vendôme'.

[55] Note Alexander's endorsement, 1.103 'Nescio enim si ante ab aliquo tam magnum inuentum fuerit adiutorium' (=Greek II, 55, 7–8).

key medical compendia (in **v3** presumably after the two manuscripts, both originally beginning with the *Liber Esculapii*, had been joined?). As for the selection of the subjects copied by **v1**, it is perhaps noteworthy that three substantial sections (ff. 63v–70v, on diseases of the nose and teeth, and *reuma uentris*) are not in the Greek Alexander: the appeal they held for the makers of the Latin Alexander was evidently still felt, and their incorporation vindicated.

While in **v2** Alexander is represented only by the tacking on of the *Mulsa Alexandri* to the front of the text of and commentary on the Latin Hippocratic *Aphorisms*, **v1** and **v3** (the latter of which contains apart from the *Mulsa* modest extracts from 1.136, 1.140, 2.238, and 2.267) both transmit Alexander together with Esculapius and Theodorus Priscianus, and **v1** also with other elements of the Galenic and pseudo-Galenic pre-Gariopontean ensemble that accompanies the Latin Alexander both in complete copies and in other sets of excerpts (see 3.2.5 below). The first 86 folios of **v1** could be seen as a sort of prototype of this corpus, resembling the later compendia also in ending with Alexander on gout, but with the important difference that the *De podagra* in **v1** is a faithful copy of the complete text and shows no signs of the radical recension represented by the *De podagra* described in 3.2.5 below.[56]

There are elements of this corpus (excerpts from Gal., *Ad Glauc.* 1, the *Liber tertius*) also in **u**, which curiously, in a large collection of remedies towards the end of the manuscript, has Alex. Trall. 2.36 *De cardiaca passione* in common with **v1**, evidently (as in **v1**) copied without editorial intervention, and made from a mainstream copy closely related to the source of **v1** and to the mainstream manuscripts **M** and **P1** (on the place of **u**'s source within the tradition, see 4.2 below).

vat1 (p. 97) is important above all for Theod. Prisc., *Eup.* 2 and 3 and Vindic., *Epist. ad Pentad.*, but it also contains a superior text of a portion (smaller than that implied by Beccaria or Pellegrin *et al. Vaticane*) of Alex. Trall. 3.66. Given that **P1** breaks off in 3.63, **vat1** (a century older than **M**) is our oldest witness for these recipes. Since 3.66, the last chapter of the Latin Alexander, is not in the Greek text (and in relatively few of the mainstream Latin manuscripts), but for the Explicit in **vat1** at this point, we may well have reckoned with the use of a common source by the Latin Alexander and the maker of (an ancestor of?) **vat1**. The Explicit, however, makes clear that the maker of **vat1** thought he was copying the end of Alex. Trall. Book 3, and so that, if it was not in the original translation-compilation, 3.66 had been added to at least one copy of the Latin Alexander by the early ninth century.

As for the value for editorial purposes of these first sets of 'miscellaneous excerpts', the age, the text quality, and the probable genetic relations of **v1**, **v2**, **v3**, **u**, and **vat1** — and the fact that none shows any sign of editorial intervention in the text of their excerpts from the Latin Alexander — all these factors make them important witnesses, whose testimony should — and will — certainly be used in the editing of the chapters that they transmit. In at least five other sets of excerpts, the Latin Alexander has been used as a source for other works, each of which shows, although to different degrees, its own editorial intent and consequent readiness to modify the excerpted text. Nevertheless, quite apart from their evidently important role in the medieval 'reception' of the Latin Alexander, and in the constitution of medieval Latin medical literature more generally, soundings indicate that even these more

[56] On **v1** and the pre-Gariopontean ensemble, see now Glaze, '*Passionarius*' and 'Galen refashioned'.

independent branches of the secondary tradition are not without value for the textual criticism and the editing of the Latin Alexander itself.[57]

3.2.2. *Liber passionalis*

The *Liber passionalis* (henceforth *Lib. pass.*) is a compendium in eighty-one chapters setting out diagnosis and therapy of about the same number of diseases. Its main concern is with internal medicine (nervous or mental diseases, diseases of the head, the chest, the gastro-intestinal tract, the abdomen). It has some notably elaborate chapters on gynaecology, but nothing on fevers (infectious diseases) or surgical treatment. The fact that each chapter begins with the diagnosis or clinical picture of the disease suggests that it was intended for readers with some medical experience.[58]

The *Lib. pass.* is known from three manuscripts, namely Berlin, Phillipps 1790 (**be**, p. 92) beginning with the end of ch. 21, St Gall 752 (**s**, p. 96, below) more or less complete, and Rouen 1407 (O. 55; late eleventh century) containing chs 1–11 only.[59] The *Lib. pass.* was discovered by Valentin Rose, who compared **s** with **be** — a remarkable discovery, given the disarray of **be** (see below); the presence of the work in Rouen 1407 was identified by Klaus-Dietrich Fischer.

Alex. Trall. serves as the sole or main source for fourteen chapters of the *Lib. pass.* (which altogether draws on twenty-six chapters of Alex. Trall., entirely from Book 1, save 2.50[60] and 3.46–7[61]). Table 3.2 offers an overview of the Alexander material in the chapter order of *Lib. pass.*, comparing in some detail the contents of **be** and **s**.

Table 3.2: The Latin Alexander and the Liber passionalis

Alex. Trall. lat. *ed.* (**M**)	**be**, ff. 51, 53, 82–87, 43–44	**s**, pp. 231–233, 236–237, 305–320
2.50 De his qui satis <spuunt> et humidum habent stomachum	51r (XXI.) (begins with last line of 2.50: see Table 3.4)	231–3 XX. . . . stomachum humidum habent (=2.50 minus last clause)
1.59 De litargico .i. obliuioso	53rv XXIIII. De litargo uerus quippe litargicus(?) (=1.59: see Table 3.3)	236–7 XXIII. De lytargicis
3.46 De ethicis febribus	82r LXXIII. De hicteticis(?) febribus (=3.46–47 complete)	305–6 LXXII. De hictericis febribus
3.47 De marosmode	82v De marasmodus	De marismodis in text

[57] Compare Fischer's demonstration (in 'Wer liest') of the importance of the secondary tradition for the editing of Cassius Felix and Gargilius Martialis, respectively. Cf. Fraisse, LXXV f. on Cass. Fel., and Maire, LI–LXV on Pliny and Garg. Mart.

[58] On the nature, contents, and transmission of the *Lib. pass.*, see above all Rose, *Verzeichnis . . . Berlin*, 362–9; Baader, 'Phill. 1790'; Fischer, 'Dr Monk'; Fischer, '*Lib. Byz.*', 276, 285–6; Fischer, '*Lib. tert.*', 105.

[59] On Rouen 1407, see Beccaria, *Codici*, 183–5; Wickersheimer, *Manuscrits*, 159–71; Glaze, '*Passionarius*'. In the Rouen manuscript only chs 1–11 are preserved, which contain nothing from Alex. Trall. The chapters drawn from Caelius Aurelianus reveal that the text of Rouen, although two centuries younger, is probably more conservative than that of **be** (I am indebted to Cloudy Fischer for this information).

[60] Rose, *Verzeichnis . . . Berlin*, 368 compares *Lib. pass.* ch. XXVIIII *De tenismon* (**s**, pp. 246–8) with Alex. Trall. 2.102–3 *De tenasmone*, but the two versions really have very little in common.

[61] Both 2.50 and 3.46–7 are also in *Ter.* (as are Alex. Trall. 1.1–4, 1.17 & 19–20, 1.59, 1.107). On the closeness of *Lib. pass.* and *Ter.* also with regard to material shared with the *Liber Byzantii*, see Fischer, '*Lib. Byz.*', 286.

Table 3.2: Continued

1.1 De allopitia et ophiasi	82v LXXIIII. De alopicia et ofiosis(?) (=1.1–4; 1.5 line 9 to the end; 1.13 lines 1–8; 1.14)	306–9 LXXIII. De alopicia et ofiasis
1.2 Signa ex quo humore allopitia generata sit	1.2.t. in text (minus allopitia)	1.2.t. in text (... humore generata sit alopicia)
1.3 Cura ad tineam capitis	Curatio ad alopiciam capitis uel tinia	Curatio alopitiae
1.4 De simplicibus medicamentis	t. as *ed.*	De simplicibus medicaminibus
1.5 De compositis medicamentis ad tineam capitis	1.5.t. absent	1.5.t. absent
1.13 Ad capillos auro similes faciendos (Vt capill() auro simil() facias M)	Vt capill() auro facies colore	Vt capillos auro facias similes
1.14 Ad capillos albos faciendos (Vt capill() aluos facias M)	Vt capill() albus facias	Vt capillos albos facias
1.17 Ad psidracia et (et *om.* M) exantimata in capite facta	83v-84r LXX(?) De sidracia exantimata in capite facta sidracia (=1.17 complete, incl. the penult. recipe om. by *ed.*)	309 LXXIIII. De sideratia exantimata ...
1.19 De acore signis	84rv LXXVI De acorus signa (=1.19 lines 1–10; 1.20 complete but modified)	310–11 LXXV. De acoras
1.20 Curatio achorarum	Curatio acoras in text	1.20.t. absent
1.124 De parotidis	84v-86r LXXVII De parotidas (=1.124 complete; 1.125 complete but much modified; 1.126–128 much shortened)	311–14 LXXVI. De parotidas
1.125 Curatio si ex plenitudine sanguinis fiant parotide	1.125.t. garbled in text	Curatio eorum talis est
1.126 Curatio in quibus parotide sunt scirotidis tumoris	1.126.t. absent	1.126.t. absent
1.127 Signa si in pus conuertantur parotide et cura	Si in pus conuertantur parotidas	Si in fus conuertantur parotidas
1. 128 Curatio si ex colerico humore fiant parotide (humore reuma fiat M)	Curatio. Si ex colerico et reuma fiat parotidas	Curatio si ex colerico et reuma fuerit parotidas
1.131 De narium passione	86rv LXXVIII De narium passiones (=1.131 shortened in the middle)	314–16 LXXVII. De narium passione
1.107 Ad egylops	86v-87r LXXVIIII Ad elilopas (=1.107 complete)	316–17 LXXVIII. De elilopas
1.64 De apozimis et cathaputiis dandis	43r LXXX De apozimis et catarticis (=1.64 complete)	
1.65 De catarticis	43rv LXXXI De catarticis (=1.65 complete)	
1.66 De apoflegmatismis	43v LXXXII De apoflecmatismis (=1.66 complete)	
1.67 De uomitu	LXXXIII De uomito (=1.67 complete)	
1.32 (1.31^{bis}) Si ex uino caput doluerit	LXXXIIII. Si ex uino capud dolet facile sanus fit (=1.32 complete)	319–20 LXXX. t. as *ed.*

The only significant difference between these two copies of the *Lib. pass.* is that Alex. Trall. 1.64–7 on the treatment of epilepsy, complete in **be**, is absent from **s.**[62] The maker of *Lib. pass.* has for thc most part tricd to make an exact copy of the model that he was excerpting, although frequently he either omits complete sentences (e.g. from 1.5, 1.13) or modifies the original in order to shorten it while retaining the gist at least of the content (e.g. the penultimate recipe in 1.17, 1.20, 1.125, 1.131). His procedure is well illustrated in his use of 1.59 and 2.50, for each of which I give side by side the versions of both *Lib. pass.* and *Ter.*, together with a full text of the Latin and the Greek originals (see Tables 3.3 and 3.4 below).

As for the genetic relations of the copy of Alex. Trall. used by the maker of *Lib. pass.*, I have not undertaken an extensive systematic collation, but in what little I have compared there are clear hints that the source here shares errors with **M** and **P1** and so belongs on the right-hand side of the stemma (**Plate XII**), possibly as a descendant of γ (4.2.2. below). Note, for example, the agreements signalled in the footnotes in Tables 3.3 and 3.4 below, in the former, n. 1 and in the latter in nn. 3 and 5–9; in Table 3.2 (above), note that the *Lib. pass.* titles corresponding to Alex. Trall. 1.13 and 1.14 agree wih those in **M**, and that **M** agrees with *Lib. pass.* also in omitting *et* in the title of 1.17 (cf. also 1.128. t.).[63]

3.2.3. '*Tereoperica*', Attributed to Petroncellus of Salerno

The work known as '*Tereoperica*' (=*Therapeutica*; henceforth *Ter.*), ascribed in the High Middle Ages to Petroncellus of Salerno,[64] is an extensive compilation in two(?) books drawing on various late antique and early medieval Latin medical texts,[65] and prefaced by a doxographical 'letter' about the beginnings of medicine and the several medical schools or sects, the *Epistula peri hereseon*; it too was compiled from several sources including Isidore and Agnellus of Ravenna.[66] The principal sources used by the maker of *Ter.* are on the one hand some of the ensemble of texts used by Gariopontus (3.2.6 below), especially the *Liber tertius* (but excluding Theodorus Priscianus and the *De*

[62] An odd feature of this excerpt is that there is no indication of the disease being treated until an oblique reference at the end of 1.65 ('non solum autem epilepticos scio iuuisse sed ...').

[63] *Lib. pass.* also has 1.19.2 *interdum etiam et* (recte; om. cett.) in common only with γ and γ′(and hence **C**, **P3** and ϕ); 1.19.5 *nihil hoc* (for *nihil horum*) in common only with **M**; 1.19.5 *durior* (for *duriora*) in common only with γ and **P3**; 1.19.5 *constrictione*: cf. *constrictio* **P1**, *constricti* **M**, *constricta* cett.

[64] The ascription is retained by De Renzi. If Petroncellus of Salerno was responsible at all for *Ter.*, then at most for a later recension, for Petroncellus (=Petrus Musandinus?) lived in the twelfth century (see Bloedner and Glaze, *Medical Books*, 50–1 n. 73). In the oldest manuscripts, *Ter.* is anonymous.

[65] For information on this text, I am indebted in particular to Monica Green and Cloudy Fischer, who is preparing a study of the sources and transmission of the *Ter.* which he has kindly allowed me to see. Cf. *BTML* no. 568, p. 148; Fischer, '*Lib. Byz.*', 285 and n. 34; Glaze, *Medical Books*, 47ff., 297ff., eadem, '*Passionarius*'; Schubring, 'Epistula'; Schubring, 'Petrizoneli'.

[66] On the *Epistula peri hereseon*, see *BTML*, p. 79, and especially Glaze, *Medical Books*, 47ff., 297ff., who estimates (p. 50 and n. 73) that it was put together in northern Italy in the late seventh century.

Table 3.3: A sample comparison of the mainstream Latin Alexander (1.59) with the Liber passionalis *and the* Tereoperica

Alex. Trall., I, 527, 20 Περὶ ληθάργου	(**Alex. Trall. lat. 1.59 P1, f. 154ra**)	(***Lib. pass.* ch. 24 be 53rv (ch. 23 s 236–7)**	(***Ter.* 2.6 Sloane 2839, ff. 82v-83r; cf. Vat. Reg. lat. 1004, f. 59r**)
1–Ὁ γνήσιος λήθαργος, ὥσπερ ἡ φρενῖτις,	LVI. 1- Verus quippe lithargus quemadmodum et frene<ti>cus fit.	XXIIII De litargo. 1- Verus quippe litargicus quemadmodum et freneticus sit	De litargia passione. Litargia prope similis est frenesin[4] ...
2– ἔχει μὲν τόπον ἐγκεφάλου, ὕλην δ'ἐναντίαν τῇ φρενίτιδι.	2- abit enim et ipse locum[1] in cerebro leden*d*i, materia autem contraria flenetica:	2- habet enim et ipse locum in cerebro litendi materia his amerario[3] frenetico	2- ipse locus cerebri contrariam habet materiam ... -2 5- si flegmaticus humor fuerit solus -5
3– ἐπὶ φλέγματι γὰρ πλεονάζοντι γίνεται ὑγραίνοντι αὐτὸν καὶ διαβρέχοντι ἰσχυρῶς, ὡς μὴ δύνασθαι μεμνῆσθαι τῶν λεγομένων, ἀλλὰ μύειν ἀεὶ ἐθέλειν τὰ βλέφαρα 4– καὶ ἡσυχάζειν ἢ δι' ὅλου καρουμένους ὑπὸ τῆς καταπνιγούσης καὶ ναρκούσης τὸ ψυχικὸν πνεῦμα ὑγρότητος ἅμα καὶ ψύξεως.	3- ex fleumate enim efficitur humectandum et infundendum fortiter cerebro ut non possit nec rememorare ut aliquid loquatur sed clausas palpebras abens 4- tacit[2] quietus et in toto grauato uel oppresso stopore animo ostenditur humectatus et infrigdatus esse cerebrus.	3- ex fleomate enim efficitur humectando et infundendo fortiter cerebrum et non possit nec rememorare ut aliquid loquatur sed causas palphebras habens 4- iacet quietus et in toto grauatus uel oppressus stupore animus tenditur humectatus et infrigdatus esse cerebrus.	3- litargicum facit humectando et infrigdando fortiter cerebro et non possunt rememorare ut aliquid loquantur et clausas habent palpebras -3
5– ἐὰν οὖν φλεγματικὸς ᾖ μόνον ὁ τὸν λήθαργον ἐργαζόμενος χυμὸς, ὁ γνήσιος λήθαργος γίνεται ...	5- Si enim fleumaticus humor fuit solus lithargus facit uerum. +– –+	5- Si enim fleumaticus humor fuerit solus litargum facit uerum |	9- clamantibus eis. Interdum aperiunt oculos et reclaudunt.-9
	1 ipse locum **MP1** locum ipse **A** *ed.* 2 tacet **A** iacet ***ed.*** pro tacit quietus habet cacochime **M**(!)	3 materiam est contraria **s**	4 Ad litargicos Quippe habet. similitudinem frenetici **Vat**.

(*continued*)

Table 3.3: Continued

6– εἰ δὲ μὴ μόνον εἴη τὸ φλέγμα ἐν τῇ κεφαλῇ, ἀλλὰ καὶ χολή, ἀνάγκη καὶ τὰ συμπτώματα μικτὰ γίνεσθαι,	6- Si autem non solus fuerit fleumaticus humor putridus in capite sed et colericus simul <cum> illo mixtus accedat <et> accedentias sint +– –+	6- si autem non solus fuerit fleumaticus humor putredo in capite sed et colericus simul cum illo mixtus accedit et accedentia sit	6- Si flegmaticus humor solus non fuerit sed colericus humor mixtus fuerit[5] accidentia sit putredinem in capite -6 et in cerebro est manifestum et non sinit periculum.
7– ὡς ποτὲ μὲν ἀγρυπνεῖν, ποτὲ δὲ ὑπὸ βαθυτάτου ὕπνου ἔχεσθαι, ποτὲ δὲ παραφρονεῖν.	7- ita ut modo uigilias paciuntur modo etiam graui oppraemantur somno et modo alienentur	7- ita ut modo uigilias patiuntur modo etiam grauior p(re)mantur somnos et modo alienentur	4- quieti iacent et in toto grauantur. uel oppressi stupore animi sunt –4
8– ἀμφότερα γὰρ πράττουσι μύουσι τε τὰ βλέφαρα καὶ τὰς χεῖρας κινοῦσιν, ὥσπερ ψηλαφῶντές τινα καὶ αὐτὰ σχεῖν οὐ δυνάμενοι.	8- utrumque agentes simul et claudentes palpebras et manus sicut qui euellere uel pelis(?) auferrere uult continere manus non possunt.	8- utrumque etiam agentis simul et gludentis palphebras et manus sicut qui euellere pilos aut auferre uult continere manus non possunt	7- ita ut modo uigilias patiantur modo graui somno opprimantur[6] et modo alienentur. –7
9– ὅσοι μὲν οὖν μετριώτερον διάγουσιν, ἐμβοώντων αὐτοῖς τινων ἀνοίγουσιν ἔσθ᾽ ὅτε τὰ βλέφαρα καὶ πάλιν μύουσιν. . . .	9-Quecumque ergo mediocriter agunt clamantibus eis ab aliquibus apperiuntur interdum oculus et iterum recludunt. . . .	9- clamantibus eis aperiunt interdum oculos et iterum recludunt . . .	8- utrumque agentes. aut insimul oculos claudunt et manus continere[7] non possunt que euellere aut auferre[8] uolunt pilos ex oculis. . . .

5 fuerit *om.* **Vat**.
6 graui oppresso somno **Vat**.
7 contempnere **Vat**.
8 ferre **Vat**.

Table 3.4: A sample comparison of the mainstream Latin Alexander (2.50) with the Liber passionalis *and the* Tereoperica

Alex Trall. II, 311, 19–313, 3	(**Alex. Trall. lat. 2.50** A, **ff. 66vb–67ra; cf. P1, ff. 189vb–190ra**) XLVII. De his qui satis spuunt[1] et humidum habent stomachum	(***Lib. pass.*** **ch. 20 s pp. 231–3** (ch. 21 **be** f. 51r with only the last few words of this ch.)) De his qui satis spuunt et stomachum humidum habent	(***Ter.*** **1.47 Par. 11219, f. 65rb–va; cf. Sl = Sloane 2839, f. 29r** XLVIII. Ad eos qui nimia expuunt saliuam et humidum habent sthomacho
1– ὥσπερ πάλιν δεῖ λογίζεσθαί καὶ ἐπὶ τῶν ἀποπτυόντων πλείονα καὶ ψυχρὸν οἰομένων ἔχειν τὸν στόμαχον· 2– οὐ γὰρ πάντως ὑπὸ πολλῆς ὑγρότητος γίνεται τὸ τοιοῦτον· ἐνδέχεται γὰρ καὶ διὰ θερμότητα συμβαίνειν·	1- Oportet iterum eos p(er)uidere qui multum | expuunt et humidum habent stomachum. 2- Non enim omnibus sub multa stomachi humectatione hec contingunt. quia possibile est et ex calore contingere.	1- Oportet igitur preuidere. qui multum spuunt et stomachum humidum habent. 2- non enim omnibus sed multa humectatio stomachi contingit.	1- Oportet eos prouidere 2- quia non omnibus <>[5] contigit haec passio. <?>[6] Aliquibus ex calore contigit.
3– <οἱ γοῦν (**M**)> νηστεύοντες γὰρ καὶ ὀλιγοσιτοῦντες πάσχουσι τοῦτο πολλάκις καὶ οὐ παύονται σιελίζοντες καὶ ἀποπτύοντες πολλὰ, ἕως οὗ τροφὴν προσενέγκωνται.	3- Qui ergo ieiuni et modicum cibum accipientes[2] hec frequenter patiuntur et non pulsant[3] (παύονται!) saliuas p(ro)iciendo donec cibum accipiant	3- Quibus ergo ieiunis et modicum accipientibus frequenter paciuntur et non pausant saliuas proiciendo donec cibum accipiant.	3- Aliquando ieiunus et modico cibo accepto euenit. Haec frequenter patiuntur et non resument[7] saliuas proiciendo donec cibum accipiant.
4– δῆλον δὲ, ὅτι τῆς θερμασίας ἀναλυούσης τὰ ἐν τῷ βάθει ὑγρὰ συνέβαινε τοῦτο· ...	4- manifestum est quia calor resoluit qui in p(ro)fundo sunt humores.[4] +– Gk II, 311, 25–27 –+	4- Manifestum est quia calor resoluit qui est in profundo stomachi.	4- Manifestum est qui ex calore soluit saliuam[8] ex profundo

1 *om. ed.*
2 Quibus ... ieiunis ... accipientibus **P1**
3 pausant **P1** *ed.*
4 est humor **P1**

5 uniter **Sl**
6 sed aliquibus ex flegma capitis **Sl**
7 resument hoc est cessant **Sl**
8 manifestum quippe est quando ex calore soluitur saliua quia **Sl**

(*continued*)

Table 3.4: Continued

5– ὅτι δὲ διὰ θερμότητα γίνεται τὸ πτυαλίζειν αὐτοὺς πλέον, ἔνεστιν ἰδεῖν κἀπὶ τῶν καιομένων ξύλων· ἀποστάζουσι γὰρ καὶ αὐτὰ ὑγρὸν δηλονότι τοῦ πυρὸς ἐκκενοῦντος τὸ ἐν τῷ ξύλῳ περιεχόμενον ὑδατῶδες.	5- Nam ex calore fit saliuarum effusio quemadmodum in lignis ardentibus fit quomodo ex ipsis defluit humor qui in ipsis est aquosus.	5- Nam ex calore fit saliuarum effusio quemadmodum et in lignis ardentibus fit quomodo ex ipsis defluit humidum quod in ipsis est aquosum.	5- euenit effusio caloris quemadmodum in lignis ardentibus defluit humor aquosus.
6– τὸ αὐτὸ δὲ καὶ ἐπὶ τῶν ὀπτωμένων κρεῶν μάλιστά ἐστι συμβαῖνον θεάσασθαι.	6- Similit(er) autem et in carnibus fit quando assantur.	6- Similit autem et in carnibus fit quando assantur.	
7– θεραπεύειν οὖν χρὴ τοὺς διὰ θέρμην[9] πολλὰ πτύοντας διά τε τῶν ἐμψυχόντων καὶ δυσκατεργάστων τροφῶν, ὥσπερ πάλιν τοὺς δι' ὑγρότητα τοῖς θερμάινουσιν <καὶ ξηραίνουσιν (**M**)>	7- Curare autem[10] eos oportet qui de calore multo saliuarum effusione laborant cibos qui-infrigdare possunt[11] et non faciledigerunturdando,[12] quem-admodum et eos qui ex humectatione multa proiciunt saliuas ex his[13] que calefaciunt et desiccant, +–quia contraria contrariis curabuntur.–+ (*Alex. Trall. lat. omits the end of this chapter=Gk II, 313, 3-13*)	7- Curare eos oportet qui de calore multum saliuarum effus[s]ione laborant quiinfrig-dare possit cibum et non facile diierere. Conuenit autem et dare quemadmodum et eos qui ex humec<ta>tione proiciunt saliuas que calefaciunt et desiccant <quia non curabuntur **be**>	7- Curare eos oportet | qui de calore multum saliuarum effu-sione laborant ex medicamine qui in frigore[14] possint uiscera interioris et cibis qui non facile degeruntur oportet dare eis. Similiter eos qui ex humecta-tione proiciunt saliuam ex medicaminibus calidis et cibis dissicatiuis curabuntur
9 θερμότητα **L M**	10 *om.* **P1** 11 qui infrigdare possunt cibus **P1** 12 dare **P1** 13 ex his *om.* **P1**		14 medicaminibus que infrigdare **Sl**

podagra), and on the other hand Cassius Felix.[67] The manuscripts of the *Ter.* start early, the four oldest copies currently known being as follows:[68]

Paris, lat. 11219, ff. 42ra–103ra (*c.* 850, France, perhaps Saint Denis) (Book 1 only);[69]

London, Harley 4977, ff. 1ra–120vb (11th cent.);[70]

London, Sloane 2839, ff. 5v–112v (end 11th/beginning 12th cent., perhaps England);[71]

Munich, clm 29698 (formerly 29137), ff. 1r–2v, fragments only of incipit, capitula, and chapters 2–5 (early 10th cent.).[72]

The version of *Ter.* transmitted by a later manuscript, Paris, lat. 14025, ff. 1ra–101vb (end 12th/beginning 13th cent., Glaze), was reproduced by De Renzi, under the title (taken from the manuscript) *Practica Petrocelli Salernitani*, in vol. IV of his *Collectio Salernitana.*[73]

Several chapters of *Ter.* draw on the Latin Alexander, and there may be more to be found. It is possible that in some sections the direct source was not Alexander but an earlier compilation akin, say, to the *Liber passionalis*, with which *Ter.* has at least six Alexander-based excerpts in common, namely those from Alex. Trall. 1.1–4, 1.17 & 19–20, 1.59, 1.107, 2.50, and 3.46–7 (for a summary of other points of contact between *Ter.* and Alex. Trall., see Table 3.1 above). The distance between the texts of *Ter.* and Alexander, however, varies enormously. On the one hand, it is clear from collation of Par. lat. 11219 with the mainstream tradition of Alexander for 1.17 & 19–20 that the source of *Ter.* 1.12–13 is a faithful copy of the text of Alexander without editorial modification (one moreover which shares frequent errors with **P1** and **M** and may therefore be a descendant of β: see 4.2 below). On the other hand, it is immediately apparent from the *Ter.* versions of Alex. Trall. 1.59 and 2.50 set out in Tables 3.3 and 3.4 above that here the maker of *Ter.*, or his source, was excerpting Alexander with much modification sentence by sentence, and in 1.59 even changing the order of certain sentences and phrases. Likewise, if the extract *De icticis febribus* (London, Harley 4977, f. 113rv), obviously based on Alex. Trall. 3.46–7, is in fact from *Ter.*, it is very different both from the Latin Alexander and from the version in *Lib. pass.* For the reconstruction of the original text of such passages, then, *Ter.* will be a witness of at most marginal interest. Nevertheless, given the presence in the tradition of *Ter.* of the faithful and important early copy of Alex. Trall. 1.17 & 19–20, this is clearly a witness that deserves to be evaluated on a case-by-case basis.

[67] cf. Sabbah, 'Cassius Felix', 23–7; Fraisse, LXXV f. It emerges, however, from Fischer's work (n. 65 above) that Cassius Felix is not the main source of *Ter.* Book1, and that Theod. Prisc. is used by *Ter.*, e.g. in the chapter on spasm.

[68] Referred to by Fraisse in her edition of Cass. Fel. as T1, T2, T3, and T4, respectively. See also Talbot.

[69] See Beccaria, *Codici*, 166–73; Wickersheimer, 'Un manuscrit', 10–11; Wickersheimer, *Manuscrits*, 112–23; Glaze, *Medical Books*, 50–1 n. 73.

[70] (Autopsy January 2003.) In spite of the eleventh-century dating (*Cat. Harley*, III, 235; Sabbah, 23, n. 50), not in Beccaria, *Codici*.

[71] See Beccaria, *Codici*, 261–3; Glaze, *Medical Books*, 50–1 n. 73; Wickersheimer, 'Un manuscrit', 10, dates it to the fifteenth century!

[72] See Beccaria, *Codici*, no. 65.

[73] On pp. 185–286, with extracts from Books 2 (pp. 287–90) and 3 (pp. 290–1). On Paris 14025, see Fischer, 'Pseudo-Democritus', 49; Wickersheimer, 'Un manuscrit', 10, dates it emphatically to the fourteenth century! *Ter.* is transmitted also in Vat. lat. 4421, ff. 1r–54v (twelfth/thirteenth century, Glaze), and in extracts in Chartres 70, Montpellier 185, Cambridge Gg 5. 35, Vienna 10, Salisburg. Mus. Carolino-Augustei 2169, London, Harley 1585 (twelfth century), and (from Book 2) Vat. reg. lat. 1004, Flor. Aedil. 165. I owe this information to Cloudy Fischer.

3.2.4. *Liber diaetarum diversorum medicorum*

The *Liber diaetarum diuersorum medicorum hoc est Alexandri et aliorum*[74] (henceforth *Lib. diaet.*) is a compilation of some forty-five chapters containing dietetic recommendations for the treatment of about the same number of diseases. It is drawn very largely from the Latin Alexander, excerpts being taken from twelve chapters of Book 1 and twenty-five chapters of Book 2. Although Alex. Trall. Book 3 contains extensive dietetic sections (e.g. 3.20, 36, 58), the maker of *Lib. diaet.* evidently turned to another source (or sources) for his last few chapters, on diet in fevers. All of the Alexander chapters stand in *Lib. diaet.* in their original order, and presumably represent the fruit of a single pass through a complete copy of Alex. Trall. Books 1 and 2.

The *Lib. diaet.* is perhaps better known as Book 5 of the thirteenth/fourteenth-century recension of the *Physica Plinii* (the so-called *Physica Plinii Florentino-Pragensis*), in which excerpts from Q. Gargilius Martialis, *Medicinae ex oleribus et pomis* were made to constitute Book 4.[75] It is in this context that it was first edited by Tommaso Pighinucci (*C. Plinii Secundi Medicina*, Rome 1509, ff. u 2r–x 6r).[76] However, the *Lib. diaet.* appears also on the one hand in manuscripts containing the *Medicina Plinii*, rather than the *Physica Plinii*, and on the other hand independently of any of the 'Pliny books'. In the earliest surviving copy, **s**, and in **l2**, the *Lib. diaet.* immediately follows the *Medicina Plinii* and the Gargilius book,[77] while **v1** and **co** transmit the *Lib. diaet.* alone of this Plinian corpus.[78]

Table 3.5 gives an overview of the use made of the Latin Alexander by the maker of *Lib. diaet.*, collating **v1**, **co**, **l2** (and Pighinucci's edition of Book 5 of the *Physica Plinii Flor.-Prag.*) against **s**.

Again, I have not undertaken a systematic collation of this tradition, but in this case it is at once evident that we have to reckon with (at least) two branches: **s**, **v1** and **l2** are united in error against **co** in omitting the extract from Alex. Trall. 2.187 (between chapters XXXII and XXXIII Pighinucci), and **s** and **v1** (and the *Phys. Plin. Flor.-Prag.*) compound the error by retaining the title of the missing chapter (2.187) in place of that properly belonging with the next chapter, from Alex. Trall. 2.200. It is apparent

[74] So it is called in **v1**, **l2**, and **co** (**co** lacks the word *medicorum*); **s** has only *Liber diaetarum diuersorum medicorum*.

[75] Each of the several versions of the *Physica Plinii* is named after the location of its (chief) manuscript(s). The oldest, the *Bambergensis*, is a (probably fifth/sixth-century) recension in three books, including some additional material, of the *Medicina Plinii*, a compilation (from around A.D. 300) of *euporista* in three books taken very largely from Pliny, *Nat.* 20–32. See *BTML*, 113–14 and 127–9, and Langslow, *Medical Latin*, 64 and 68–9 for further references.

[76] The title of Pighinucci's edition — with *medicina* rather than *physica* — is misleading. His edition was closely followed by that of Alban Thorer, in *De re medica* (1528), ff. 92v–98v (repr. in *Medici antiqui omnes* (1547), ff. 207v–211r). See *BTML*, 111 nos 389–90, and Önnerfors, *Med. Plin.*, XXXIII.

[77] This sequence is found also in other manuscripts, including Herten, Bibl. Nesselrode-Reichenstein 192 (eleventh/twelfth century; Beccaria, *Codici*, 208–13); Prague, lat. 2425 (fourteenth/fifteenth century; Rose, *Anecdota*, II, 61, 107; Önnerfors, *Med. Plin.*, XXIII); and Leiden, Voss. lat. O. 92 (ninth or early tenth century; Rose, *Anecdota*, II, 108; Beccaria, *Codici*, 338–40; Önnerfors, *Med. Plin.*, XIX), where two short medical pieces separate the end of the *Med. Plin.* from Garg. Mart. and the *Lib. diaet.* cf. Maire, LXVIII ff.

[78] Beccaria also reports that extracts of the *Lib. diaet.* are transmitted in St Gall, Stiftsbibliothek 44, pp. 268–276 (later ninth century; Beccaria, *Codici*, 364–8), Siena, Bibl. comunale degli Intronati F. V. 8, ff. 173–175 (tenth/eleventh century; Beccaria, *Codici*, 331–2), and St Gall, Stiftsbibliothek 878, p. 374 (earlier eleventh century).

Table 3.5: The Latin Alexander and the Liber diaetarum

(§ indicates that text and unnumbered title are present pretty much as in **s***;* under **l2**, *(2) indicates that the whole original title was overwritten)*

Alex. Trall. ***ed.***	**s,** pp. 133–159	**v1,** ff. 134v–137v, 140r–142v	**co,** ff. 61r–66v	**l2,** ff. 146v–151v	***Phys. Plin.*** **Bk 5, ed. Pighinucci**
1.6 med.	I. De capillis cadentibus	§	§	Dieta illorum quibus capilli cadunt (2)	I. . . . fluentibus
1.25	II. Si de epate caput dolet	Dieta si . . .	. . . dolet caput	§	II.
1.32(1.31^{bis}) fin.	III. Si ex uino caput dolet	Dieta si . . .	§	§	III. Si de . . .
1.33 med.	IIII. Si de percussione caput dolet	Dieta si de percussura . . .	. . . percussura . . .	§	IIII.
1.58	V. De cibis freneticis	Dieta freneticorum	§	. . . freneticorum	V.
1.60 fin.	VI. De letargicis	Dieta de litargicis	Dieta de lithargicis	Dieta lithargicorum (2)	VI. Dieta de lythargicis
1.63 med.-fin.	VII. De epelempsia	Dieta de epilempticis	De epilempsia	Dieta epilempticorum (2)	VII. Dieta de epilenticis
1.81 init.-fin.	VIII. De melancolia	Dieta de . . .	De melancolia	Dieta melancolicorum (2)	VIII. De melancolicis
1.91	VIIII. De oculorum passione	Dieta de . . .	§	§	IX.
1.130	X. De aurium passione	Dieta de . . .	§	§	X.
1.142	XI. Dieta sinancti<c>is	. . . sinancis	. . . sinancis	. . . sinancicorum	XI. . . . synanticis
	XII. De catarro Yppocratis	§	§	§	XII. Dieta de catarro
1.145	XIII. Dieta de pleureticis	Dieta p.	Dieta p.	§	XIII. De p.
	XIII. *bis* Dieta Sorani ad pleuresin	Dieta S. pleureticis	§	§ (2)	XIIII. Ad pleuresim

(continued)

Table 3.5: Continued

Alex. Trall. *ed.*	**s,** pp. 133–159	**v1,** ff. 134v–137v, 140r–142v	**co,** ff. 61r–66v	**l2,** ff. 146v–151v	***Phys. Plin.*** **Bk 5, ed. Pighinucci**
2.18, 2.21	<XIIII.> Dieta ad stomachum frigidum	. . . de stomacho frigido	§	§	XV. . . . de stomacho frigido
2.22	XV. Si de calore nimio	Dieta si . . . nimio stomachus dolet	XVI. Si de calore uino	Dieta infirmi de calore (2)	XVI. . . . nimio fiat fastidium
2.26	XVI. Si de glutinosis et pinguibus <humoribus> fiat fastidium	Dieta si . . . humoribus . . .	XVII.	§ (2)	XVII. *om.* fastidium
2.27	XVII. Si de calida distemperantia fit fastidium	Dieta si . . .	XVIII. . . . fiat fastidium	§	XVIII. . . . fiat fastidium
2.37	XVIII. Dieta ad cardiacos	§	XVIIII.	§	XIX.
2.40 init.	XVIIII. Dieta si melancolicus humor uomicam exierit	Dieta melancolicis que de colerico humore uomitum exegerit	XX. Dieta melanchol() qui de colerico humore nomin() exierit	. . . exegerit (si . . . uomicam overwritten)	XX. Si . . . exegerit
2.55	<XX.> Si ex colerum plenitudine effusio uentris cum uomitu fuerit	Dieta si . . . effusio nimia uentris uel uomitus fuerit	XXI. Dieta si de . . . effusio nimia uentris cum uomitum fuerit	§ (Si . . . cum overwritten)	XXI. . . . effusio nimia uentris uel uomitus sit
	XXI. Dieta de peripleumonicis secundum Soranum	D. Sorani de p.	XXII. De pleumonicis dieta Sorani	§	XXII. Dieta Sorani de peripleumodicis
	<XXII.> Dieta tetanis	. . . tetanicis	XXIII. . . . tetanicis	. . . de titanis	XXIII. . . . tetanicis
2.61, 2.62	XXIII. Dieta de epaticis	Dieta epaticis	XXIIII. Dieta epaticis	§	XXIIII. De epaticis
2.73 fin.	XXIIII. Dieta epatis calide distemperantie	. . . epaticis . . .	XXV. . . . epaticis . . .	§	XXV. . . . epaticis . . .
2.74, 2.79	Dieta frigide distemperantie epatis siue uentris	. . . epatis si uenter emiserit	XXVI. . . . distemperantie si uentre emiserint	§	XXVI.

Table 3.5: Continued

2.86, 2.94	De sintericis	Dieta disintericis	Dieta disintericis	Dieta de disentericis	XXVII. Dieta dissintericis
2.108	Dieta spleneticis frigide distemperantie	§	. . . distemperantie frigide	§	XXVIII.
2.109, 2.135	De calida distemperantia splenis	§	. . . spleneticis	§	XXIX. Dieta calidae d-ae s.
2.156	Item dieta de ydropicis siue epar patientibus	. . . de epar . . .	XXX. Dieta udropem siue quidem epate male aliquid patitur	De ydropicis siue de epate patientibus	XXX. Dieta hydropicis . . .
2.164	Dieta de emoptoicis	. . . diemoptoicis	XXXI. De e. dieta	§	XXXI. Dieta emoptoicis
2.184. med.-fin.	D<i>eta nefreticis	§	XXXII. De freneticis	Dieta nefreticorum (n. overwritten)	XXXII.
2.187			Dieta ad renum inflammationem		
2.200	Dieta ad renium inflammationem	§	Dieta cum urina multum funditur	Dieta multum fundentium urinam (2)	XXXIII. . . . renum . . .
2.205	Dieta de coli passione que ex frigore fit	§	. . . qui ex frigdore est	§	XXXIIII.
2.222	Si de colerico humore coli patiuntur dieta est ordinanda	§	. . . patiuntur (ch. begins Dieta est ordinanda)	. . . colum patiatur: dieta ordinanda est (-um and -atur overwritten)	XXXV. . . .: quomodo dieta . . .
2.241 med.	Dieta podagricis ex colerico <humore>	§	§	§	XXXVI. . . . humore

from autopsy that **l2** corrects this title and adds the missing chapter with the correct title a few folios later.[79] (Many titles in **l2** have been overwritten in whole or in part (indicated by '(2)' in Table 3.5). In some cases it is clear that they were thereby changed, but often it is unclear whether the writing over was to correct them or to make more legible the fading red of the original.)

The text presented, in two parts, by **v1** is of interest. In the first place, the first part of the *Liber diaetarum* ends (f. 137v) with ch. XXVII followed by XLIIII (*Dieta ad eos qui seringiones habuerint* — not from Alex. Trall.). Secondly, while the first part shows a number of significant agreements with **co** (note chs IIII, VI, XI, XIII, XXIII–XXVII), the second part (f. 140vff.) diverges from **co** (including in the matter of the extract from 2.187 mentioned above) and agrees very closely with **s** in every chapter-title (XXVIII–XXXVI). Evidently, the maker of **v1** had two versions of the *Liber diaetarum* at his disposal. It is possible that he regarded the first one (close to **co**, used for chs I–XXVII and XLIIII) as complete, for he adds an Explicit after ch. XLIIII on f. 137v. That he realized that he had a second copy of the same work is suggested by the fact that he resumed copying (from the second version, close to **s**) at the point where his first version gave out.

These two branches in the earlier (i.e. pre-*Physica Plinii*) tradition of the *Lib. diaet.* are further characterized in the sample piece of text in Table 3.6 below; this passage, relating to the dietetic treatment of gout, was chosen deliberately to allow further comparison between the *Lib. diaet.* and the *De podagra* (3.2.5 below).

Even in such a short extract, we see in several places that **s**, **v1** and **l2** agree against **co** (and are in general closer than **co** to the ancestor of *Phys. Plin.*). For example, **co** alone retains *ut inimicum* at the end of §2, *carnes* at the start of §5, a particle at the end of §6; in §1, for *qualia sunt*, **co** alone has *qualis est*; in §5, for *bouinas* **co** alone has *bubulas*, and from the pair of co-ordinated adjectives, originally *tenuis atque subtilis*, at the end of §5, **co** alone has *utiles* (presumably reflecting *su(b)tiles*; cf. the reading of **po** in Table 3.8 below), the others all *tenues*.

This extract gives a pretty representative idea of how the maker of *Lib. diaet.* set about excerpting his source. His aim was evidently to reduce the text to a fairly minimal set of lists of things to take and things to avoid. The extent to which he has shortened this chapter is readily seen from Table 3.8, where the original is reproduced in full. Given this ruthless approach to any remotely dispensable material, it is remarkable that the strictly otiose intensifier *ut inimicum* survived in the version preserved in **co**. The earlier tradition of the *Lib. diaet.* contains a terrible error in §1 in banning all the foods there listed, an error corrected by the addition of *dandus est* in the *Phys. Plin.*, but only partly corrected, in that it remains unclear where the list of banned substances begins.

Finally, this passage — again, in spite of its modest length — contains one clear indication, and two possible further hints, that the source of the *Lib. diaet.*, unlike that of the *De podagra* (3.2.5 below), was an Alexander manuscript within the mainstream tradition. The manuscript used by the maker of *Lib. diaet.* evidently contained the error *duras* (§4), an error shared with all the mainstream manuscripts, in place of correct *albas* (for Greek λευκή) transmitted by the *De podagra* tradition (and **v1**). That the source of *Lib. diaet.* was a descendant of α is consistent also with the shared error

[79] After (2.184) *Dieta nefreticorum* in **l2**, there is a circle with an upright cross, which refers the reader to f. 154r *Dieta ad renum inflammationem*.

Table 3.6: A sample comparison of the mainstream Latin Alexander (2.241) with the two branches of the (earlier) tradition of the Liber diaetarum *(and with* Phys. Plin. Flor.-Prag. *Book 5)*

Alex. Trall. lat. 2.241 (based on v1, 76vb–77rb; cf. Table 3.8)	***Lib. diaet.*, co, 65v**	***Lib. diaet.*, v1, 141vab (cf. s, p. 153; l2, 150v)**	***Phys. Plin. Flor.-Prag.*, ed. Pighinucci, Bk 5, cap. xxxvi**
DE DIETA 1- . . . sed ea sunt offerenda que infrigdent et humectent corpus qualia sunt.[1]	Dieta podagricis ex colerico 1- +— —+ Omnis cybus qui infrigdant et humectat qualis est	Dieta podagricis ex colerico 1- Omnis cibus qui infrigidat et humectat: qualia sunt intuba, lactuca, malua, bletus, grisola canabrasica, cardamomum, eruca, porrum, allium et cepa fugiendus est.[6]	Dieta podagricis ex colerico humore 1- Omnis cibus qui infrigidat et humectat dandus est: qualia sunt intuba, lactuca, malua, blita, brassica, chrysolaca, cardamum, eruca, porrum, allium et cepe fugienda sunt.
2- DE OLERIBVS. Olera danda sunt intuba lactucas maluas et si delectentur blitus Crisolacana succos[2] et ea quecunque sunt que infrigdare et humectare possunt. Brassica autem et cardamum[3] et erucam et porrum et allium et cepas ut inimica sunt fugienda.	intuba, lactuca, malua, bletus, grisolacana, +— —+ brassica, cardamomum, eruca, porrus, allium, cepe ut inimicum ista omnia sunt fugienda.		
3- DE VOLATILIBVS. Volatilia danda sunt fasiani et domestici pulli et[4] non saginati, perdicis, turdos, merulas, gattiolas, fecitulas.	3- De uolatilibus dabis fasianos et domesticos pullos, perdices, turdos, merulas, gantas, ficetiulas	3- Volatilia dabis fasianos et domesticos pullos, perdices, turdos, merulas, gantulas, facetulas.[7]	3- Volatilia dabis phasianos ac domesticos pullos, perdices, turdos, merulas, cantulas, ficedulas.
4- DE PISCIBVS Pisces uero aspratiles, et maxime eos qui albas[5] habent carnes	4- Pisces aspratiles et maxime qui duras carnes habent +— —+	4- Pisces aspratiles et maxime qui duras habent carnes.[8]	4- Pisces aspratiles et maxime qui duras carnes habent.

1 corpus qualia sunt *om. ed.*
2 crisola cansogcus **P1** crisolocanne succus *ed.* crisocolla **A**
3 cardamomum **α**
4 sed **α**
5 duras **α**

6 -a sunt **l2**
7 fic- **l2**
8 carnes habent **s**

(*continued*)

Table 3.6: Continued

Alex. Trall. lat. 2.241 (based on v1, 76vb–77rb; cf. Table 3.8)	***Lib. diaet.*, co, 65v**	***Lib. diaet.*, v1, 141vab (cf. s, p. 153; l2, 150v)**	***Phys. Plin. Flor.-Prag.*, ed. Pighinucci, Bk 5, cap. xxxvi**
. . . (Et ysicia . . .)			
5- DE CARNIBVS Berbicina manducent iuscellata et maxime uentres et bouinas similiter. . . . Quando autem nimius est dolor in pedibus, tunc tenues atque subtiles dieta danda est. . . .	5- Carnes berbicinas manducent iuscellatos maxime uentres, et bubulas similiter et quando grauis est dolor hec non sunt danda set utiles cibi +– –+	5- bouinas[9] manducent iuscellata: et maxime uentres ac[10] bouina similiter; quando grauis est dolor[11] hec non sunt danda, sed tenues cibi.	5- Veruecinas uero carnes manducent uiscellatas: et maxime ex his uentres ac bouinas similiter; quando autem grauis est dolor hec non sunt danda, sed tenues cibi.
6- DE LEGVMINIBVS. Fabas uirides et siccas sed ante infusas in aqua et fasiolus alexandrinus et maxime infusus . . . Alia autem legumina prohibenda sunt.	6- Legumina dabis fauas uirides et siccas sed in aqua ante infusas fasioli similiter infusos. +– + Nam alia legumina sunt fugienda. +– –+	6- Legumina dabis fabas uirides et siccas (*corr. ex* -is) sed in aqua ante infusas[12] et fasiolos (*corr. ex* fass-) similiter infusos. Alia legumina prohibenda sunt.	6- Legumina dabis fabas uirides et siccas sed in aqua ante infusas et faseolos similiter infusos. Alia legumina prohibenda sunt.

9 Berbicinas (-a **l2**) **s l2**
10 et **s l2**
11 dolor est **l2**
12 infusas ante in aqua **l2**

cardamomum (§2) for correct *cardamum* (the latter in *De podagra* and **v1**; Greek κάρδαμον), although this error could easily be polygenetic. It is interesting also that *Lib. diaet.* like α (and in this case **v1**) lists five kinds of bird at the end of §3, while the Greek text and *De podagra* have only four.

From this small sample comparison one may provisionally conclude that *Lib. diaet.* was not made from *De podagra*, nor from a source derived from other than the mainstream tradition, and that — also in view of the radical excerpting methods employed by its maker — it need be called as a witness for the reconstruction of the chapters that it excerpts only *in extremis*.

3.2.5. *De podagra*[80]

The *De podagra*, in the manuscripts sometimes ascribed to Galen, is drawn entirely from the Latin Alexander, and represents a selection with some rearrangement of part or all of twenty-seven of the thirty-seven chapters on gout at the end of Book 2 (235–71). I include **v1** here (and in Table 3.7 below) because these chapters are excerpted also in this manuscript, but it is important to note that the section on gout in **v1** is not a recension but a faithful copy from a mainstream manuscript closely related to **M** and **P1** of chs 235–70 in their entirety; this is demonstrated *in extenso* in the fact that in Table 3.8 below the text of Alex. Trall. 2.241 is actually based on that of **v1** (with select comparisons with **P1**, **A** and ***ed.***). It is not clear why ch. 271 was not copied by the maker of **v1**. The excerptor may have been led to regard 271 as of marginal importance by its preamble announcing remedies for those patients unable to keep down medicines taken by mouth; or he may have been put off by the long final recipe calling for flesh of stingray and blood of mole. We cannot know. Nor is it clear whether any significance is to be attached to the fact that 271 is ignored also by the *De podagra*, which does make use of 270.

Table 3.1 (above) allows more easily than Table 3.7 (below) a swift overview of the content and arrangement of the *De podagra*. The chapters are excerpted in the following order: 235–6, 261–70, 237–51 (omitting 242), 242. After the optimistic introduction on the curability of gout (235) and the survey of the various types of cause of the disease (236), we jump to the treatment of gout caused by the blood (261). This could be seen as a (perfectly defensible) decision to treat the humours from which the disease arises in the order set out in 236, where *sanguis* precedes *colericus humor*, were it not for the fact that nine further, unrelated chapters are then excerpted (262–70) before we return to gout caused by the second humour, *colericus humor* (237) and thence proceed in order to 251, omitting only (by accident?) 242 *De balneo*, which is then added at the end. Chs 252–60, which detail a number of further, complex treatments for gout arising from *flegmaticus humor*, are absent from all the copies of *De podagra* known to me, whether by accident or as a result of an editorial decision, we cannot know. Overall, then, the original text is severely curtailed, but there is at least one recipe in the *De podagra* which is apparently absent from the mainstream tradition of the Latin Alexander as we know it at present, namely the *Puluis catarticus inuentus a peritis medicis* described in ch. 5 of *De pod.* (=*Pass.* 4.6 Cura^2) but absent from ***ed.*** and **A**.[81]

[80] cf. Thorndike and Kibre, 1056, nos 8 (=**v1**) and 9 where this text is said to form 'part of Galen, *De febribus ad Glauconem*'. Cf. also 3.2.6 below.

[81] This is correctly observed by Wickersheimer, *Manuscrits*, 151 in his comments on **po**. Note, however, that the preceding recipe, the *Leptocarion*, which Wickersheimer says is also lacking from *ed.*, is in fact present in the mainstream tradition, including in *ed.*, where only the title is missing.

Table 3.7: The Latin Alexander, the pre-Gariopontean De podagra *and Gariopontus*, Pass. *4.4–18*

Alex. Trall. ***ed.***, 2. 235–271	**A,** ff. 116va–129va	**v1,** ff. 75v–86v	**po,** ff. 60v–67r	**l2,** ff. 107r–111	**vat2,** ff. 109r–112v	**vat3,** ff. 80v–85v & **vat4**, ff. 101v–107v	**Gar.** ***Pass***. Bk 4, chs 4–18
2.235 De podagra 2.236 De podagre causis	CXXXIIII. De podagra	f. 75va, (line 1 badly damaged; black caps boxed in red) ?PODAGRA? DE LIBRO — ?ALONI?	De podagro (m2) (lacks end of 2.236; 2.261 follows)	I. De podagricis (2.261 follows)	no t. (2.261 follows)	no t. (ornate init. P- in **vat3**) (2.261 follows)	4.4 Podagra (includes 2.261)
2.237 Signa si de colerico humore podagra fuerit generata	CXXXV. t. as *ed.*	CXXXV. t. as *ed.*	(following 2.270) De eodem (m2) big initial	(following 2.270) VI. De podagra generata ex colerico humore	(following 2.270) as *ed.*	(following 2.270) no t., big initial	(following 2.270) 4.7 Podagra
2.238 Curatio podagre calide de coleribus adhibenda	CXXXVI. . . .de coleribus cathartica	. . .de coleribus catartica De catarticis	De eodem (m2)	VII. De humore colerico qui fit in articulis pedum	. . .de coleribus in articulis	no t., big initial	Cura
2.239 Podagricis que sunt extrinsecus adhibenda	Que sunt podagricis extrinsecus adhibenda		De eodem (m2)	VIII. De diuersitate podagre curat(ionum)	. . . ntrinsecus . . .	no t., big initial	Variatio curae (2.238 mid. – 2.239 end)
2.240 De embrocis	De embrocis	De embrocas	De eodem (m2)	IX. De diuersitate rosacei olei ad pedes ung(endos)	De embrocha	no t., big initial	Cura
2.241 De dieta	De dieta	De dieta	De eodem (m2)	X. De dieta podagricorum	no t.	no t., big initial	4.8 De dieta

De oleribus	De oleribus	De oleribus	De oleribus	XI. De holeribus	De oleribus	De oleribus	4.9 De oleribus
De uolatilibus	De uolatilibus	De uolatilibus	no t., big initial	XII. De uolatilibus	De uolatilibus	no t., big initial	4.10 De uolatilibus
De piscibus	De piscibus	De piscibus	no t., big initial	XIII. De piscibus	De piscibus	no t., big initial	4.11 De piscibus
De carnibus	De carnibus	De carnibus	no t., big initial	XIIII. De carnibus	De carnibus	De carnibus	4.12 De carnibus
De leguminibus	De leguminibus	De legumini-bus	no t., big initial	<X>V. De leguminibus	De leguminibus	no t., big initial	4.13 De fabis
De pomis	De pomis	De pomis	no t., big initial	XVI. De pomis	De pomis	no t., big initial	4.14 De pomis (to end of 2.241)
De tragimatibus	De tragimati-bus	De tragimata	no t., big initial	XVII. De dragaematibus	De dragoematibus	no t., big initial	
De gestatione	De gestatione	De uectatione	no t., big initial (2.248 follows)	XVIII. De egestatione (2.248 follows)	Idegestatione (2.248 follows)	no t., big initial (2.248 follows)	
2.242 De balneis	De balneis	De balneis			(following 2.251) De balneis (1st half only)	(following 2.251) no t., big initial (1st half only)	(following 2.251) 4.18 De balneis (2.242 1st half only)
2.243 Que oportet podagricis extrin-secus adhibere ad dolorem mitigan-dum…	…adhiberi.	2.243.t. in text					

(continued)

Table 3.7: Continued

Alex. Trall. *ed*., 2. 235–271	**A,** ff. 116va–129va	**v1,** ff. 75v–86v	**po,** ff. 60v–67r	**l2,** ff. 107r–111	**vat2,** ff. 109r–112v	**vat3,** ff. 80v–85v & **vat4**, ff. 101v–107v	**Gar.** ***Pass***. Bk 4, chs 4–18
2.244 Confectio dyaltee caceltice	. . .dialteas calastici	. . .dialteas calasticum					
2.245 De emplastris	Exemplar fenicis	Emplaustrum finicine 2.246.t. in text					
2.246 De linimentis	De lenimentis						
2.247 Signa si de flegmatico humore podagra generetur	CXXXVII. . . . odagra fuerit generata	. . .fleumatico (hum(ore) s.s.) fuerint (-n- s.s.) generata					
2.248 Curatio flegmatice podagre	Curatio si de flegmatico humore podagra generatur	Curatio si de fleumatico et frigido hum(ore) podagra generatur	(following 2.241) no t., big initial	(following 2.241) XIX. Cur podagre de flegmatico humore generantur	(following 2.241) Curatio si de flegmatico humore podagra generatur	(following 2.241) no t., big initial (**vat3** lacks the last three words)	(following 2.241) 4.15 De pod. ex phleg. generata (minus last sentence of 2.248) Cura
2.249 De catarticis	De catarticis	De catarticis	no t., big initial	XIX.[bis] De catarticis dandis	De catarticis	no t., big initial	
2.250 Oximel Iuliani catarticum	Oximelle Iuliani catarticum	Catarticus oximelli Iuliani	no t., big initial (stops in v. 3 without reason)	XX. De oximelle Iuliani	no t.	**vat3** no t., big initial **vat4** Deocximelle	4.16 De oxymelle

2.251 De cathaputiis dandis	De catapotiis dandis	De cataputias dandas (no new heading)		XXI. De cataputiis dandis (incomplete, loss of folio)	De cataputias danda (2.242 follows)	no t., big initial (2.242 follows)	4.17 De catapotiis .i. pilulis (2.242 follows)
2.252 De antidoto dyacorallion	De antidotis podagricis aptis	De antidotis podagricos					
		Confectio de antidotis					
2.253 Item de antidoto Trachii (Ἡρακλείδου)	Antidotum Eraclii (*corr. ex* -tlii *uel* -dii) philosophi	Antidotus autem est et aliter dandus 2.253.t. in text					
2.254 De potionibus							
2.255 De localibus curis. . .	as *ed.*	as *ed.*					
		De calefactionibus					
2.256 De calefacientibus potenter	Item aliud cataplasma	Item cataplasma					
2.257 De balneis	De balneo	De balneo					
2.258 De unguentis dyaforeticis	De unguentis	De unguentis					

(*continued*)

Table 3.7: Continued

Alex. Trall. ***ed.***, 2. 235–271	**A,** ff. 116va–129va	**v1,** ff. 75v–86v	**po,** ff. 60v–67r	**l2,** ff. 107r–111	**vat2,** ff. 109r–112v	**vat3,** ff. 80v–85v & **vat4,** ff. 101v–107v	**Gar.** ***Pass***. Bk 4, chs 4–18
2.259 Ad eos qui in pedibus de flegmatico humore nimios habent tumores	CXXXVIII. t. as *ed.*	as *ed.*					
2.260Psilotrum podagricis	Psilotron podagricis	Psilotra poda-gricis in text					
2.261 Curatio podagre ex sanguine generate	CXXXVIIII. Si ex sanguine fuerint generata	De podagra. Si ex sanguine fuerit generata	(following 2.236) De eodem (m2) no t., big initial	(following 2.236) II. De cura eorum (in marg., edge of f. cut: Signa podagre qu[sanguine fit et cur[)	(following 2.236) Podagra si ex sanguine fuerit generata	(following 2.236) no t., big initial	(following 2.236) (4.4) Cura
2.262 De localibus curis	t. as *ed.*	t. as *ed.*	De eodem (m2) no t., big initial	III. De reumatizato loco	t. as *ed.*	no t., big initial	4.5 De rheumatismo et eius cura
2.263 Ad porros, hoc est si in nodis tumores fuerint et lapides	CXL. . . . si in nodis tuberes fecerit	In text: Ad poros hoc est si in nudos tubos fecerit aut lapis	In text: as **vat2** (. . . nodos tuuos . . .)	IIII. Ad poros soluendos (minus the last 6 lines of 2.263; 2.264 complete)	In text: Ad poros hoc est si in nodo tubos fecerit aut lapides (minus the end of 2.263; 2.264 complete)	In text: as **vat2** (. . . feceri ut . . . **vat3**) (minus the end of 2.263; 2.264 complete)	4.6 De porris (minus the last 6 lines of 2.263; 2.264 complete)
2.264 De antidotis	De antidoto	in text					

2.265 Ad porros	De cerotis ad poros	De cerotis ad poros	no t., big initial (4 recipes + 1 not in *ed.*)	V. Curatio eorum (a selection of the remedies in 2.265, the last third of 267 and all of 270)	De cerotis ad poros	no t., big initial (4 recipes (3 in **vat4**) +1 not in *ed.*)	Cura[1] (2.265 in part)
2.266 De anodinis antidotis et catarticis dandis	CXLI. t. as *ed.*	t. as *ed.*					
2.267 Catarticum de hermodactilis	CXLII. Catarticum de hermodactilo	Catarticum de hermodactilo	(the last third only)	(V. cont.) (the last third only)	(2.270 follows)	(the last third only)	Cura[3] (2.267 mid.-end, minus last sentence)
		Qualiter nutriendus est qui hermodactili antidotum sunt accepturi (in text in *ed.* & A)	(2.270 follows)	(2.270 follows)		**vat4** (ornate I-) Iter qualiter nutriendi sunt qui, etc. as **v1** (2.270 follows)	(2.270 follows)
2.268 De cathaputiis	CXLIII. De catapotiis	De cataputiis					
2.269 Potio de coronopodium	CXLIIII. Potiones de coronopodio et diamiro	Potiones de coronopodion et diamirum					
	CXLV. Antidotum de coronopodio	De duobus antidotis ad podagricos (in text in *ed.*)					

(*continued*)

Table 3.7: Continued

Alex. Trall. *ed*., 2. 235–271	**A,** ff. 116va–129va	**v1,** ff. 75v–86v	**po,** ff. 60v–67r	**l2,** ff. 107r–111	**vat2,** ff. 109r–112v	**vat3,** ff. 80v–85v & **vat4**, ff. 101v–107v	**Gar. *Pass*.** Bk 4, chs 4–18
2.270 De antidoto alio podagricis dando per totum annum	Item antidotum aliud quod datur in anno integro podagricis (in text)	Item aliud antidotum qui datur in anno integro	In text as **v1** (2.237 follows)	(V. cont.) (2.237 follows)	(2.237 follows)	**vat3** no t., big initial; **vat4** (ornate I-) Iter antidotum aliud quodatur in anno integro podagricis (2.237 follows)	(Cura[3] cont.) (2.270 complete) (2.237 follows)
2.271 De localibus adiutoriis mitigatiuis	CXLVI. t. as *ed.*						

Table 3.7 (above) offers a detailed comparison of the form and arrangement of the *De podagra* in five eleventh-century manuscripts with on the one hand the chapters on gout in the mainstream tradition and in **v1**, which evidently belong together, and on the other hand the chapters devoted to the disease in Book 4 of the *Passionarius* of Gariopontus.

Precisely because the *De podagra* is transmitted also in the *Passionarius* of Gariopontus (and seems indeed to be the only point of contact between the Latin Alexander and Gariopontus), I save further comment on the text of the *De podagra* until I have introduced the latter work.

3.2.6. Gariopontus of Salerno, *Passionarius*

The *Passionarius Garioponti* (or, as in some manuscripts, *Galeni*; henceforth *Pass.*) is an important 'synthetic redaction'[82] in seven books, made in the second quarter of the eleventh century by the Salernitan medical author Gariopontus (Gari(m)potus/ Guarampotus).[83] The raw material for Gariopontus' work as redactor was a collection of late antique/early medieval Latin medical texts, including the two books of the Latin Galen, *Ad Glauconem* with the so-called *Liber tertius*, parts of Theodorus Priscianus,[84] the books of Aurelius and Esculapius, and the *De podagra* drawn from the Latin Alexander (3.2.5 above).[85] Glaze rightly emphasizes the importance of distinguishing the 'unsynthesized', pre-Gariopontean ensemble of these texts,[86] often transmitted in sequence together,[87] from the 'synthesized, *redacted* version' properly identified with Gariopontus. Gariopontus' contribution was by excerpting and rearranging, and a certain amount of rewriting, to produce from this popular but unwieldy early medieval ensemble a single work in seven books (each with a table of contents), organized largely by the affected body-parts,[88] and in which all varieties of a given disease, regardless of the theoretical orientation of the original source,[89] are taken together.

The *Passionarius* was a best-selling success. No fewer than fifty-seven manuscript copies of the work are currently known (eleventh–sixteenth century),[90] of which the earliest is probably Vienna 2425 (late eleventh century),[91] and of which nearly half are from the twelfth century.[92] Gariopontus' work was printed three times in the second

[82] Glaze, *Medical Books*, 39.

[83] Bibliography: Fischer, '*Lib. Byz.*', 282 and n. 21; Gar. ed. (1536); Glaze, *Medical Books*, especially 39, 171ff.; Glaze, 'Galen refashioned', 53f. and n.2; Kristeller, 'School of Salerno', 147ff.; Rose, *Anecdota*, 2, 105ff., 176ff.; *Theod. Prisc.*, xiii–xiv; Thorndike, *History*, I, 733ff.

[84] See Rose, *Theod. Prisc.*, xiii–xv.

[85] On the ensemble, see Rose, *Theod. Prisc.*, xii–xiii; Beccaria, *Codici*, 35–6; Stoffregen, 10–16; Baader, 'Die Anfänge', 694–7; Stok, 268; Glaze, '*Passionarius*'; Glaze 'Galen refashioned', 54 and n.3, and note Fischer, *ed. pr.* Lib. tert.

[86] Glaze, *Medical Books*, 173 n. 23.

[87] Glaze, '*Passionarius*', notes that 'many of the manuscripts containing the ensemble seem to have originated in Italy, though they ... were apparently disseminated at an early date'.

[88] Roughly speaking, Books 1–4 proceed from head to foot; Book 5 deals with skin-diseases; Books 6–7 are devoted to fevers.

[89] On the importance of this step of ignoring the long-obsolete and barely understood theoretical differences between the texts of the earlier 'ensemble', see Glaze, '*Passionarius*'.

[90] See Schmid, *Caelius Aurelianus*, 67–71; Baader, 'Überlieferung', 141; Glaze, *Medical Books*, 309ff.; eadem, '*Passionarius*'. As Glaze notes (last ref.), there is as yet no complete list of the manuscripts of Gariopontus.

[91] cf. Rose, *Anecdota*, II, 113; Glaze, *Medical Books*, 177 n. 29.

[92] See Glaze, '*Passionarius*'.

quarter of the sixteenth century,[93] and held in the highest regard until the early twentieth century. It has been more recently the victim of scholarly neglect, but its importance is now being positively re-evaluated in the work of Eliza Glaze.

For present purposes, we are concerned with Book 4 of the *Pass.*, which, after three chapters from the *Liber Esculapii*,[94] consists entirely of the *De podagra*, more or less complete (although with some additions and some subtractions) and with the chapters selected and ordered as in **po**, **l2**, **vat2**, **vat3**, and **vat4**. Given that the *De podagra* is not attested before the eleventh century, the question arises in principle whether we owe it in the first place to the editorial activity of Gariopontus, or whether he incorporated it more or less as he found it in a pre-existing redaction. The latter is made a priori more likely if, as seems to be the case, the *De podagra* is the only point of contact between the Latin Alexander and the *Passionarius*, and the collation of a single chapter in its three versions in, respectively, the mainstream Latin Alexander, the *De podagra*, and the *Passionarius* puts it, to my mind, beyond doubt. Table 3.8 (below) sets side by side Gariopontus (the 1536 Basel edition compared with Zurich, Zentralbibliothek, C. 128 (early twelfth century)[95] and Paris, Arsenal 867 (late twelfth century)[96]), the Greek Alexander, the Latin Alexander (based on the text of **v1** compared with **P1**, **A** and *ed.*), and the *De podagra* (based on the text of **po** compared with **l2** and the three Vatican manuscripts), all on the subject of the dietetic treatment of gout.[97] From this comparison a number of important points emerge with clarity.

In the first place, to begin with the question raised a moment ago, the text of Gariopontus represents consistently and frequently a further recension of the version of the Latin Alexander transmitted in the *De podagra*; this is true already of the manuscript versions of the *Passionarius*, and the distance is increased by the 1536 edition.[98] It is never the case that the *De podagra* must owe its form to a Gariopontean reworking of Alexander, but it is frequently the case that the text of Gariopontus appears to reflect an attempt to tidy up, and improve the Latinity of, the *De podagra*. For example, at the end of §5 Gariopontus must have found something like the text of the *De podagra*, 'si ipse qui patitur *estum aut ardorem calidus* iuuenis aut medie etatis sit', which obviously contains in the underlined words a corruption of *est natura calidus* (Greek θερμὸς τὴν κρᾶσιν), but which he rewrites as 'qui patiuntur aestum aut ardorem si calidi iuuenes aut media aetate sunt'. Here, although he smoothes the Latin, he compounds the error in the text of the *De podagra*. Elsewhere, he appears to correct it successfully, e.g. §5 'de tenui et acri rheumate' for *detenuisse acra reuma*, §5 'nimium rhuma' ('nimium dolor' in the Paris ms.!) for *minor dolor*, §6 'alicas' for *aliquantas*. The last three examples may suggest that he had access to a superior text, but this is often not the case. His text

[93] First by Bartholemi Trot as *Passionarius Galeni* (Lyons, 1526), and then twice by Henricus Petrus as *Garioponti vetusti admodum medici ad totius corporis aegritudines remediorum praxeon libri v* (Basel, 1531), and as *Habes sincerioris medicinae amator, iterum renatos viii de morborum causis, accidentibus et curationibus libros Garioponti medici, qui usu et successu artis nemini ex ueteribus cedit, testibus qui usi sunt eius remediorum ratione indicationeue* (Basel, 1536). On the confusion, in the Renaissance and since, over the authorship of *Pass.*, see Glaze, 'Galen refashioned', 58ff.

[94] *Pass.* 4.1 *De sciatica=Esculapius* 44; 4.2 *De psialgia=Esc.* 45; 4.3 *De podagra=Esc.* 47. I owe this information to Cloudy Fischer.

[95] On this manuscript, see Glaze, '*Passionarius*'.

[96] On Paris, Arsenal 867, cf. 3.1.4 above.

[97] This particular chapter (2.241) was chosen for this purpose partly in order to allow an easy further comparison between the *De podagra* and the *Liber diaetarum* (3.2.4 above).

[98] Note e.g. *adiutum* for *iuuatum* in the first part of §5; the addition of *porcellorum*, and the loss of *quales sunt* (or *id est*), at the end of §5; the loss of *autem expediunt* at the start of §8.

Table 3.8: A sample comparison of the mainstream Latin Alexander (2.241) with the earlier tradition of the De podagra, *and with the use of the latter in the* Passionarius

Alex. Trall. II, 509, 2 ff.	**Alex. Trall. lat. 2.241, based on v1, ff. 76vb–77rb (compared with P1, A, *ed.*)**	**po, 65v–66v (cf. l2, 110v–111r *vs* vat2, 111v–112r; vat3, 84rv; vat4, 105v–106v: *f*=vat2 vat3 vat4)**	**Gar. *Pass.* 4. 7–14 (*ed.* Basel 1536) (cf. Zurich, C.128, 48rv [capp. XII–XVI]; Paris, Arsenal 867, 123rv)**
τὰ νῦν δ᾽ἀπὸ τῆς διαίτης ἀρξώμεθα διδάσκοντες, ὡς δεῖ καὶ αὐτὴν μηδὲν ἔχειν θερμὸν ἤτοι χολὴν ὅλως τίκτειν δυνάμενον. οὕτω μὲν οὖν προνοεῖσθαι δεῖ τοῦ τε ὅλου καὶ τῶν πεπονθότων μορίων, λοιπὸν δὲ καὶ τῇ διαίτῃ προσέχειν, ὥστε καὶ αὐτὴν ἐμψύχουσάν τε καὶ ὑγραίνουσαν εἶναι, παραιτεῖσθαι δὲ πᾶν, ὅ τι ἂν θερμαῖνον πάνυ τι χολῶδες τίκτειν δύνηται.	DE DIETA. Nunc autem de dieta dicendum est. Hi ergo[1] qui de colerico hum(ore) pedes dolent oportet eos obseruare[2] ut non utantur ea que calorem colerico humori augmentand*o* generare possunt sed ea sunt offerenda que infrigdent et humectent corpus qualia sunt.[3]	Nunc autem de dieta dicendum est. Hi *autem*[6] qui de colerico humore pedes dolent, oportet eos obseruare ut non adhibeant[7] ea que calore colericum humorem augmentando generare possunt, sed ea sunt offerenda que infrigdent et humectent corpus.	nunc autem de dieta[12] dicendum est. VIII. De dieta. Quibus[13] ex cholerico humore pedes dolent, obseruandum est ne offerantur ea quae calore suo[14] cholericum humorem augmentando generare possint, sed offerenda sunt quae infrigidant et humectant corpus.
Περὶ λαχάνων. Λαχάνων δὲ προσφερέσθωσαν ἴντυβόν τε καὶ θριδακίνην καὶ μαλάχην, εἰ δὲ ἡδέως ἔχοιεν, καὶ βλίτον καὶ χρυσολάχανον καὶ σόγχον καὶ πᾶν ὁτιοῦν ψύχειν (ἐμψύχειν M) τε καὶ ὑγραίνειν δυνάμενον. κράμβην δὲ καὶ κάρδαμον καὶ εὔζωμον καὶ πράσον καὶ σκόρδον ὡς πολέμια φεύγειν δεῖ.	2- DE OLERIBVS. Olera danda sunt intuba lactucas maluas et si delectentur blitus crisolacana succos[4] et ea quecunque sunt que infrigdare et humectare possunt. Brassica autem et cardamum[5] et erucam et porrum et allium et cepas ut inimica sunt fugienda.	De oleribus uero danda sunt intiba, lactuce, malue et si delectantur blitus, chrisolo chana[8] et quecunque humectare et[9] infrigdare nouerit[10] corpus. Brassica autem et cardamum et erucam et porrum et allium ueluti inimica sunt fugienda.[11]	IX. De oleribus. De oleribus danda sunt intiba, lactuca, malua et si delectantur blitis[15] chrysolocanna.[16] Brassica autem[17] et cardamum et eruca et porrum et allium[18] plus inimico fugienda sunt.
	1 Ergo quibus **A** ***ed.*** 2 seruare ***ed.*** 3 corpus qualia sunt *om.* ***ed.*** 4 crisola cansogcus **P1** crisolocanne succus *ed.* crisocolla **A** 5 cardamomum **α**	6 ergo **l2** ***f*** Peterh. 251 7 utantur *f* 8 chrisolocana **l2** grisolacana *f* 9 uel **l2** 10 -int (mouerint **vat4**) **l2** ***f*** 11 alliu(m) *inimicitius* sunt fugiende *f*	12 dieta podagricorum **P** 13 Quibus autem **Z P** 14 suo calore **Z P** 15 blitus **Z P** 16 et crisolachana **Z** grisocanna **P** 17 autem *om.* **P** 18 et allium *om.* **P**

(*continued*)

Περὶ ὀρνίθων. Τῶν δὲ ὀρνίθων προσφερέσθωσαν τῶν τε φασιανῶν καὶ τῶν κατοικιδίων ὀρνίθων τὰ μὴ λιπαρὰ καὶ ἀτταγῆνας καὶ πέρδικας καὶ κοσσύφους καὶ κίχλας.	3- DE VOLATILIBVS. Volatilia danda sunt fasiani et domestici pulli et[19] non saginati, perdicis, turdos, merulas, gattiolas, fecitulas.	Volatilia danda sunt pulli, fasiani sed non saginati, perdices, turdus, merula, ficedula.	X. De uolatilibus. Volatilium[57] dandi sunt pulli, phasiani, sed non saginati, perdices, turdus, merula, ficedula.[58]
Περὶ ἰχθύων. Καὶ τῶν ἰχθύων τοὺς πετραίους μάλιστα καὶ τῶν ἄλλων, οἷς ἡ οὐσία λευκὴ καὶ ψαφαρὰ κατὰ φύσιν καὶ οὐδὲν ἔχουσα πιμελῶδες. τὰ μέντοι ἐκ λίμνης παραιτείσθωσαν· ἔστωσαν δὲ πάντων αἱ ἀρτύσεις ἀπέριττοι μήτε ἐλαίου πολὺ μήτε τῶν δριμέων (δριμυτέρων L M) σπερμάτων προσλαμβάνουσαι.	4- DE PISCIBVS Pisces uero aspratiles, et maxime eos qui albas[20] habent carnes et nichil in se habent pinguedinem.[21] Que autem in stagnis et limosis locis capiuntur[22] prohibendi sunt. Sit autem conditura piscium sine aliqua superfluitate et neque oleum multum neque acri aliquod sementis admisceantur	Pisces[30] aspratiles et maxime hos[31] qui albam abent carnem[32] nichilque habent in se pinguidinis.[33] Qui autem in stagnis et in limosis locis capiuntur prohibendi sunt. Sit[34] conditura piscium cum hac qualitate ut neque oleo multo condiantur[35] neque aliquibus acris seminibus[36]	XI. De piscibus. Pisces[59] aspratiles et maxime qui albas carnes habent[60] et nihil pingue sumantur.[61] Qui autem in stagnis uel[62] in limosis locis capiuntur prohibendi sunt. Condiantur autem pisces neque ex multo oleo neque acris[63] seminibus
Περὶ ἰσικοῦ. Καὶ ὁ ἰσικός δὲ ὁ ἐκ τούτων ὠφελιμώτατός ἐστι καὶ μάλιστα ὁ ἐκ τῶν σκληροτέρων (ἰχθύων *add.* L M), οἷον ὀρφοῦ, κηρίδος, τευθίδος, σηπίας, κτενίων, καὶ τῶν ὀστρακοδέρμων δὲ μὴ φοβεῖσθαι ἐπιδοῦναι.	et ysicia ex eis facta iuuare possunt eos et maxime ex durioribus piscibus qualia sunt orfon, cyrida tentidas, sepias, pectines, sed et ostreas et concilia non timeas dare.	ut eum desiccando iuuare possunt, maxime durioribus piscibus, quales sunt orfi, cirides, dentices, sippie, pectines, etiam[37] ostreas et cocleas non timeas dare.	ut possint desiccando iuuare. Duriores quoque maxime pisces[64] orphos,[65] cirides, dentices, sipias, pectines non dabis,[66] sed et ostreas et cochleas non timeas dare.
Περὶ κρεῶν. Καὶ τῶν προβατείων δὲ κρεῶν προσφερέσθωσαν τὸ ἀπόζεμα καὶ μάλιστα τῆς κοιλίας τῶν βοῶν. ὁμοίως γοῦν οἶδά τινας τῶν οὕτω ῥευματιζομένων ἐπὶ πλείστῳ καὶ δριμεῖ ῥεύματι μέγιστα ὠφελουμένους ὑπὸ τῶν βοείων κρεῶν.	5- DE CARNIBVS Berbicina manducent iuscellata et maxime uentres et bouinas similiter. Ego igitur[23] scio quendam reumatizantem de cumia et crireuma et[24] quam maxime bubula carne manducando fuisse iuuatum. Sed hec non frequenter danda est.	Ceruinam[38] manducent iuscellatam et maxime uentres, et bouinam similiter. Ego enim[39] scio quendam reumatizantem tenuisse[40] acra reuma, et quam maxime buuulinam[41] carnem manducando[42] fuisse iuuatum. Sed hec[43] non frequenter dande sunt.	XII. De carnibus. Ceruinam manducent iusselatam,[67] et maxime uentres, et bouinam[68] similiter. Ego igitur scio quendam reumatizantem de tenui et acri[69] rheumate et quam maxime bubulinam carnem manducando fuisse adiutum.[70] Sed haec frequenter non danda[71] sunt.
οὐκέτι γὰρ οὔτε συνεχῶς οὔτε σφοδρῶς τις ἔλεγεν ἀλγεῖν τοὺς πόδας, ὥσπερ ὅτε τῇ λεπτυνούσῃ διαίτῃ κεχρημένος ἦν. ἐσθίειν δὲ τοὺς πόδας αὐτῶν μᾶλλον καὶ τὰς κοιλίας ἀποζέματος. ἦν δὲ οὗτος ἀκμάζων τὴν ἡλικίαν καὶ θερμὸς τὴν κρᾶσιν.	Quando autem nimius est dolor in pedibus, tunc tenues atque subtiles dieta danda est. Comedant autem pedes eorum magis et uentres[25] in iuscello et ipse qui patitur si est natura calidus et iuuenis et media etate.	Quando autem minor[44] est dolor a[45] pedibus, tunc tenuis ac[46] su<b>tilis dieta danda est. Comedant autem pedes eorum magis et uentres[47] in iuscello si ipse[48] qui patitur estum aut ardorem[49] calidus iuuenis[50] aut medie etatis sit.[51]	Quando autem nimium est rhuma[72] in pedibus, tunc tenuis et subtilis dieta danda est. Comedant autem pedes porcellorum[73] et magis uentres in iusselo[74] qui patiuntur[75] aestum aut ardorem si[76] calidi[77] iuuenes aut media aetate[78] sunt.
Περὶ ὀσπρίων. Τῶν δὲ ὀσπρίων προσφερέσθωσαν αὐτούς τε τοὺς	6- DE LEGVMINIBVS Fabas uirides et siccas sed ante infusas in	Fabas uirides et siccas sed antea infusas in aqua et faselum[52]	XIII. De fabis.[79] Fabas uirides et siccas sed antea infusas in aqua aut

κυάμους χλωροὺς καὶ τῶν ξηρῶν τοὺς ἀκροζέστους καὶ τοῦ φασιόλου τοῦ Ἀλεξανδρινοῦ, μάλιστα τοῦ ἀποβραχέντος καὶ τῆς τήλεως τοὺς βλαστοὺς, ἄλικος καὶ πτισάνης, οὐδὲν ἄτοπόν ἐστιν αὐτοὺς προσφέρεσθαι. τὰ δ' ἄλλα τῶν ὀσπρίων κάλλιόν ἐστιν αὐτοὺς παραιτεῖσθαι.	aqua et fasiolus Alexandrinus et maxime infusus et fenigreci cimas et aliqua[26] et ptisanas accipiant. Alia autem legumina prohibenda sunt.	Alexandrinum et maxime infusum et fenigreci cimas <et aliquantas ptisanas>[53] accipiat. Alia autem legumina prohibenda sunt.	phasellum[80] Alexandrinum et maxime infusum et foenugraeci cimas et alicas[81] ptisanas accipiant, alia autem legumina prohibeantur.
Περὶ ὀπωρῶν. Καὶ τῶν ὀπωρῶν τὴν πάνυ γλυκεῖαν καὶ πέπειρον συμβουλεύω προσφέρεσθαι περὶ ὥραν δευτέραν ἢ τρίτην, μάλιστα τῶν περσικῶν ἢ ῥοδακίνων καὶ σταφυλῆς τῆς σκληρᾶς καὶ ἀστύφους ἐχούσης τὰς ῥωγὰς καὶ δαμασκηνῶν καὶ μήλων τῶν	7- DE POMIS Poma que multa sunt dulcia et maturas ualde[27] accipere eas secunda aut tertia hora[28] et maxime persica si sint duracina et uuas duracinas sed non stipticas et damascinas et mela dulcia et citro mundato et purgata[29] bene. pera et mela granata et alia omnia poma	Poma que multum dulcia sunt natura[54] suadeo accipere hora secunda aut tertia, maxime persicca si sint duracina aut uuas duracinas sed non stipticas et damascenas et mala dulcia et citonia purgata mundataque bene,[55] pira et mala granata. alia uero poma omnia[56] aut rare aut nullo	XIIII. De pomis.[82] Poma quae multum sunt dulcia natura suadeo accipere hora secunda aut tertia, maxime si persica sunt duracina aut uuae duracinae sed non stipticae et damascena et mala dulcia et citonia purgata et mundata bene pira[83] et mala gran-

19 sed **α**
20 duras **α**
21 pingue **α**
22 pascuntur ***ed***
23 autem **α**
24 de tenuae et acra reuma et **P1** de tenui et acro reumate **A *ed.***
25 et maxime *ed.*
26 alicam **α**
27 suadeo **α**
28 hora *ante* secunda **A** ***ed***. *om.* **P1**
29 p. et m. **α**

30 Pisces uero *f*
31 hi *f*
32 alba habens carnes **vat4** albas habent carnes **l2**
33 in se nichil pinguedinis habentes **l2** et nichil habent (habeant **vat4**) in se pinguem *f*
34 Sit autem *f*
35 *post* seminibus *f*
36 seminibus condiantur *f*
37 et **l2** sed (set **vat4**) *f*
38 De carnibus ueruicinis (uerb- **vat4**) *f*
39 enim *om.* **l2** igitur *f*
40 detinuisse **l2** detenuisset *f*
41 bubulam **l2** *f*
42 bubulam manducando carnem **l2**
43 he **l2**
44 minus *f*
45 in cett.
46 aut *f*
47 uentres eorum **l2**
48 supse **vat2** subse **vat4**
49 odorem **vat4**
50 ardorem habeat aut si sit iuuenis **l2**
51 sit *om.* **l2**
52 fasiolum *f*
53 <et aliquantas ptisanas> **l2** *f* (faselum . . . ptisanas] fasiolum et aliquantanta ptisanas **vat4**)
54 dulcia sunt et matura **l2** sunt dulcia natura *f*
55 et bene mundata **l2** citonias purgatas et mundatas (purgatas **vat4**) bene *f*
56 omnia poma **l2** *f*

57 De uolatilibus **P**
58 ficetula **Z P**
59 Pisces uero **Z P**
60 habent albas carnes **Z P**
61 sumant **P**
62 et **Z**
63 acribus **Z P**
64 pisces maxime **Z P**
65 .i. orfos **Z** quales sunt orfi **P**
66 non dabis] dabis **Z** *om.* **P**
67 iuscellatam **Z** iuscellatas **P**
68 -a **Z** -as **P**
69 acro **Z**
70 iuuatum **Z P**
71 he . . . dande **P**
72 reuma **Z** dolor **P**
73 porcellorum *om.* **P** eorum boum **Z**
74 iuscello **Z P**
75 patitur **P**
76 Si *.i. primum uerbum cap. XV* **Z**
77 colerici **P**
78 medie etatis **Z P**
79 leguminibus (lug- **P!**) **Z P**
80 phaselum Z faseolum **P**
81 alicas et **Z P**
82 fructibus **P**
83 et m. bene pira *om.* **P**

(*continued*)

Table 3.3: Continued

γλυκέων καὶ κιτρίων καθαρθέντων καὶ λελεπισμένων καλῶς ποιεῖν. ἀπίων δὲ καὶ ῥοιῶν καὶ τῶν ἄλλων ἁπάντων σπανίως ἢ μηδὲ ὅλως προσφέρεσθαι δεῖ.	raro aut nullo modo sunt gustanda.	modo gustanda sunt.[91]	ata. Alia uero omnia poma aut raro aut nullo modo sunt gustanda.
Περὶ τραγημάτων. Τῶν δὲ τραγημάτων συμφέρει μάλιστα τὰ κάστανα λαμβάνειν μήτε καρύων ἢ στροβίλων ἢ ἀμυγδάλων ἐσθίειν, ἀλλὰ μηδὲ πλακούντων ἢ κοπτῶν· ἅπαντα γὰρ ταῦτα βλαβερὰ τοῖς διὰ χολῶδες περίττωμα ῥευματιζομένοις τὰ ἄρθρα.	8- DE TRAGIMATA Tragimata autem expediunt maxime castaneas neque uero nuces aut nucli pinium[84] aut amigdalas acci | piant. Sed neque placonta aut(?) comesa.[85] Omnia enim hec nociua sunt his qui de colerico reumatizant humore articuli.[86]	Tragoemata autem expediunt[92] maxime castanee, aut[93] nuces uel nucleos pineos accipiant aut amigdalas,[94] sed neque placentas aut crustula <s>edant. Omnia enim hec nociua sunt eis qui de colerico reumatizant in[95] articulis.	De tragematibus[104] maxime castaneas aut nuces uel nucleos pinearum aut amygdalas accipiant sed neque placenta[105] aut crustula aedantur.[106] Omnia[107] haec nociua sunt quibus ex cholerico[108] rheumatizant articuli.
Περὶ κινήσεως. Κινείσθωσαν δὲ μετρίως ἄνευ κόπου πολλοῦ καὶ πρὸ τροφῆς μᾶλλον ἢ μετὰ τροφήν· ὁ γὰρ κόπος ἐναντιώτατός ἐστι τούτοις ἐκθερμαίνων ἐπὶ πλέον καὶ ἐκπυρῶν τὰ ἄρθρα ἕλκειν τε παρασκευάζων εἰς αὐτὰ καὶ ἐπισπᾶσθαι πάλιν ἑτέραν ἐκ τῶν πορρωτέρω μορίων ὕλην αἴτιός τε διὰ τοῦτο γινόμενος ῥευματισμῶν.	9- DE VECTATIONE Vectare[87] autem mediocriter debent, et absque labore multum et magis ante[88] cibum quam post cibum. Labor quoque est illis contrarius quia ex eo plus calefiunt[89] et accendunt [*corr. ex* accedunt][90] articuli et trahunt ad se de longinquis locis alios hum(ores) ex quibus mox nascitur reumatismus.	Gestare[96] autem mediocriter et absque labore multo magis ante cybum. Labor quoque est[97] illis contrarius quia[98] ex eo plus[99] calefaciunt et accendunt<ur>[100] articuli[101] et trahunt ad se de longis[102]<inqu> locis alios humores ex quibus mox nascitur reumatismus.[103]	Gestentur autem mediocriter et absque labore multo magis ante cibum. Labor quoque est illis inutilis[109] quia ex eo plus calefiunt et accenduntur articuli et trahunt ad se de longinquis locis humores ex quibus nascitur rheumatismus.

84 nucleos pineos **A** *ed.*
85 contusa **α**
86 articulis **α**
87 De gestatione Gestare **α**
88 absque **P1 A**
89 calefaciunt **P1**
90 accenduntur **A** *ed.* adtenduntur **P1**

91 sunt gustanda *f*
92 expetunt **l2** Peterh. 251
93 et **l2**
94 aut amigdalas accipiant *f*
95 in *om. f*
96 Egestare **l2** Peterh. 251
97 labore . . . est *om.* **vat4**
98 que *f*
99 plus *om.* **l2**
100 acceduntur *f* accedent(?) **l2**
101 articulis **l2 vat2 vat4**
102 longinquis **l2** *f*
103 reumatismus nascitur **l2**

104 De tragematibus] De t. autem pomis **Z** Tragemata aut expediunt **P**
105 plantata **P**
106 edant **Z P**
107 Omnia autem Z Omnia enim **P**
108 colerico humore **Z**
109 illis inutilis est **Z** illis contrarius est **P**

evidently contained §5 *ceruinam* (in common with **po** and **l2**), which he accepts for correct *ueruecinam* (so in the Vatican copies); in the second part of §4 he is obviously working from a text in which the sentence beginning 'Et ysicia ex eis facta' is corrupt in the same way as the archetype of the five *De podagra* manuscripts here considered; in §7 he finds and accepts, in common again with these five *De podagra* manuscripts, the erroneous new sentence-opening *alia uero*; in §2 he may have found *inimicitius* (as in the Vatican copies), of which his 'plus inimico' looks like a correction. For a clear example of an attempt by Gariopontus to improve the Latin of the *De podagra* (and the Latin Alexander), note his construction in §1 'obseruandum est ne offerantur' replacing 'oportet eos obseruare ut non+subjunctive', or his insertion/reconfiguring of the imperatival main verbs 'sumantur', 'condiantur', 'non dabis' in §4, and 'gestentur' at the start of §9.[99]

Secondly, as for the tradition of the *De podagra*, it is immediately evident from the text of the chapter *De diaeta* (which is not clear from the comparison of the overall arrangement of the work in Table 3.7, above), that, while there are innovations common to all the manuscripts so far studied (e.g. §2 'humectare et infrigdare nouerint corpus' for *infrigdare et humectare possunt*, §4 the intrusion of 'condiantur', §4 the terrible mess in the sentence beginning 'Et ysicia ex eis facta', §5 'minus/minor' for *nimius*, §6 'aliquantas' for *alicam*, §7 'natura' for *matura*), we must reckon with at least two branches. One is represented by the three Vatican manuscripts, which are almost identical, and derive from a superior copy, but which share errors such as §2 'inimicitius' for *ut inimica*, §9 'que' for *quia*. The other branch is represented by **po** and **l2**, which show more divergences between themselves, but share important errors including §1 'adhibeant' for *utantur*, §2 'ueluti' for *ut*, §5 'ceruinam' for *ueruecinam*.[100]

For the history of the text of the Latin Alexander, the *De podagra* is of direct interest and importance in transmitting (in the short section that I have collated) at least one good reading lost from the mainstream tradition. In 2.241, in the section *De piscibus*, where the mainstream tradition (and the *Lib. diaet.*, 3.2.4 above) has 'duras',[101] the *De podagra* and the *Passionarius* have 'albas', which in view of the Greek λευκή (II, 509, 19) is surely to be preferred. It is particularly nice that at this point **v1**, which as I have already noted was evidently copying a lost complete manuscript, also has *albas*.[102] This provides, on the one hand, further characterization of the archetype of the mainstream tradition (α in the stemma), and, on the other, proof of the need to take this part of the secondary tradition into account when reconstructing the full text of the Latin Alexander on gout.

3.2.7. '*Bamberg Surgery*'

Finally, let me make brief mention of a third medical compilation made probably in Salerno which contains at least one passage drawn from the Latin Alexander. This is the so-called '*Bamberg Surgery*', dated by Sudhoff[103] to the period 1080–1160, and

[99] Cameron, 72, speaks of Book 4 of the *Passionarius* as 'virtually a direct copy' of the *De podagra*. This is, it seems, an exaggeration, but the dependence-relation is correctly stated.

[100] Cambridge, Peterhouse 251 evidently belongs to the latter group, and is closer to **l2** than to **po**. It has §5 *ceruinam* for *ueruecinam* in common with both, but §8 *expetunt* for *expediunt* and §9 *egestare* for *gestare* in common with **l2** alone. I owe these readings to Eliza Glaze, pers. comm.

[101] I have collated **P1**, **M**, **A**, **P3** and **P2** with *ed.*

[102] Note also the divergent translations of σπερμάτων in §4 between *sementis* in α (this time with **v1**) and *seminibus* in *De pod./Pass.* Which is likely to be correct, I cannot yet say.

[103] Sudhoff, *Chirurgie*, II, 106. On the '*Bamberg Surgery*', see especially Corner.

probably to the second quarter of the twelfth century. It is transmitted in at least seven manuscripts including the following (which I have checked):[104]

Bamberg, Staatsbibliothek, med. 3 (L. III. 11), ff. 158r–173v (mid-12th cent., made in the monastery of Michelsberg, today part of Bamberg);[105]

Cambridge, Gonville and Caius 400 (=**C** above), ff. 84r–90v (early 13th cent.);

Bamberg, Staatsbibliothek, med. 7 (L. III. 10; mid-13th cent.);

New York, Acad. of Med, ms. SAFE, ff. 3vb–8vb (mid-13th cent., France) (incomplete).[106]

On the basis of the two Bamberg manuscripts, Sudhoff prints an edition of the complete text of the *Bamberg Surgery*, in 1,242 lines.[107] Lines 267–74 of his edition represent a shortened and otherwise altered version of Alex. Trall. 1.119 (the Latin Alexander at this point being a shortened version of Greek II, 95, 23–97, 11). In Table 3.9 below I reproduce side-by-side the Greek Alexander, the Latin Alexander, and Sudhoff's text of the *Bamberg Surgery* (which I have checked against Bamberg, med. 3, and compared with the New York manuscript).

This short extract illustrates nicely a very selective and abbreviating use of Alexander. It also shows us the work of an excerptor who was not concerned to change the wording of his source. Apparently he adds the occasional phrase to clarify his text (e.g. 'si aliquid intus cecidit' at the end), but, as far as I can see, all the lexical divergences are most probably due to corruption, sometimes fairly dramatic ('interius' > 'inferius' for *mitius*; 'cum in occulos' somehow for *aulisco in*; even, I would suggest, 'uulnere' for *uolueris*), conceivably reflecting unfamiliarity with the letter-forms of the (Beneventan?) exemplar.[108] This extract also reminds us, if reminder was needed, how very different versions of a practical text can arise within a relatively short time: Sudhoff's text based on the oldest manuscript represents, at least to judge from these few lines, a recension of the version in the New York manuscript, which, although a century younger than Bamberg, med. 3, transmits a text significantly closer to that of the original source (compare the New York readings that I have picked out in the small apparatus to Table 3.9, nn. 2–10).

3.3. Conspectus of the More Important Manuscripts of the Secondary Tradition

ba Barcelona, Archivo de la Corona de Aragón, Ripoll 181
(García, 624–5; Green, 'Handlist I', 140; Green, '*Trotula*' (=*Women's Healthcare*, V), 134–5; Kristeller IV, 483a)

Early thirteenth century, Spain or Catalonia (Green). Parchment, ff. 211, 160×210mm, in various hands, the part containing Alex. Trall. being written in 2 columns of 30 lines.

[104] On the first three, see Sudhoff, *Chirurgie* II, 103–7. Thorndike and Kibre list also Oxford, Bodleian Library, Digby 79, ff. 194r–212 (13th cent.) (cf. Green, 'Handlist' I, no. 72, p. 160); London, British Library, Royal 12. D. XII, ff. 99r–103v (14th cent.); and [*Constantini chirurgia*:] Leyden 37, ff. 1r–13v (14th cent.). I owe this reference to Cloudy Fischer. The *Bamberg Surgery* is also in Yale University, Cushing Medical Library, ms. 10 (12th cent.), I owe this information to Eliza Glaze.

[105] On this manuscript, see Glaze, '*Passionarius*'.

[106] On this manuscript, drawn to my attention by Cloudy Fischer, see Green, 'Handlist' I, no. 64, p. 157f.

[107] Sudhoff, *Chirurgie*, II, 108–47.

[108] An idea I owe to Eliza Glaze.

Table 3.9: An extract of the Latin Alexander (1.119) in the Bamberg Surgery

Alex. Trall. II, 95, 23 ff.	**Alex. Trall. lat. 1.119, A 39vab**	***Bamberg Surgery*, vv. 267–74 Sudh. (cf. New York, ms. SAFE)**
Περὶ τῶν ἐμπιπτόντων εἰς τὴν ἀκοὴν λιθαριδίων ἢ ἄλλων τινῶν. Λιθαριδίου ἢ κυάμου ἢ ἄλλου τινὸς ἐμπίπτοντος εἰς τὴν ἀκοὴν εἰλήσας τὴν μηλωτίδα ἐρίῳ βάψον ῥητίνῃ τερεβινθίνῃ ἤ τινι τῶν ἐχεκόλλων καὶ καθεὶς πρᾴως ἐπισπῶ. καὶ πταρμὸν δὲ κινῶν ἔμφραττε τὸ στόμα καὶ τὰς ῥῖνας· κατὰ γὰρ τὴν γινομένην τοῦ πνεύματος ἔντασιν ἐκρίπτεται τὸ ἔνδον σφηνωθέν. ποίει δὲ τοῦτο συνεχῶς καὶ σπούδαζε ὡς ταχέως ἐκπεμφθῆναι.	CXVII. Si in aures aliquid fuerit ingressum. siue faba siue lapillus. Si autem lapillus aut faba aut aliquid aliud in aurem fuerit ingressum; inuolues circa spatomele lanam. et intinges in resina terebintina. aut in aliquo glutinoso medicamine. et depones mitius; et tacto q(uo)d incidit extrahes. Sternutamenta quidem adhibita mouent aperiendo meatus auris sp(irit)u irritato; et sic p(ro)icitur. +– –+	Si in aurem ingressum fuerit aliquid sicut(?) faba uel[2] aliquis lapillus, circa aliquid lignum[3] <uel> spatumilem lanam inuolue et eam terbentinam intinge aut aliquo conglutinoso et depone inferius[4] et sic subito abstrahas[5] et sternutamenta adhibeas. Mouet enim aperiendo auris meatum spiritumque irritat et sic proicitur.
εἰ δὲ μή γε, φλεγμονῆς ἐπιγενομένης σπασμοὶ πολλάκις ἐπακολουθοῦσιν, ὡς καὶ κινδυνεύειν αὐτοὺς ἀπολέσθαι. δεῖ οὖν καὶ ἔλαιον πολλάκις ἐγχεῖν χλιαρόν· οὕτω γὰρ τῶν τόπων ἀφλεγμάντων γενομένων τὸ ἐγκείμενον ῥᾳδίως ἐξελεύσεται.	Q(uo)dsi ex indignatione flegmon accesserit; sepius spasmi subsequuntur. ita ut in periculo sint; et exinde moriantur. Oportet ergo oleum tepidum infundi sepius in aurem. Sic enim poterit locus sine tumore esse; et facile factus liquor exire.	
καὶ κλύζειν δὲ μελικράτῳ καλόν ἐστιν αὐτοὺς, ὅταν χαυνωθῶσιν αἱ φλεγμοναί· ἀναπτύεται γὰρ διὰ τοῦ ὑγροῦ πολλάκις τὸ ἐμπεσὸν καὶ διὰ τριχολαβίου εὐχερῶς ἕλκεται.	Et ex mulsa lauari bonum est quando molesti humores in aure surrexerint; 1 et exit sepius q(uo)d incidit. et diatrecolabon id est uertibella facile trahitur.	
καὶ αὐλίδιόν τινες ἐμβαλόντες τῇ ἀκοῇ, εἶτα τῷ στόματι ἐκμυζήσαντες ἠδυνήθησαν τῷ τρόπῳ τούτῳ ἐπισπασάμενοι ἑλκύσαι. δεῖ δὲ πρό γε πάντων ἐλαίῳ χλιαρῷ κεχρῆσθαι καὶ τοῖς πταρμικοῖς, ὡς εἴρηται, καὶ μελικράτῳ· οὕτω γὰρ ἡμῶν πραξάντων εὐχερῶς καὶ μετὰ μηλωτίδος καὶ μεθ' οἱουδήποτε βουληθείης τῶν εἰρημένων ἐκ τοῦ βάθους ἀνενεχθήσεται.	Sed et aulisco in aure misso; quidam sucando traxerunt. Oportet enim oleo tepido ante uti; et sternutamentis sicut dictum est et mulsa. Sic enim nobis agentibus; facilius et cum spatomele et quomodo uolueris ut dictum est facile ex alto extrahitur.[1]	Et cum in occulos uel aures missum fuerit adherendo potest abstrahi. Oportet autem oleo tepido uti ante[6] et post sternutamento ut dictum est. Sic etiam[7] <agentibus nobis cum spatumelle facilius abstrahitur aut>[8] ex uulnere si aliquid intus cecidit [9] a profundo[10] extrahitur.

1 cf. Oribas., *Eup.* 4.40, p. 558 Aa / p. 557 La, both versions with *lythargirus* for λιθαρίδιον(!); cf. the much shorter and very different paragraph in the Greek Oribasius (p. 453, 1–5 Raeder).
2 sicut(?) ... uel] siue ... siue NY
3 circa ... lignum] aut aliud tale cura NY
4 interius NY
5 et ... abstrahas] et cum ceciderit extrahis NY
6 ante uti NY
7 enim NY
8 *suppl. ex* NY
9 facilis NY
10 ex alto NY

Contents:
(I quote Green) 'medical texts, including Johannes Afflacius, *Liber aureus*; Alexander of Tralles; and several Salernitan authors', and a version of the *Liber de sinthomatibus mulierum* (cf. Green):
108rb–130r Alex. Trall., Book 3 + an excerpt from Book 1
131r–134v Incipit prologus libelli Warbodi (Marbodi?) *de ornamentis uerborum* (!)
135r–210v the *Practica* of Magister Bartholomeus

Alex. Trall.: 108rb–109rb 74 unnumbered *capitula* to Book 3, 109vb blank, 110ra 'Incipit prologus tercii uel quinti libri alexandri de Tralles yatros sophiste' (emphasis mine). There follow (110ra–130ra) the prologue and all sixty-six chapters of Book 3, including the lines at the end of 3.19, 3.59,[109] and 3.64 missing from *ed.*, and omitting (like **M**, **G1**, and **C**) only the very last recipe at the end of 3.66, and then (130ra), without any sign of a break, the last six lines of 1.144 (*De cura pleureticorum*), without the first word of the sentence '(periculum): maximum infert ita ut difficultatem faciat ad prohibendos humores ... si autem infirmior uirtute fuerit fug(er)e omnino narcoticas passiones dare pleureticis!'[110]

be Berlin, Staatsbibliothek Preußischer Kulturbesitz, Phillipps lat. 1790 (Baader, 'Phill.'; Beccaria, *Codici*, 199–202; Bischoff, *Katalog*, no. 429, p. 90; Fischer, '*Lib. Byz.*', 276, 285–6; Fischer, 'Dr Monk', 240; Rose, *Verzeichnis ... Berlin*, 362–9)

Second to fourth quarter of ninth century (Bischoff) (ninth century, Rose; first half ninth century, Beccaria), made probably in eastern France (Bischoff). Parchment, ff. 111,[111] 218 × 132mm; written in minuscule of various hands of slightly different ages ('wohl generationsmäßig verschieden', Bischoff), in single columns of 26–27 lines, with titles, numbers and some initials in red; some additions in later hands. Many folios have been lost, and the surviving parts are in disarray, possibly from a very early date.[112]

Contents: 1r–29r medical recipes
29r–32r Galen, *Epistula de febribus*; 32v–33v Hippocrates, *Epistula de uirginibus*
34ra–35vb part of the *capitula* for a large medical compendium
36rv Isidore, *Etymologiae* 4, brief extracts
37–42 and 47–50 medical recipes and a series of medical and astrological fragments
43–47v, 51r–69v and 78r–87r *Liber passionalis*[113]

[109] Just before the lacuna in (probably) ε (see end of Section 4.3), **ba** has for *tardandus est*: 'trahendus est uel moretur'!

[110] cf. the wording of **A**: '(Periculum enim) maximum infert ita ut uix difficultatem faciat ad p(ro)iciendos liquores ... Si autem infirmior uirtute fuerit fuge omnino narcoticas potiones.'

[111] This volume was formerly part of the Meerman collection, at which point it had ff. 169.

[112] See Rose, *Verzeichnis ... Berlin*, 362, and Beccaria, *Codici*, 202.

[113] The first section in **be** (43–47v) actually contains the end of the collection. The first twenty chapters are lost, so that f. 51 begins with the end of XXI=XX of the version in the Sangallensis 752 (**s** below). See Rose, *Verzeichnis ... Berlin*, 364, 367–9.

89r–103v Galen, *Ad Glauconem*, extracts from Book 1
104r–111r medical recipes

Alex. Trall.: *Liber passionalis*: on the use made of Alex. Trall. in the *Liber passionalis*, see Section 3.2.2 above and Table 3.2; note that **be** contains Book 1, chs 64–7, which are not in the version of the *Liber passionalis* in **s**.

Cambridge, Peterhouse 251 (*non uidi*[114])
(Gameson, 68; James)

Six mss., all medical, in a single (twelfth/thirteenth-century) binding. Our concern here is with No. 6 (ff. 106–191), smaller than the others. *c.* 1090–1110, made in St Augustine's, Canterbury (Gameson). Vellum, 242×162mm, written in a 'beautiful round clear hand' (Glaze, pers. comm.) in single columns of 37 lines, with book-initials (at least the first excised); *capitula*- and chapter-initials alternating in red, blue, green, and purple throughout.

Contents: the pre-Gariopontean ensemble (minus Theod. Prisc.), in six books, 'but lacking any attributions to Galen, Aurelius, Esculapius or Alexander' (Glaze, pers. comm.):
106r–129v Book 1 and 129v–142r Book 2 (Galen, *Ad Glauconem* 1–2)
142v–158r Book 3 (*Liber tertius*)
158v–167r Book 4 (Aurelius)
167v–186r Book 5 (Esculapius)
and as Book 6: **186r–191r *De podagra***, entitled 'De podagricis'
191rv miscellaneous medical prescriptions

Alex. Trall.: *De podagra*: see Section 3.2.5 and Table 3.7 above; contains 22 *capitula* complete, from (1) 'Podagricorum causas scire oportet quia ...' to (22) 'De balneis quomodo uti debeant ... si fri<gi>dum tempus est'.[115]

co Copenhagen, Kongelige Bibliotek, Gamle Kongelige Samling 1653
(Beccaria, *Codici*, 119–24; Bischoff, *Nachlass*, Fiche 2, 1.5; Fischer, '*Lib. Byz.*', 278–9; Newton, *Monte Cassino*, *passim* (cf. index, p. 405); Rose, *Anecdota*, II, 107)

Eleventh century, made in Italy (from fourteenth century, in England for a time). Parchment, ff. 220, 210×138mm, written in Beneventan minuscule by several hands, in single columns of 39 lines, with here and there titles, numbers, and initials in red; with insertions in the text and margins in contemporary ordinary minuscule and with other, less frequent, insertions in a fourteenth-century hand.

Contents: 3r–28v Mustio, *Gynaecia*
28v–31v Cleopatra, <*Gynaecia*>
31v–60r Galen, *Alphabetum ad Paternum*; 60rv Galen, <*De dinamidiis*>
61r–66v *Liber diaetarum*
66v–67r *Diaeta Hippocratis*; 67r–71v *Diaeta Theodori*
72r–75v *Liber artis medicinae*; 75v–76v *Dogma Hippocratis*; 76v astrological fragments

114 For the following information on this ms. I am indebted and extremely grateful to Eliza Glaze.
115 For this information, again, I am indebted to Eliza Glaze.

77r–147v Oribasius, *Synopsis* 1–6 (including 109r isolated recipes): note that Book 5 is the *Liber Byzantii* (see Fischer)
148r–149r *De succedaneis* (on substitute ingredients)
149r–181v medical recipes, especially antidotes
181v–182r and 182r–183v two treatises on weights and measures
183v–184r four short treatises on prognosis and therapeutics
184r–185r an alphabetical (A–I) index of medical recipes
185r–188v medical recipes
189r–215v medical recipes from Oribasius in alphabetical order

Alex. Trall.: *Liber diaetarum*: on the use of Alex. Trall. in the *Liber diaetarum*, see Section 3.2.4 above and Table 3.5; note that **co** alone contains the extract from 2.187 in its rightful place.

l2 London, British Library, Royal 12. E. XX (autopsy January 2003) (Beccaria, 'Sulle tracce', II, 29; Gameson, 118; Glaze, '*Passionarius*'; Kibre, *Hipp. Lat.*, 38–9; Kibre, 'Repertorium II'; Önnerfors, *Med. Plin.*, XX; *Stud. phil.* 117–27; Rose, *Anecdota*, II, 107; Warner and Gilson, II, 56–7 (with illustrations of ff. 33, 136 in IV, pl. 73b, 73c))

Mid- to late twelfth century (Glaze), 1110–1130 (Gameson), made in England (Beccaria, Kibre, Önnerfors), ?Rochester (Gameson). Vellum, ff. 164 (orig. 162, ff. 163–164 being added later), 178×121mm. Written in England in several good small hands, in single columns (save in lists of *capitula*, which are in 2 columns) of 38 or 39 lines, with chapter-numbers and titles in red and chapter-initials alternately in red and green, with fine ornamental book-initials, but not all of them coloured in (including that at the start of the *De podagra*, f. 107v).

Contents: 1r–32v commentary on Hippocrates, *Aphorisms* (to 7.87) (Lat. B)
33r–111v the complete pre-Gariopontean ensemble,[116] minus Theod. Prisc.:
- 33r Gal., *Ad Glauc.* 1–2
- 68v *Liber tertius*
- 82v Aurelius
- 91r Esculapius

and, as Book 6: **107r–111v *De podagra***
112r–114r some minor medical tracts and recipes
114r–116v Ps. Oribasius commentary on Hippocrates, *Aphorisms* (Lat. A), extracts
117r–118v miscellaneous medical notes, recipes for powders, pessaries, etc.
119r–146v *Physica Plinii* 1–4[117]
146v–151v (+ 154r) *Liber diaetarum*[118]
151v–154r Isidore, *Etymologiae* 4 (not quite complete)

[116] Compare Warner and Gilson's note of the contents of 33r–111v, 'a compilation (in six books, incomplete because of loss of leaves after f. 111) perhaps meant to be taken for a work of Galen, as it begins with part of the preface to the treatise *Ad Glauconem de medendi methodo*, but containing really a different recension of the *Passionarius* of Gariopontus of Salerno'; this is to be corrected.
[117] Correct Gameson's 'Pliny the Elder, extract on medicine from *Historia naturalis*'.
[118] Correct Gameson's 'Latin abridgement of Alexander Trallianus, *Therapeutika*'.

154r–156r miscellaneous commonplaces of medicine (beginning with *Dieta ad renum inflammationem* misplaced from the *Liber diaetarum*)
156r–162v a collection of antidotes

Alex. Trall.: *De podagra*: see Section 3.2.5 and Table 3.7 above; **l2** has a list of 22 *capitula*, but, because of the loss of a folio or more after f. 111,[119] it lacks the end of (2.251) *De catapuciis dandis* and the last chapter, which should have been (2.242) *De balneis quomodo uti debent.*
Liber diaetarum: see Section 3.2.4 and Table 3.5 above; note that **l2** contains on a later folio the extract from 2.187 correctly preserved in **co** but lost in the common ancestor of **s** and **v1**.

Madrid, El Escorial N. iii. 17 (*non uidi*[120])
(*Cat. Escorial*, III, 155; Diels, *Handschriften*, I, 94, 130; Glaze, '*Passionarius*'; Diels, *Nachtrag*, 34, 44)

Twelfth century (Diels), written in 'a puny, spindly, ungainly 12th-c. minuscule with an excess of abbreviations' (Glaze, pers. comm.).

Contents: 41r ff. the pre-Gariopontean ensemble, minus Theod. Prisc.:
41r Galen, *Ad Glauconem* 1–2
81r *Liber tertius*
99r *Liber Aurelii*
109v *Liber Esculapii*
130v–136r *De podagra*

Alex. Trall.: 130v 22 numbered *capitula* to *De podagra*, the last three being *De oximelle Iuliani*, *De catapuciis dandis*, and *De balneis*; the *De podagra* is apparently complete, and ends 136r after the last chapter, *De balneis.*

po Poitiers, Bibliothèque municipale 184
(Beccaria, *Codici*, 181–3; *Cat. gén. Dép.*, XXV, 54–5; Fischer, '*Lib. Byz.*', 279; Glaze, '*Passionarius*'; Sigerist, 'A summer', 590; Wickersheimer, *Manuscrits*, 147–54 (including pl. of f. 68v))

Eleventh century (Wickersheimer, Sigerist), late eleventh or early twelfth century (Beccaria), made in France.[121] Parchment, ff. 81 (originally of two parts, or two manuscripts, of the same age, joined very early), 198 × 132mm, written in single columns of 27 lines, with titles and initials in red, with contemporary marginalia.

Contents: (A) the pre-Gariopontean ensemble minus Theod. Prisc.:[122]
1r–27r Galen, *De medendi methodo ad Glauconem* 1–2
27r–46r *Liber tertius*
46r–54v *Liber Aurelii*
54v–60v *Liber Esculapii*, fragments, on melancholy
60v–67r Alex. Trall., *De podagra*
67r–69v varia: *De diebus aegyptiacis uersus*; *Calendarium diaeteticum*; *De macrocosmo et microcosmo*; *De diebus aegyptiacis*; *Medicamenta ad guttam*

[119] f. 111v ends: 'melius enim si non semel sub una potione purgentur sed sepius et paulatim oportet' followed by anacoluthon and abrupt change of subject.
[120] I depend for the description of this ms. on the works listed and the generous assistance of Eliza Glaze.
[121] And fifteenth-century French marginalia on ff. 67v–68 suggest that it was at that time in France.
[122] Sigerist's description of 27r–67r as 'the first four books of Gariopontus' is to be corrected; cf. Glaze.

70r–73v Grimaldus, *De dieta… ancipitrum*

(B) 74–81v *Liber Esculapii*, fragments, 12 chapters, with a chapter of the *Liber Byzantii* appended to ch. 4 (see Fischer)

Alex. Trall.: *De podagra*: see Section 3.2.5 and Table 3.7 above; no Incipit, 20 *capitula*; breaks off mid-folio without apparent cause (with 'et tenues educit') after only three lines of XVIII. *De oximelle Iuliani* (=2.250, line 3) and so lacks (2.251) XVIIII. *De catapuciis dandis* and (2.242) XX. *De balneis*.

s Sankt Gallen, Stiftsbibliothek 752 (autopsy January 2001) **Plate XI**
(*Verzeichnis … St. Gallen*; Beccaria, *Codici*, 381–3; Glaze, '*Passionarius*'; Önnerfors, *Med. Plin.*, XIX; idem, *Stud. phil.*, 83; Rose, *Anecdota*, II, 108–9, 130, 171; Rose, *Verzeichnis … Berlin*, 364–5, 367; Sigerist, 'The Sphere', (including a facsimile of p. 82 on p. 295); Sudhoff, *Chirurgie*, II, 621)

Parchment, pp. 326 (comprising two manuscripts, 5–160, 161–326), 245×190mm, perhaps both from the St Gallen scriptorium; both written in single columns, with titles, numbers and initials in red. (A) (pp. 5–160) second half ninth century (Bischoff *apud* Önnerfors)/end ninth century (Beccaria, Sudhoff); (B) (pp. 161–326) tenth century (Beccaria, Rose), but generally the manuscript is dated to tenth–eleventh century (see Beccaria, *Codici*, 383).

Contents: (A) 6–159 *Physica Plinii Sangallensis*, in five books:

6–80 *Medicina Plinii* 1–3

83–133 Gargilius Martialis, *Medicinae ex oleribus et pomis*

133–159 *Liber diaetarum diuersorum medicorum*

80–81 Hippocrates, *Epistula ad Antiochum regem*

82 *Sphaera Apulei Platonici de uita*

(B) 161–178 Isidore, *Etymologiae* 4

179–326 *Liber passionalis*: 'Incipiunt oxea et chronia passiones yppocratis gallieni et urani (Sorani) — Explicit liber passionalis'.

Alex. Trall.: *Liber diaetarum*: see Section 3.2.4 and Table 3.5 above; the version of the *Lib. diaet.* in **s** is very close to that contained in **v1**.

Liber passionalis: see Section 3.2.2 and Table 3.2 above; note that **s** lacks Alex. Trall. 1.64–7 (=chs 80–3 in **be**).

u Uppsala, Universitetsbibliotek, (Carolina) C 664
(Andersson-Schmitt, 239–43; Beccaria, *Codici*, 344–50; Bracciotti, 62, n. 8; Glaze, '*Passionarius*')

Parchment, ff. i+179+i (more recently paginated 1–358) (originally in several parts: see Beccaria):

(A) pp. 1–84 and 101–358: first half ninth century (Beccaria) or second half (Bischoff *apud* Önnerfors, *Eranos* 58 (1960), 147–9; Andersson-Schmitt), or 'un periodo di transizione fra i secc. X e XI' (Bracciotti), made probably in northern Italy, 240×170mm. Written by various hands, in single columns of 26–27 lines, with numbers, titles, initials, and sometimes capoversi in red, and with later insertions by several hands (including in Old High German of twelfth/thirteenth century). Many of the texts are incomplete through loss of, or damage to, ff.

(B) pp. 85–100: ninth century, northern Italy, 207×147mm. Written by a single hand in 2 columns of 29 lines.

Contents: (A) numerous small medical works, including:
8–10 Vindicianus, *Epistula ad Pentadium*
10–14 Hippocrates, *Epistola ad Antiochum regem*
14–22 Vindicianus, *Epitome altera*, incomplete
25–30 Ps. Alexander, *De pulsibus et urinis*
32–54, 79–80 Galen, *Ad Glauconem* 1, excerpts
55–78, 81–84 *Liber tertius*
(B) 85–97 a collection of recipes
97–100 Ps. Alexander, *De pulsibus uel urinis. ... De effimeris febribus* (incomplete)
(A) 127–156 Ps. Apuleius, *Herbarius*
157–175 *Curae herbarum*
185–186 *Curae ex hominibus*
187–260 *Curae ex animalibus*
293–330, 335–336, 331–334, 337–338 a collection of medical recipes numbered up to 140, including:
320–322 Alex. Trall. 2.36
339–340 *Diaeta Theodori*, fragment

Alex. Trall.: this important medical manuscript contains just one extract from Alexander, namely (2.36) 'CXXVIIII. Cardica passio stomachi causa est. Contigit autem his quibus pessimi et uenenosi cum mordicationem stomachi ibidem colliguntur humores ... aut ex egritudinibus diuersis augmentantibus'.

vat1 Città del Vaticano, Bibl. apostolica vaticana, regin. lat. 1143 **Plate IX** (Beccaria, *Codici*, 319–22; Pellegrin *et al.*, *Vaticane* II.1, 149–50)

First half ninth century (with OHG words of tenth and eleventh century), made in Germany, perhaps in the neighbourhood of Mainz (Bischoff *apud* Pellegrin *et al.*). Parchment, originally in three parts, ff. 202 (with altogether four quaternions and other folios lost), 210×130mm; written in single columns, with occasional titles and numbers in red and initials decorated and highlighted in red, with additions by other, slightly later hands. Some folios have been damaged by moisture.

Contents: 1r–80v Theodorus Priscianus, *Euporista* 2–3
80v–86v miscellaneous recipes and extracts, ending with the start of the *Epistula ex quatuor humoribus* which comes in its entirety at 193r–196r; other miscellaneous medical recipes also at 105v–109v, 118–125, 129v–134v, 141r–187v, 190r–193r, 196r–200r
86rv Isidore, *Etymologiae* 4.5
87v–88v Alex. Trall., part of 3.66[123]
88v–101v, 110r–117v, 102r–105v a medical compendium of pseudonymous letters and therapeutic texts
125r–129v Vindicianus, *Epistula ad Pentadium*

[123] I am unable to identify the 'Antidotus Theodosion' (87rv), implicitly ascribed to Alex. Trall. by Beccaria and Pellegrin *et al.*, *Vaticane* (cf. the 'Antidotum Theodotion' at the end of the collection of recipes in **vat3** (below), ff. 98r–108r). An antidote recommended for gout at Alex. Trall. 2.266 (Greek II, 565, 16ff.) is ascribed to 'Theodosius philosophus'.

135r–140r Hippocrates, *Epistula ad Antiochum regem*; 140rv a Hippocratic letter on blood-letting
200rv, 187v Latin–OHG glossary of plant-names (eleventh century)

Alex. Trall.: 87v–88v 'Item ad eos quibus in profundo sunt febres ... oleo uetus sext. I, aqua sext. I'=Alex. Trall. 3.66, f. 93r vv. 18–37 (i.e. omitting the instructions for the last recipe, and without the last three recipes in *ed.*).[124] Then: 'Alexandri adrofistae de effemiras et icticas et maramodis febribus et de orrore et frigdore liber explicit feliciter.'

vat2 Città del Vaticano, Bibl. apostolica vaticana, cod. Barberinianus lat. 160 (Beccaria, *Codici*, 324–31; Beccaria, 'Sulle tracce', I, 44, II, 28ff.; Diels, *Nachtrag*, 34, 44; Glaze, '*Passionarius*'; Kristeller VI, 388a; Newton, *Monte Cassino*, 311, 389–90 (pl. 208=f. 8v); Pellegrin *et al.*, *Vaticane* I, 189–91; Silverstein, 34–6)

Eleventh century, probably from Apulia (Beccaria, Kristeller, Pellegrin *et al.*); the 1060s, from Monte Cassino (Newton). Parchment, ff. ii+289 (+ 5 ff. unnumbered or wrongly numbered), 334×230mm, originally in several parts (ff. 1–142; 143–198; 199–235; 236–289). Written partly in Beneventan (ff. 1–129, 143–253) and partly in ordinary contemporary minuscule, in both cases in several hands, mainly in single columns, with *intestazioni*, numbers, and smaller initials in red and some larger ones decorated in red or yellow, and with beautiful illustrations of the herbs and animals in the opening books.

Contents: 1r–6v Apuleius, *Herbarius* (*capitula*)
6v–8r Hippocrates, *Epistula ad Maecenatem*
8r–10r Antonius Musa, *De herba uettonica*
10r–27v Apuleius, *Herbarius*
27v–38r Sextus Placitus, *Liber medicinae ex animalibus*
38r–48v Dioscorides, *Liber medicinae ex herbis femininis*
48vff. the pre-Gariopontean ensemble minus Theod. Prisc.:
  48v–76v Galen, *Ad Glauconem* 1–2
  76v–88r Galen, *Liber tertius*
  88r–94r *Liber Aurelii*
  94r–109r *Liber Esculapii*
  109r–112v Alex. Trall., *De podagra*
113r–135v collection of medical recipes; 135v–136r a treatise on weights
136r–138v Galen, *De urinis*; 138v–141r Ps. Alexander, *De pulsibus et urinis*
141r–142r *Dogma Yppochratis*
143r–198v commentary on the Hippocratic *Aphorisms* 1–7 (Lat. A)
199r–216r Oribasius, *Synopsis ad Eustathium filium*
216r–235v Galen, *Alphabetum ad Paternum*
236r–265v Theod. Prisc. 1–3
266ra–274va Quintus Serenus, *Liber medicinalis*
274va–275va Hippocrates, *Epistula ad Antiochum regem*

[124] The last recipe in **vat1** contains three ingredients not in *ed.* and water as the last ingredient (wax in *ed.*), but no instructions as in *ed.* and Ch.

275va–276ra Vindicianus, *Epistula ad Pentadium*, incomplete (at 288rv it is complete)
276ra *Dies Aegyptiaci*
276rb–281vb three sets of medical recipes (**including some from Alex. Trall.**[125])
282rv *Sapientia artis medicinae*
282v–286r Isidore, *Etymologiae* 4
286rv–288r excerpts from: Galen, *De dinamidiis*; a medical letter; Hippocrates, *Prognostica*; Hippocrates, *Indicia ualetudinum*; *Quomodo visitare debeas infirmum*; *Quomodo febrientem curare debeas*
288r–289v Vindicianus, *Epistula ad Pentadium*; *Gynecia*, excerpt

Alex. Trall.: *De podagra*: see Section 3.2.5 and Table 3.7 above; in **vat2** this section begins: 'LVII. Incipit liber Galieni de podagra'. **vat4** has the same incipit, with the ascription to Galen; the chapter numeration follows on from that of the *Liber Esculapii*, the *capitula* of which list 57 chapters.

vat3 Città del Vaticano, Bibl. apostolica vaticana, lat. 4417
(Beccaria, *Codici*, 307–9; Fischer, 'Pseudo-Democritus', 48; Glaze, '*Passionarius*'; Goetz, *CGL*, III, xxxiii; Rose, *Theod. Prisc.*, XII)

End eleventh century or beginning twelfth century (Glaze),[126] probably from Italy (Beccaria, Glaze). Parchment, ff. 127, 307 × 178mm. Written in single columns (save lists of *capitula*, in 2 columns), with ornate and coloured interlaced/animated initials in a distinctively Beneventan style,[127] and smaller initials and some titles in red or highlighted in red; with, in the first texts, interlinear glosses in the same hand,[128] and, in the margins, titles and additions in hands of twelfth- and fourteenth-century date.

Contents: the pre-Gariopontean ensemble, minus Theod. Prisc.:
1r–37v Galen, *Ad Glauconem* 1–2
37v–54v *Liber tertius*
54v–64r *Liber Aurelii*
64r–80v *Liber Esculapii*
80v–85v Alex. Trall., *De podagra*
85v–87v various medical recipes, and two dietetic calendars
87v–95v collection of medical recipes
96r–98r Galen, *De succedaneis*
98r–108r collection of medical recipes, 'Antidotum Adriani ... Antidotum Theodotion'[129] (followed, 108r–109v, by additions in several hands)
109v–112r signs from the urine; *De pulsibus et urinis*, excerpt

[125] These include f. 276rb *Trociscus crucudes Alexandri* (from 2.97=p. 132, 19 Mih.); f. 277ra *Trociscus Alexandri spleniticis* (from 2.148=p. 190, 5 Mih.); f. 277rb *Trociscus Alexandri ad ciliacum optimum* (from 2.100=p. 144, 12 Mih.). I am grateful to Cloudy Fischer for drawing my attention to the name Alexander in these places.

[126] *c.* 1090–1120 (Eliza Glaze, personal communication to Cloudy Fischer, May 2001).

[127] I owe this information to Eliza Glaze.

[128] Some of the disease names in these tables are glossed in the same manner as by Gariopontus (e.g. f. 37v, which also contains a Gariopontus prologue, in the blank space by the *capitula* of the *Liber tertius*; other early glosses show influence of the early pharmacopeia developments following Constantine's translations (names of *materia medica* mostly) (Eliza Glaze, pers. comm.).

[129] At least one of these is from Alex. Trall., namely f. 106v *Antidotum Alexandri ad stomachum frigidum et ad eos qui non bene digerunt* (=the first recipe in 2.35). The 'Antidotum Theodotion' is similar to the 'Antidotus Theodosion' in **vat1**, f. 87rv (above, n. 123).

112r–114v on medicinal weights and measures
115r–117v Pseudo-Democritus, *Liber medicinalis* LXVIIII–LXXVII.
119r–127v medical glossary (ed. Goetz, *CGL* III, 616–30)
Alex. Trall.: *De podagra*: see Section 3.2.5 and Table 3.7 above.

vat4 Città del Vaticano, Bibl. apostolica vaticana, lat. 4418
(Beccaria, *Codici*, 309–12; Glaze, '*Passionarius*'; Rose, *Theod. Prisc.*, X, 484)
Eleventh century (Beccaria, Glaze), from central or southern Italy (Beccaria, Glaze). Parchment, originally in three parts, ff. 172, 270×163mm; written by several hands in single columns, with titles in red, a few ornate and coloured large initials, and smaller initials in red and yellow, with interlinear glosses in parts (A) and (B).
Contents: (A) the pre-Gariopontean ensemble, minus Theod. Prisc.:
1r–8v, 25r–48v, 9r–24r Galen, *Ad Glauconem* 1–2
24rv, 49r–67v *Liber tertius*
67v–79v *Liber Aurelii*
80r–101v *Liber Esculapii*
101v–107v Alex. Trall., *De podagra*
107v–109r *Sapientia artis medicinae*
109r–110r Vindicianus, *Epistula ad Pentadium*
(B) 111r–143v collection of medical recipes
143v–148v alphabetically-ordered medical glossary
149r–149v verses on the *dies Aegyptiaci*; a short diagnostic text(?); an astrological (?) text
(C) 150r–171r *Dynamidia* 1–3
Alex. Trall.: *De podagra*: see Section 3.2.5 and Table 3.7 above; as in **vat2**, this section in **vat4** begins: 'Incipit liber Galieni de podagra'.

v1 Vendôme, Bibliothèque municipale 109 (autopsy April 1999) **Plate X**
(Beccaria, *Codici*, 185–8; *Cat. gén. Dép.* III, 425f.; Glaze, '*Passionarius*'; Rose, *Theod. Prisc.*, xiii, xvii, xxiv, 256; Sigerist, 'Vendôme', 68ff. (including facsimiles of ff. 59v and 61v); Wickersheimer, *Manuscrits*, 175–81)
Eleventh century, formerly at the Abbaye de la Sainte-Trinité de Vendôme (f. 1r). Parchment, ff. 144, 306×216mm; written in neat and clear minuscule in 2 columns (250×175mm) of 37 lines. Has suffered damage in places from fire and water.

A noteworthy feature is that, f. 61rb being inexplicably blank, f. 61v (=1.114; Greek II, 83–85) shows an interlinear text running through both columns, which 'must have been copied from another, much better MS ... a good example of an early mediaeval text emendation'.[130] I have collated a few of the complete copies with the two versions of **v1** at this point and established that the interlinear text, much superior indeed (as Sigerist thought) to the original, 2-column version, is from a manuscript very similar to, if not identical with, **A** (above), the only difference worth reporting in a passage of some 400 words being one instance of *et* **v1**: *enim* **A** and one of *aliud* **v1**: *alia* **A**. More puzzling is the relation of the 2-column version to the mainstream tradition. In 2.36 and 2.235–6, **v1** frequently agrees in error with **M** and **P1**, and was probably using a descendant of γ?(see 4.2 below). Here (1.114), however, **v1** shows no significant

[130] Sigerist, 'Vendôme', 76; Sigerist reproduces both versions side by side: 'Vendôme', 76–8.

agreements in error with **M** or **P1** or **P3** (which knew a descendant of γ, γ': see 4.7.2 below) or **P2**. My impression (from **M**, **P1**, and **P3**) is that the text deriving from γ is pretty chaotic at this point, and it may be that the maker of **v1** for this reason sought another first model, the congeners of which may be revealed by further collation or may belong to another branch of the tradition.

Contents: **1r Alex. Trall., *De mulsa***
1v–58r four books of the pre-Gariopontean ensemble:[131]
Galen, *De medendi methodo ad Glauconem* 1–2
Liber tertius
extracts from Theod. Prisc. 2
58r–59r a short extract *De sincope*[132]
59r–66r Alex. Trall., extracts
66–86 Esculapius and Alex. Trall., extracts, including *De podagra*
87 Ps. Galen, *De dynamidiis*
87–88 Caelius Aurelianus, *De salutaribus praeceptis* (a short fragment)
88 a glossary, only partly medical
88v–91v Theod. Prisc. 3.1–8 and part of 3.9
92r–97v three series of medical recipes (mainly antidotes against poisons; purgatives; simples) and a short text on blood-letting
98–134v *Liber dynamidii*, altogether more than 380 recipes
134v–137v and 140r–142v *Liber diaetarum* (interrupted by a short series of medical recipes and two short texts of medical wisdom)

Alex. Trall.: 1r (1.103) *Mulsa Alexandri*
59r (2.36) 'De cardiaca passione. De secundo libro Alexandri ubi de stomacho locutus est'
59v–63r (1.108–23) 'De auribus uitia Alexander': it is noteworthy that 1.112–14 on f. 60v bear the same numeration as in **M** and **P1** (CVIIII, CX, CXI)!
63v–65r (1.131–3) 'De narium passiones'
65r–66r (1.134–5) 'De dentium causationes Galienus', and 'Ad dentium dolores'
68v–70v (2.79) 'Incipit de reuma uentris de libro Alexandri sicut ibidem testabatur ut de libro Philonium subtraxisset'
71r–73r (2.180–4) 'Incipit de secundo libro Alexandri de cura nefreticorum'
75v–86v (2.235–70) *De podagra* (with chapters in the order of the mainstream tradition): see Section 3.2.5 and Table 3.7 above
134v–137v and 140r–142v *Liber diaetarum*: see Section 3.2.4 and Table 3.5 above (the contents are summarized also by Sigerist, 'Vendôme', 84–6).

v2 Vendôme, Bibliothèque municipale 172 (autopsy April 1999)
(Beccaria, *Codici*, 188f.; Beccaria, 'Sulle tracce', II, 28; *Cat. gén. Dép.*, III, 450; Sigerist, 'Vendôme', 89–91 (including illustration of f. 3r=fig. 3); Wickersheimer, *Manuscrits*, 182–4)

[131] Rose's reference to this manuscript as 'Gar(iopontus)' is to be corrected; cf. Glaze, '*Passionarius*'.

[132] The Incipit at this point ascribes the following work to 'Alexander amicus ueritatis', and clearly links this extract with those at 59r ff., which are from Alex. Trall. Sigerist, 'Vendôme', 74–5, took this extract *De sincope* to be from a Latin version of Alexander Philalethes, head of the Herophilean school near Laodicea at the end of the first century B.C. Von Staden, *Herophilus*, 533–9, is more doubtful.

Eleventh century (Beccaria, Wickersheimer, Sigerist), from the Abbaye de la Sainte-Trinité de Vendôme. Parchment, ff. 72, 240×180mm, written in single columns (185×120mm) of 35 lines. In ff. 31 and 40ff. the ms. is badly damaged.

Contents: **1r Alex. Trall., *De mulsa***
1v–11r Hippocrates, *Aphorismi*
11r–72r Hippocrates, *Aphorismi*, with Latin commentary (Lat. A)

Alex. Trall.: 1r (1.103) *Mulsa Alexandri.*

v3 Vendôme, Bibliothèque municipale 175 (autopsy April 1999)
(Beccaria, *Codici*, 189–92; *Cat. gén. Dép.*, III, 451–2; Rose, *Theod. Prisc.*, XVIII, XXI, 257; Sigerist, 'Vendôme', 97–113 (including illustrations of f. 45=fig. 5); Wickersheimer, *Manuscrits*, 184–90)

Eleventh century (Sigerist, Wickersheimer), end eleventh century (Beccaria), from the Abbaye de la Sainte-Trinité de Vendôme. Parchment, two manuscripts bound together: (A) ff. 45 (1–45), 195×120mm, written in 2 columns of 39 lines, with titles, numbers, and initials in red; (B) ff. 105 (47–151), 180×115mm, written in single columns of 33 lines.

Contents: (A) 1r miscellaneous recipes
2rv Alex. Trall., *Mulsa*
3ra–41ra Esculapius, *De morbis*, ending with *De podagra*. LIIII
41ra–42r Cassius Felix, excerpts (11 chapters)
42r–45rb miscellaneous recipes and excerpts on the womb and menstruation

(B) 47r–93r Esculapius, *De morbis* (including, 49r, reminiscences of Alex. Trall.)
93r–94r miscellaneous recipes (incl. some from Alex. Trall.)
94r–97r Theodorus, *Diaeta*
97v–99v Theodorus Priscianus, *Gynaecia*, and (99–108) other gynaecological works
108v–133v collection of medical recipes
134r–150v *Liber ad Glauconem secundum Aurelianum de positione membrorum omnium interaneorum*, incomplete
151v miscellaneous recipes (fourteenth century)

Alex. Trall.: 2rv (1.103) *Mulsa Alexandri*

49r *Sinancis passio* bears an unmistakeable resemblance to Alex. Trall. 1.136 *De squinance uel sinance*, but is very different, and contains eight lines more on the differential diagnosis of the four types; likewise (49r) *Cura sinancis* resembles Alex. Trall. 1.140 *De flobothomia et catartico ac uentosis sinancis*: the first sentence is almost identical, but the **v3** version is then very much more compressed.

93rv two recipes from Alex. Trall. 2.238 'De libro Alexandri catartico dia[d]rodon ...' and 'Item alio dia cidonion melon.'

93v three recipes from Alex. Trall. 2.267 (vv. 21–29 *ed.*) 'Catartico de campassionem ...' and 'Item alia potio satis bona et a nobis experimentata ...', followed by some *Emplastra* which I have not been able to identify.

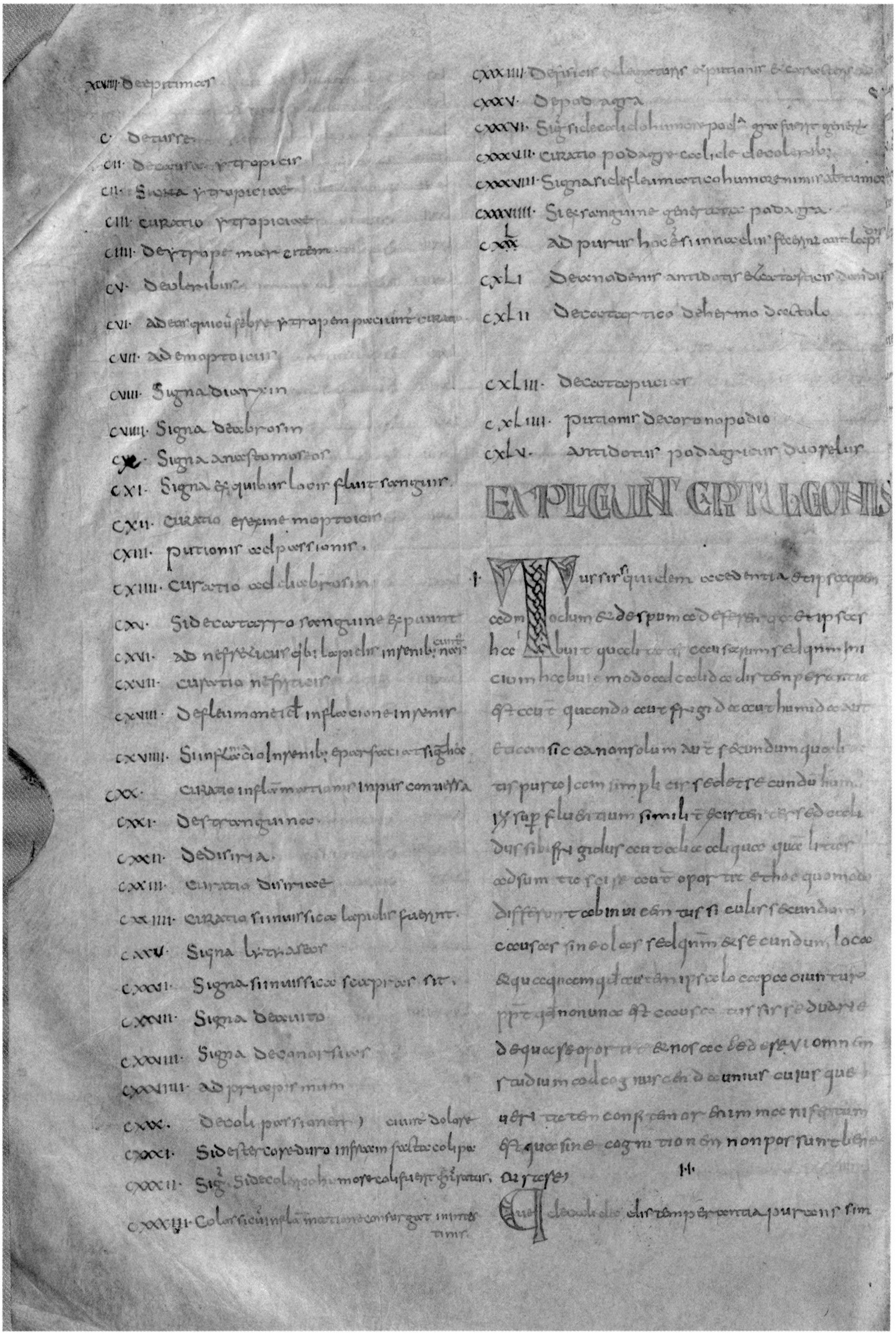

Plate I: Paris, BN, lat. 9332 (early 9th century), f. 180v

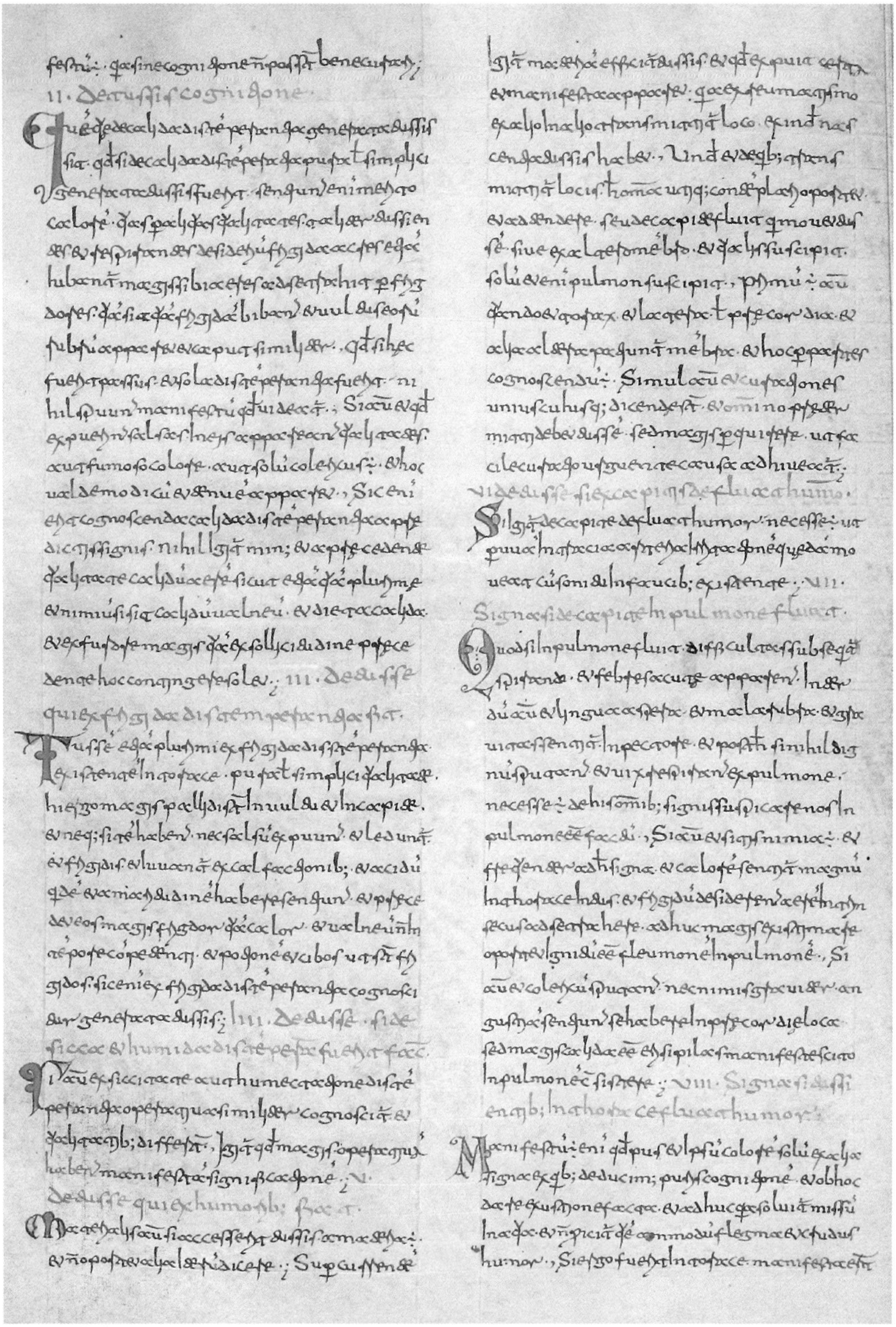

Plate II: Montecassino, Archivio della Badia 97 (early 10th century), p. 350

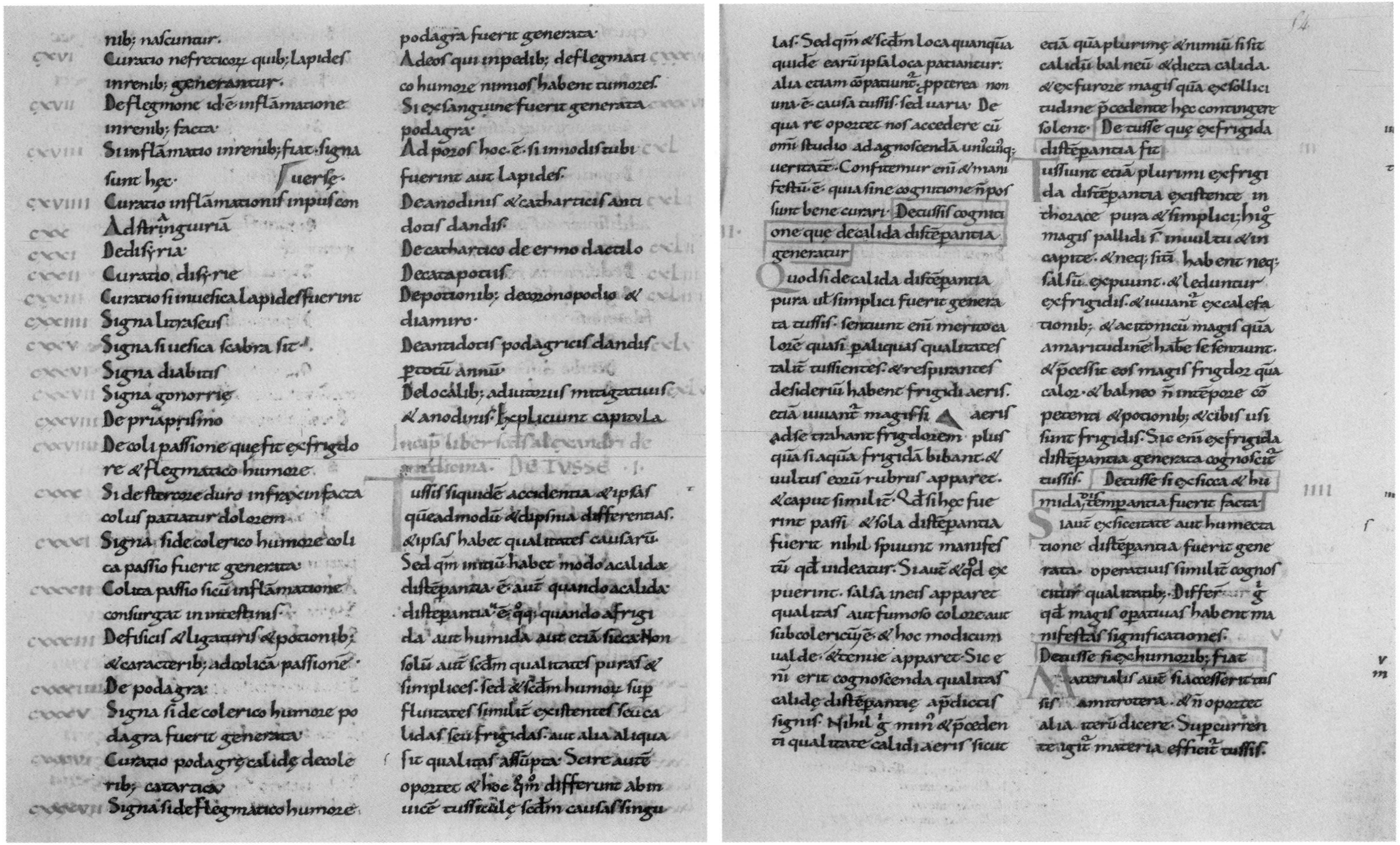

Plate III: Angers, Bibl. mun. 457 (11th century), ff. 53v–54r

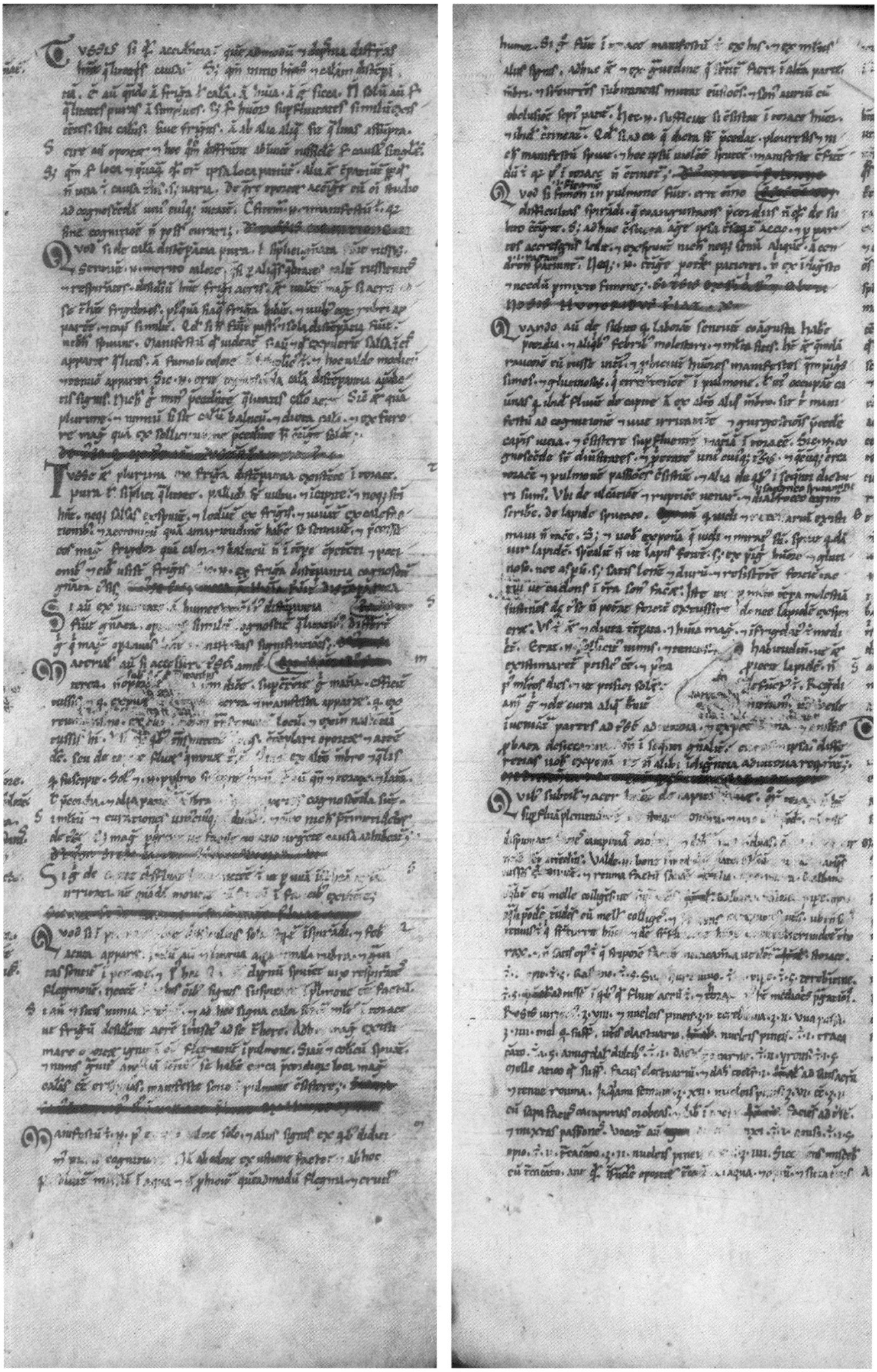

Plate IV: Orléans, Bibl. mun. 283 (end 11th century), pp. 34b–35a

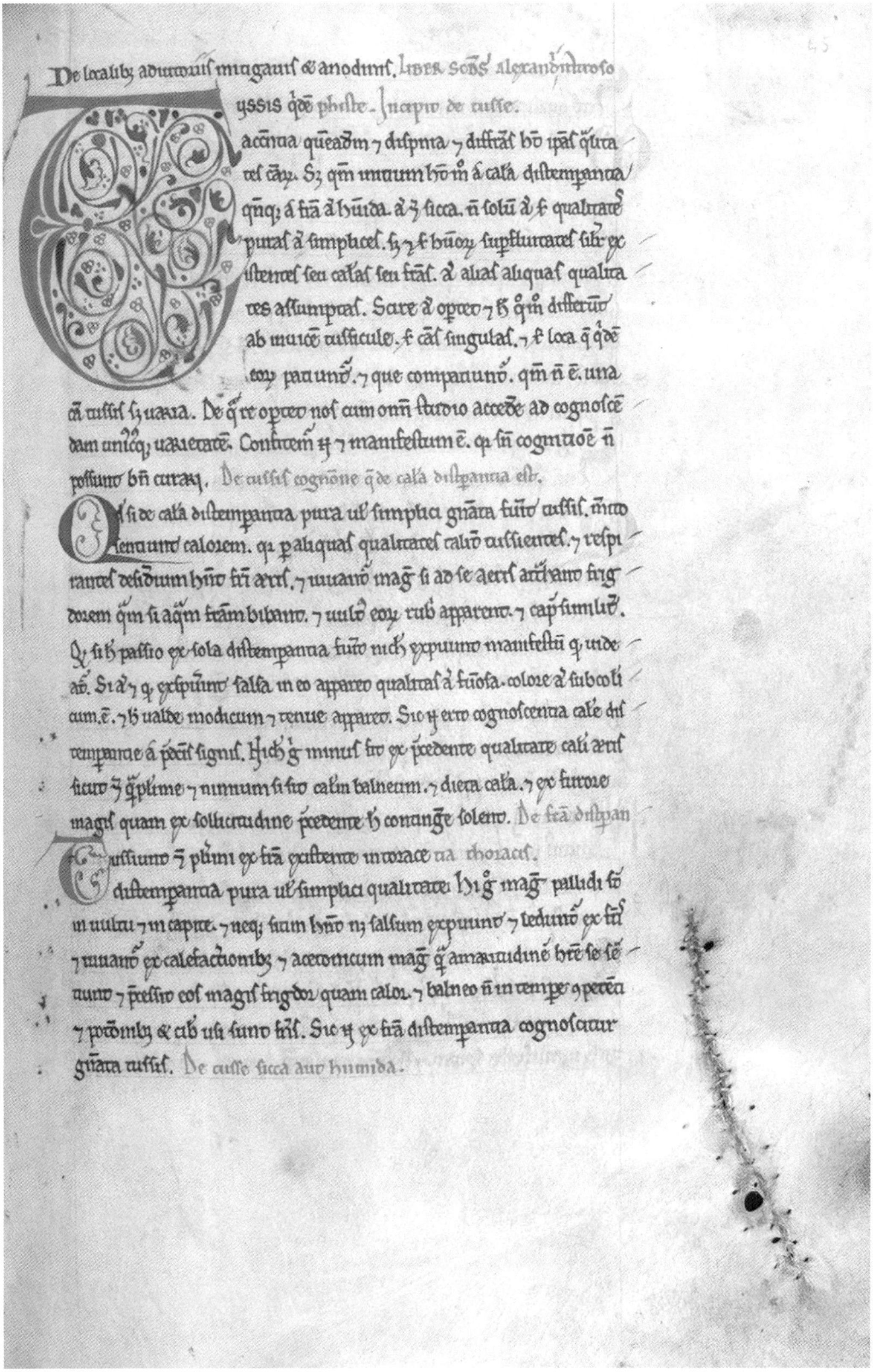

Plate V: Glasgow, University Library, Hunter 435 (12th/13th century), f. 45r

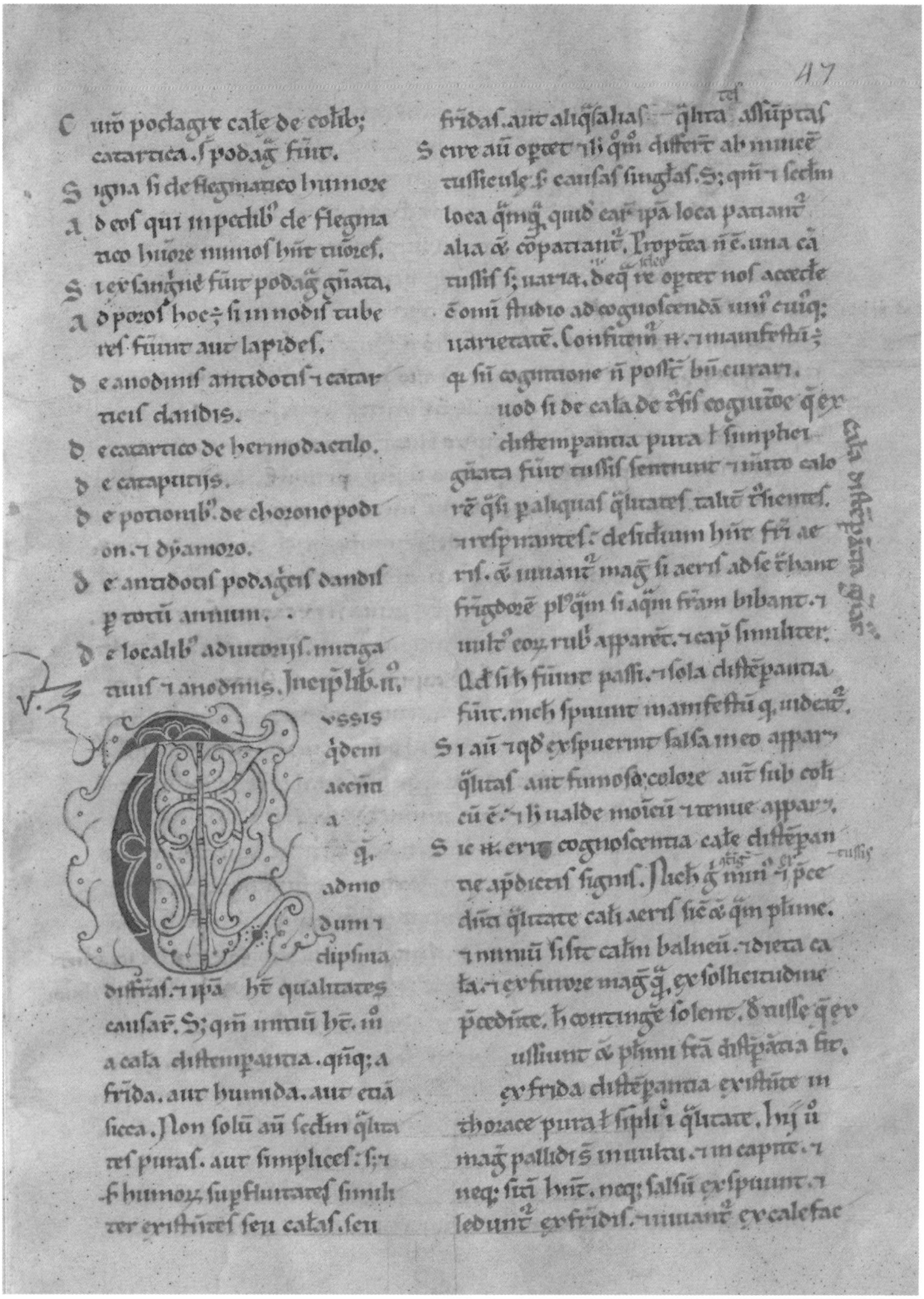

Plate VI: Paris, BN, lat. 6881 (13th century), f. 47r

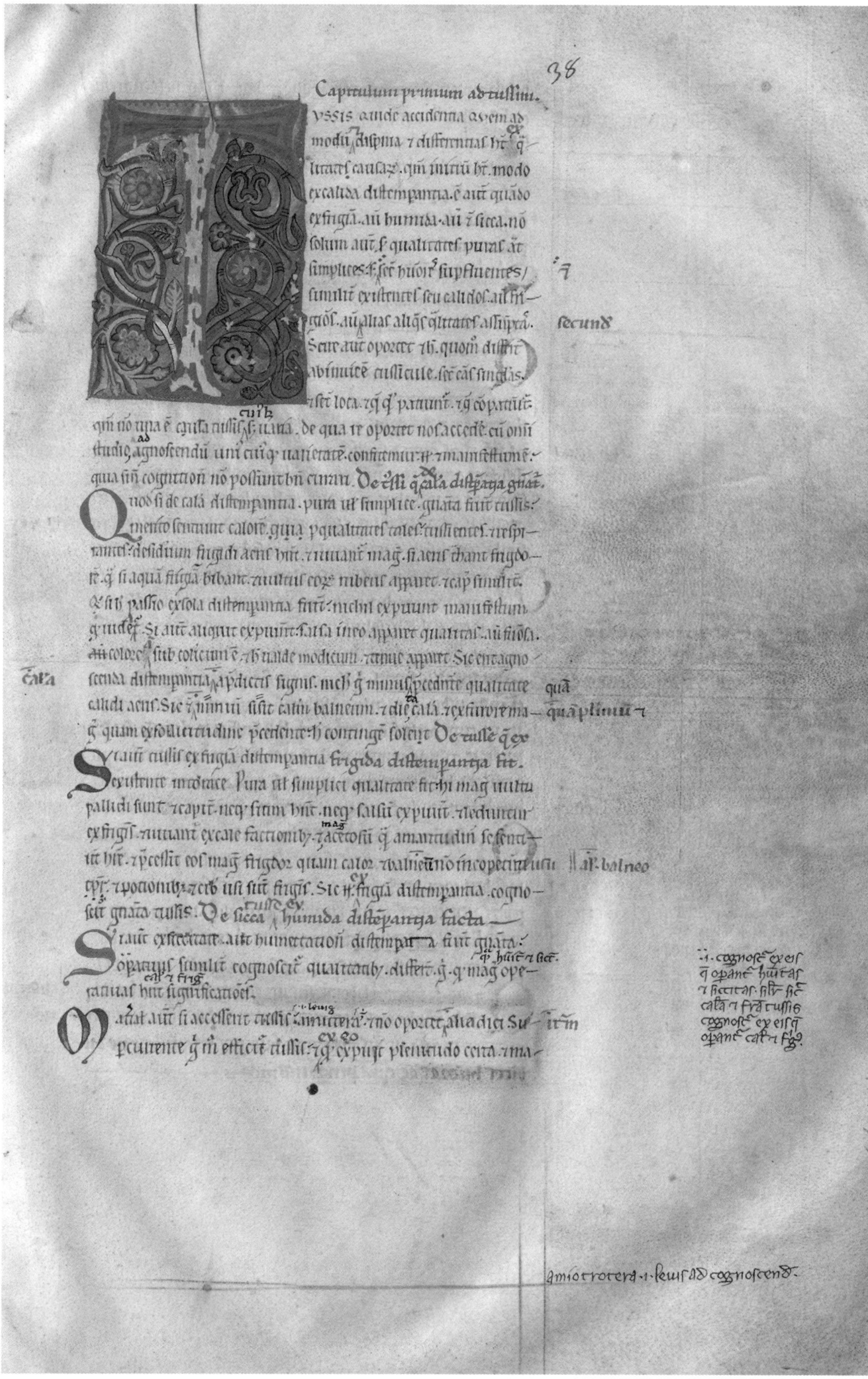

Plate VII: Paris, BN, lat. 6882 (13th century), f. 38r

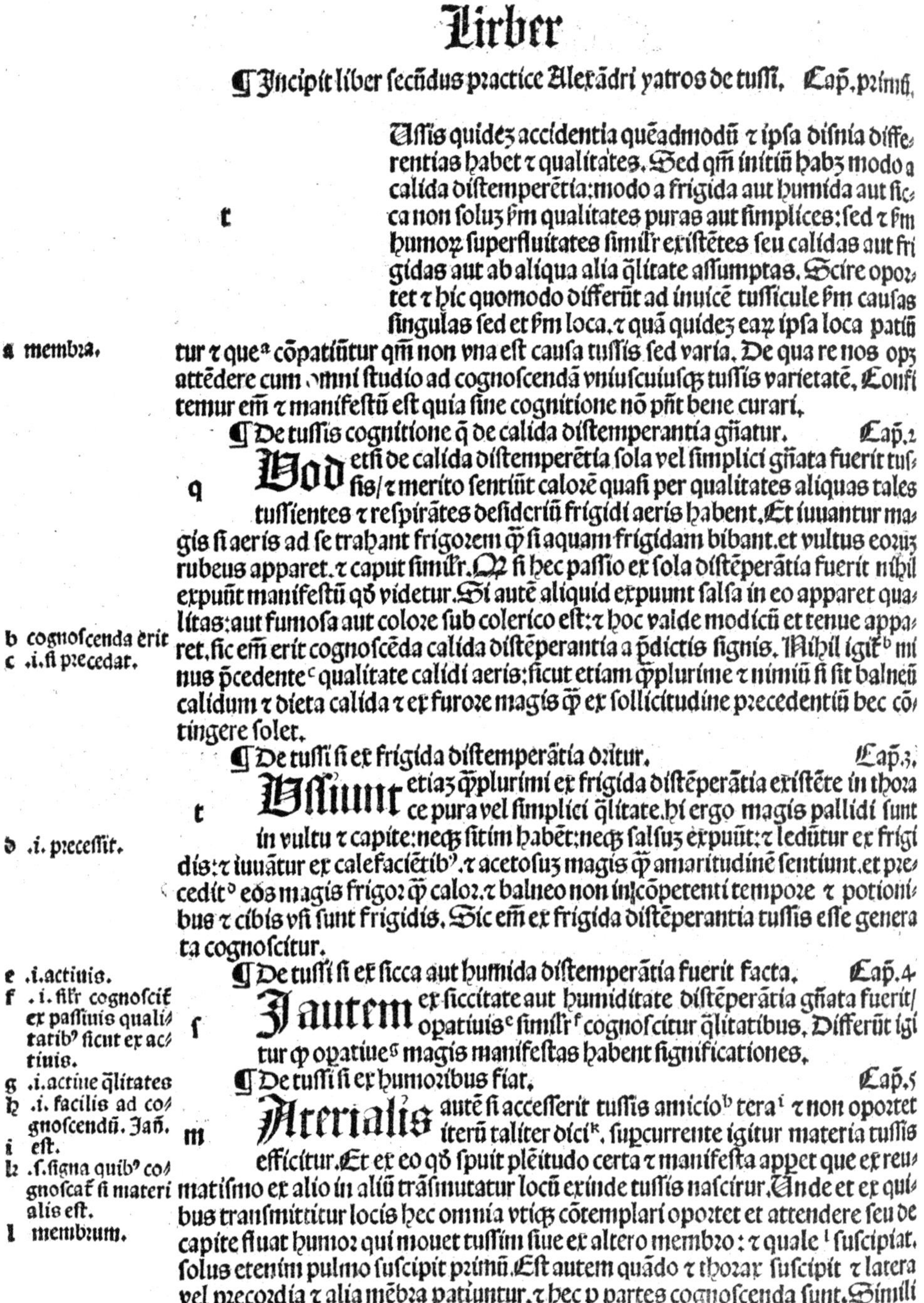

Liber

¶ Incipit liber secũdus practice Alexãdri yatros de tussi. Cap. primũ.

Tussis quidez accidentia queadmodũ z ipsa disnia differentias habet z qualitates. Sed qm̃ initiũ habz modo a calida distemperẽtia: modo a frigida aut humida aut sicca non soluz fm qualitates puras aut simplices: sed z fm humoꝝ superfluitates simil'r existẽtes seu calidas aut frigidas aut ab aliqua alia q̃litate assumptas. Scire oportet z hic quomodo differũt ad inuicẽ tussicule fm causas singulas sed et fm loca. z quã quidez eaꝝ ipsa loca patiũtur z que[a] cõpatiũtur qm̃ non vna est causa tussis sed varia. De qua re nos opz attẽdere cum omni studio ad cognoscendã vniuscuiusqꝫ tussis varietatẽ. Confitemur em̃ z manifestũ est quia sine cognitione nõ pñt bene curari.

t

a membra.

¶ De tussis cognitione q̃ de calida distemperantia gñatur. Cap. 2

Quod etsi de calida distemperẽtia sola vel simplici gñata fuerit tussis/ z merito sentiũt calorẽ quasi per qualitates aliquas tales tussientes z respirãtes desideriũ frigidi aeris habent. Et iuuantur magis si aeris ad se trahant frigorem q̃ si aquam frigidam bibant. et vultus eorũz rubeus apparet. z caput simil'r. Qꝫ si hec passio ex sola distẽperãtia fuerit nihil expuũt manifestũ qd videtur. Si autẽ aliquid expuunt salsa in eo apparet qualitas: aut fumosa aut colore sub colerico est: z hoc valde modicũ et tenue apparet. sic em̃ erit cognoscẽda calida distẽperantia a p̃dictis signis. Nihil igit[b] minus p̃cedente[c] qualitate calidi aeris: sicut etiam q̃plurime z nimiũ si sit balneũ calidum z dieta calida z ex furore magis q̃ ex sollicitudine precedentiũ hec cõtingere solet.

q

b cognoscenda erit
c .i. si precedat.

¶ De tussi si ex frigida distemperãtia oritur. Cap. 3.

Tussiunt etiaz q̃plurimi ex frigida distẽperãtia existẽte in thorace pura vel simplici q̃litate. hi ergo magis pallidi sunt in vultu z capite: neqꝫ sitim habẽt: neqꝫ salsuz expuũt: z ledũtur ex frigidis: z iuuãtur ex calefaciẽtib᷒. z acetosuz magis q̃ amaritudinẽ sentiunt. et precedit[d] eos magis frigor q̃ calor. z balneo non inꝯcõpetenti tempore z potionibus z cibis vsi sunt frigidis. Sic em̃ ex frigida distẽperantia tussis esse generata cognoscitur.

t

d .i. precessit.

¶ De tussi si ex sicca aut humida distemperãtia fuerit facta. Cap. 4

Si autem ex siccitate aut humiditate distẽperãtia gñata fuerit/ opatiuis[e] simil'r[f] cognoscitur q̃litatibus. Differũt igitur q̃ opatiue[g] magis manifestas habent significationes.

s

e .i. actiuis.
f .i. simil'r cognoscit ex passiuis qualitatib᷒ sicut ex actiuis.
g .i. actiue q̃litates

¶ De tussi si ex humoribus fiat. Cap. 5

Materialis autẽ si accesserit tussis amicio[h] tera[i] z non oportet iterũ taliter dici[k]. supcurrente igitur materia tussis efficitur. Et ex eo qd spuit plẽitudo certa z manifesta appet que ex reumatismo ex alio in aliũ trãsmutatur locũ exinde tussis nascitur. Unde et ex quibus transmittitur locis hec omnia vtiqꝫ cõtemplari oportet et attendere seu de capite fluat humor qui mouet tussim siue ex altero membro: z quale[l] suscipiat. solus etenim pulmo suscipit primũ. Est autem quãdo z thorax suscipit z latera vel precordia z alia mẽbra patiuntur. z hec p partes cognoscenda sunt. Similiter autem z curationes vniuscuiusqꝫ dicende sunt. Et omino nihil pretermittẽdum de tusse: sed magis ꝑquirere vt facilis curatio vrgente causa adhibeatur.

m

h .i. facilis ad cognoscendũ. Jañ.
i est.
k .s. signa quib᷒ cognoscat si materialis est.
l membrum.

¶ De tussi si ex capite fluat humor. Cap. 6

Plate VIII: *Practica Alexandri yatros greci cum expositione glose interlinearis Jacobi de partibus et Januensis in margine posite* (Lyons, 16 April 1504), f. 32v

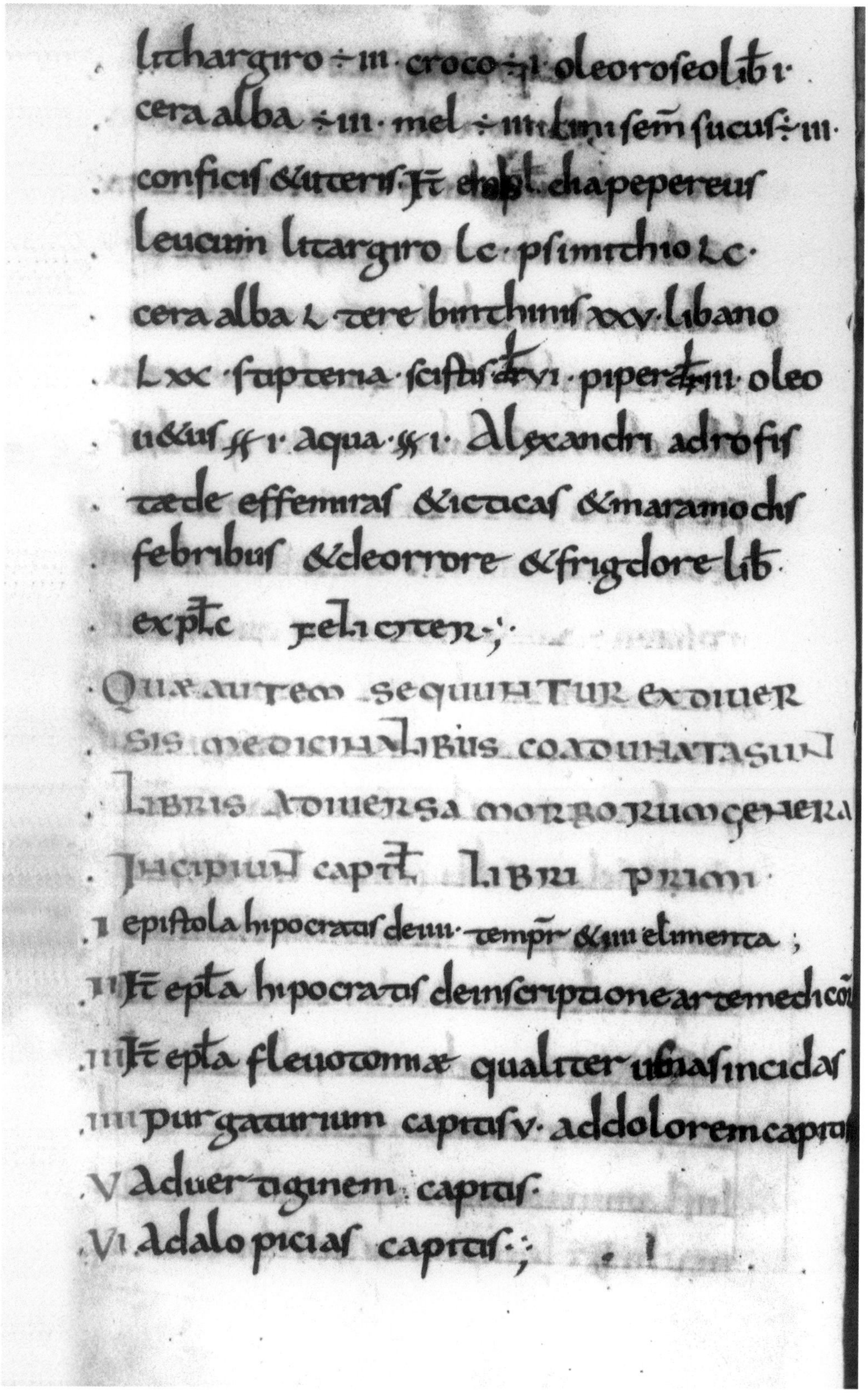
lithargiro ÷ III· croco ÷ I· oleo roseo lib I·
cera alba ÷ III· mel ÷ III· ... semen sucus ÷ III·
conficis & uteris. Item ... chapepereus
leucum litargiro L c· psimithio L c·
cera alba L tere birthinis xxv· libano
L xx· ... piper ... III· oleo
u&us ... I· aqua ... I· Alexandri adrofis
taede effemiras & ictiacas & maramochis
febribus & de orrore & frigdore lib·
explicit feliciter.
Quae autem sequuntur ex diuer
sis medicinalibus coadunata sunt
libris aduersa morborum genera
Incipiunt capitula libri primi·
I epistola hipocratis de IIII tempora & IIII elimenta ;
II Item epistula hipocratis de inscriptione artem medicina
III Item epistula fleuotomiae qualiter uenas incidas
IIII purgatorium capitis V· ad dolorem capitis
V Ad uertiginem capitis·
VI Ad alopicias capitis ;

Plate IX: Città del Vaticano, Bibl. apostolica vaticana, regin. lat. 1143 (9th century, 1st half), f. 88v

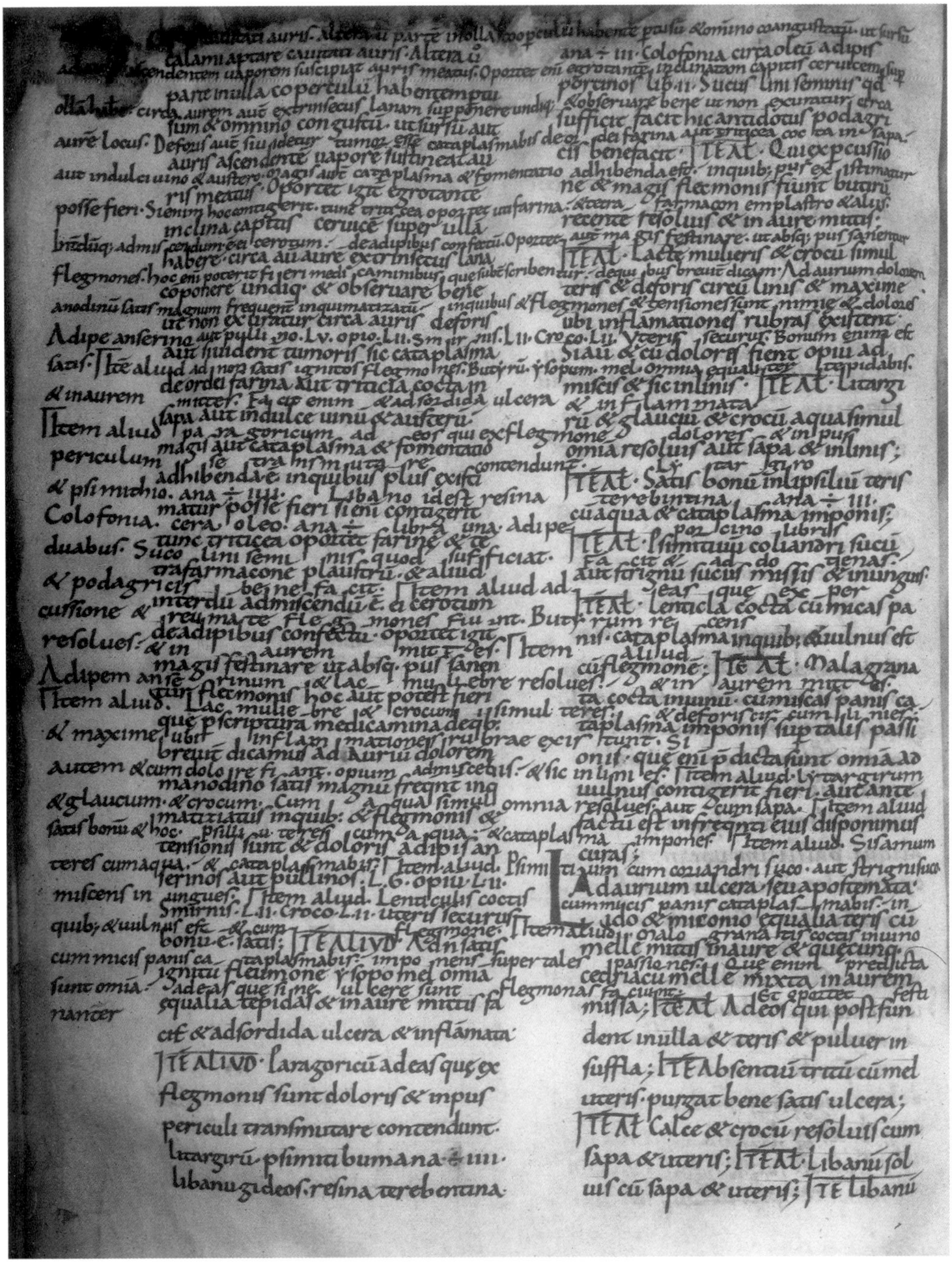

Plate X: Vendôme, Bibl. mun. 109 (11th century), f. 61v

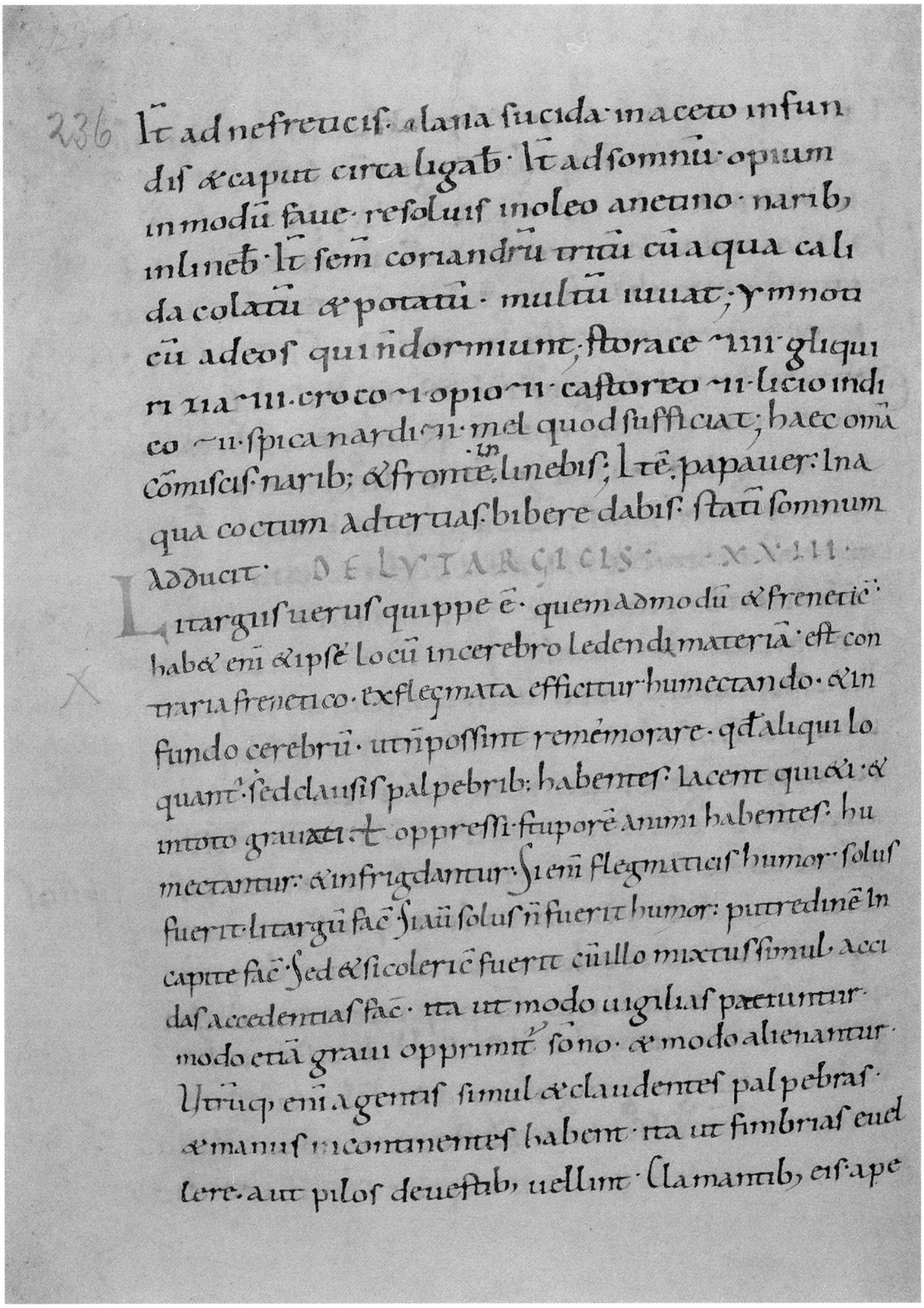
236 Itē ad nefreticis. alana sucida in aceto infun
dis & caput circa ligab. Itē ad somnū. opium
in modū faue. resoluis in oleo anetino. narib;
inlineb. Itē sem coriandrū tritū cū aqua cali
da colatū & potatū. multū iuuat; ymnon
cū ad eos qui ñ dormiunt; storace .iiii. gliqui
ri tia .iii. croco .i. opio .ii. castoreo .ii. licio indi
co .ii. spica nardi .ii. mel quod sufficiat; haec omā
comiscis narib; & fronte in linebis; Itē papauer in a
qua coctum ad tertias bibere dabis statī somnum
adducit. DE LYTARGICIS. XXIII.
Litargus uerus quippe ē. quemadmodū & frenetic.
habet enī & ipse locū in cerebro ledendi materiā est con
traria frenetico. Ex flegmata efficitur humectando. & in
fundo cerebri. ut ñ possint rememorare. qđ aliqui lo
quant. sed clausis palpebrib; habentes. Iacent quieti. &
in toto grauati. t oppressi stuporē animi habentes. hu
mectantur. & infrigdantur. Si enī flegmaticis humor solus
fuerit litargū fac. Si autē solus ñ fuerit humor. putredinē in
capite fac. Sed & si colerici fuerit cū illo mixtus simul. acci
das accedentias fac. ita ut modo uigilias patiuntur.
modo etiā graui opprimit sono. & modo alienantur.
Utrūq; enī agentas simul & claudentes palpebras.
& manus incontinentes habent. ita ut fimbrias euel
lere. aut pilos de uestib; uellint. Clamantib; eis ape

Plate XI: Sankt Gallen, Stiftsbibliothek 752 (10th century), p. 236

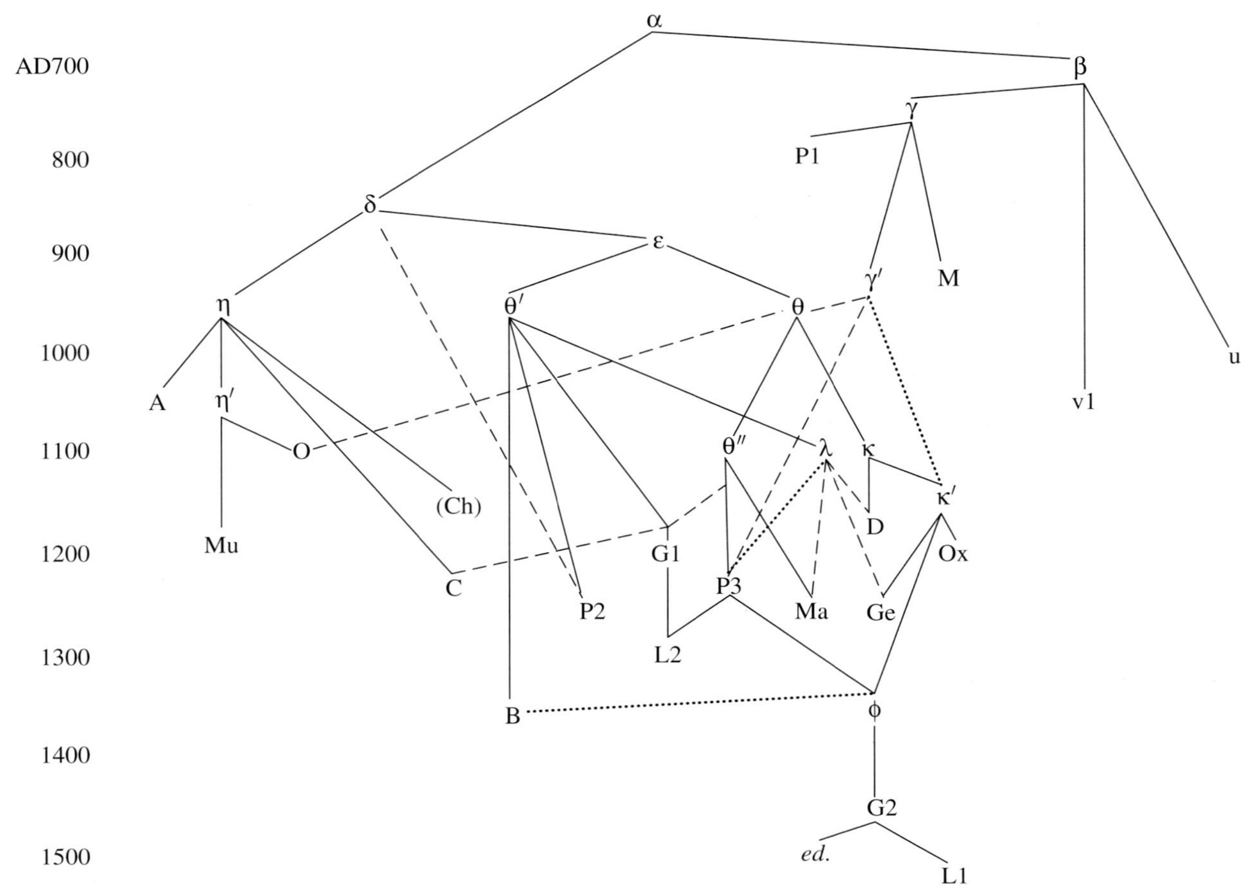

Plate XII: Stemma showing the relations between the mainstream manuscripts of the Latin Alexander (and v1 and u of the secondary tradition).
(Probable or certain use of an accessory model is indicated in dashes, possible but uncertain use in dots. The dating of lost copies is approximate only.)

CHAPTER 4. RELATING THE MANUSCRIPTS: A JUSTIFICATION OF AND COMMENTARY ON THE STEMMA

This chapter summarizes my findings and hypotheses to date regarding the genetic relations existing within the 'mainstream' tradition (i.e. between those manuscripts which contain complete copies of the text), and between the latter and the most important of the 'excerpting' manuscripts, namely Vendôme 109 (v1) (the Uppsala (u) and Poitiers (po) excerpts are also assessed in some degree). At the end of the chapter is a provisional Latin text (together with the Greek original) of those chapters collated and referred to in 4.1–4.9, apart from Book 2, chs 1–11, which are set out more fully, by way of a sample of the intended edition, in Chapter 5.

My attempts first to produce and then to explain and justify the stemma printed as **Plate XII** have yielded a long and complex chapter. The first five sections (4.1–4.5) set out what I hope are fairly clear errors characterizing lost copies of the text, moving down the tree, as it were, from the archetype, α (4.1), to the latest recension, that of ϕ, the more-or-less immediate source of the text used in the early printing of 1504, *ed.* (4.5). The next three sections (4.6–4.8) are much more tentative, dealing with questions that I do not pretend to have answered conclusively, but which are too important not to raise, namely the sources of ϕ (4.6), the principal cases of apparent contamination (4.7), and at least eight further remaining problems concerning the relations between the manuscripts (4.8). The chapter ends with impressionistic notes on the form of the text in each manuscript and brief illustration of individual secondary readings (4.9), and finally the provisional text, referred to above, of those chapters constantly referred to in Chapter 4 on the collation of which the reconstruction of the stemma is based (4.10).

4.1. α: The Question of a Single, Reconstructable Archetype

There is no reason to doubt that all the Latin manuscripts currently known derive ultimately from a single Latin translation of the Greek text. The further postulation, however, that they derive from a single archetype is made harder by the fact that supposed 'errors' common to all the Latin manuscripts may in principle originate not in unconjecturable errors in an early lost manuscript-copy, but in errors in the original translation itself (these in turn reflecting either corruption in the translator's Greek manuscript, or the translator's incompetence, or both). Thus, at e.g. 1.87.2 (see below) the translator's Greek model may have omitted (by a *saut du même au même*) the words μὲν τοῖς ἀδήκτοις καὶ πραϋτάτοις ἔξωθεν, and at 2.236.5 the negative οὐ. Again, at 2.11.3 it is arguable that the translator thought he was writing good sense and translating the Greek in front of him; in this instance, this is made less likely by his frequent and correct translation of Greek ἀπαλλαγῆναι (with *liberare*, *sanare*, *releuare*, etc.), but it is always open to the sceptic to point out that the wording of the translator's Greek manuscript may have made the crucial difference. The same applies to additions to the Greek text, such as the lines from Theodorus Priscianus at the very start of 1.1: unless we have evidence of a version without the addition — and in this case, the Theodorean material is there in the secondary tradition (the *Liber passionalis* and the *Tereoperica*,

3.2.2 and 3.2.3 above) — we have no grounds for claiming that its incorporation was not part of the original creation of the Latin Alexander.

The collation of only a small part of the Latin text has not yielded sufficient 'errors' common to all the Latin manuscripts to justify the confident postulation of a single archetype. However, that some of these shared errors are more easily explicable in terms of corruption within a Latin than a Greek tradition justifies, I hope, the reference that I make in the stemma and this chapter to an archetype (α) distinct from the original translation. In one chapter in particular (2.241), collation of the secondary tradition has revealed a small handful of errors common to all the mainstream manuscripts but avoided by the excerpting manuscripts. This is the most important example so far uncovered, offering a clear characterization of α, and nicely illustrating the importance of secondary traditions in the reconstruction of the history of texts. Collation of further parts of the text will no doubt reveal more shared errors, the quality and quantity of which will strengthen or weaken the postulation of α. For now, I list those so far discovered, separating those involving simply omission of Greek material from those requiring the assumption of more complex corruption.

4.1.1. Omissions Common to all the Latin Manuscripts

1.87.2 The obviously accidental omission of (a translation of) the words underlined in the following passage from the Greek text, II, 7, 2–4 καὶ βοηθήμασι χρῶ, ἔνδοθεν μὲν τοῖς ἀδήκτοις καὶ πραϋτάτοις ἔξωθεν δὲ τοῖς συμπέττειν δυναμένοις τὰς φλεγμονάς.[1]

2.236.5 The omission of the negative before *mediocris commotio* for Gk II, 503, 1 οὐ μετρίους ἐργάζεται τοὺς παροξυσμούς: see 4.10.6 below and note ad loc.

4.1.2. Other Forms of Apparent Corruption Common to all the Latin Manuscripts

2.4.2 The addition of *si accesserit tussis* in an effort to make sense of a Latin text rendered unintelligible by the transposition of the section-heading 2.5.t. *De tusse si ex humoribus fiat* (itself not in the Greek text either).

2.5.2 The substitution of *solus* (*solum* M) for *locus* in *qualis suscipit locus* (Gk II, 149, 19 ποῖα <μᾶλλον δέχεται μόρια M>: see 5.4 below and note ad loc.

2.11.3 The nonsensical *extussire* in *non poterat fortiter extussire* (*om.* G1 L2 Ge′) for Gk II, 153, 23–4 οὐκ ἠδυνήθη τοῦ βήσσειν ἰσχυρῶς ἀπαλλαγῆναι: see 5.4 below and note ad loc.

2.241.4 Pisces uero aspratiles, et maxime eos qui duras habent carnes et nihil in se habent pingue: albas v1 *Pod.* | pingue α *Pod.* (vat2 vat3 vat4) *Pass.* pinguedinis (-em v1) v1 *Pod.* (po l2) (Gk II, 509, 18–19 Καὶ τῶν ἰχθύων τοὺς πετραίους μάλιστα καὶ τῶν ἄλλων, οἷς ἡ οὐσία λευκὴ καὶ ψαφαρὰ κατὰ φύσιν καὶ οὐδὲν ἔχουσα πιμελῶδες)

[1] Nearly all the Latin manuscripts also ignore ἔξωθεν δέ, having just *intrinsecus qui digerere possint flegmones*; three, however, have 'inside or outside' (*intrinsecus uel extrinsecus* G1 Ma *interius uel exterius* Ge); and one, P3, has *extrinsecus* alone.

This passage came to light during my cursory study of the secondary tradition. It is important here because it shows all of the mainstream manuscripts erring together in comparison not only with the Greek text, but also with v1 and with the consensus of the manuscripts of the *De podagra* (3.2.5 above), a well-attested branch of the excerpting tradition. Whatever the truth behind the second case of variation here (*pingue* ~ *pinguedinis*: I incline to prefer the latter),[2] *albas* in v1 and the *De podagra* must be right (Greek λευκή) and *duras* in the mainstream tradition wrong (and *duras* is surely not for the second Greek adjective ψαφαρός 'friable' either). All of the surviving mainstream manuscripts (α) err where at least two lost mainstream manuscripts (the sources of v1 and the *De podagra*, respectively[3]) preserved a correct reading. (For further hints in the secondary tradition of a lost copy higher than α in the stemma, see 4.8.1 below)

Whatever the status of α, the surviving Latin manuscripts reflect two hyparchetypes, β and δ in the stemma. β is represented directly by only two complete copies, P1 and M, but additionally by the most extensive surviving set of excerpts of the Latin Alexander, that contained in v1 (and by a small excerpt in u). However, β is also represented indirectly in the other 'half' of the tradition, in that accessory use of a copy deriving from β (γ′ in the stemma) is certainly reflected in all the copies deriving from θ (especially P3 and Ox and probably O as well, which seems to have used θ as an accessory model). In what follows, I deal first with the descendants of β and then with those of δ. I note instances of contamination as they arise, but postpone a more systematic discussion of contamination to the end of the chapter, before concluding with a list of outstanding problems (and illustration of innovations exclusive to single manuscripts).

4.2. β, γ and δ: Readings Setting P1 M (and u v1) Apart from the Rest

We are in the fortunate position of being able to collate P1, M, u, and v1 — all four for 2.36 *De cardiaca passione*, and P1, M, and v1 for 2.235–6, the first two chapters of the section on gout. Many of the readings unique to these four (or three) copies are either of uncertain value or probably preferable to the alternatives offered. Still, there are sufficient shared errors to establish their descent from a common hyparchetype, β.

The passages below illustrate, first, errors in β (or γ, in passages where we do not have u or v1), secondly errors in δ, and thirdly instances where β and δ diverge but it remains as yet uncertain which is in error.

4.2.1. β Errs

2.37.1 et propter sincopos patiuntur P1 u v1 (pro hoc M): propterea *cett.* (*om.* Ma P3)
(Gk II, 281, 6 καὶ διὰ τοῦτο συγκοπῆναι κινδυνεύουσιν)

Most probably, the original had *propterea* or *propter hoc* and P1, u, and v1 reflect an error in β (partly corrected in M?). δ then has either the correct reading or an improvement of *propter hoc*.[4] We cannot rule out the possibility that the original had

[2] This variation is curiously reminiscent of 2.3.1 *salsum* (*-as* O) *salsidinem* P1 (ἁλμυρόν).
[3] As the sample collations in Tables 3.7 and 3.8 show, v1 shares with α some errors avoided by *Pod.*
[4] In Book 1, A has 8x *propterea*, 3x *propter hoc*, and this proportion is maintained in Book 2.

adverbial *propter*, although this seems less likely in view of the reasonably elevated level of the translation at this point.[5]

2.235.1 ex multis et ex diuersarum causarum (causarum *om.* P1): diuersis causis Ox P3 φ po diuersis *cett.* (Gk II, 501, 8–9 ἐκ πολλῶν καὶ διαφόρων αἰτιῶν)

The mixture of ablative and genitive after *ex* in β is bewildering and hard to parallel.[6] Presumably, *causis* was in the original and lost in δ: Ox and P3 may have found it in θ (which took it from γ′) and made it available to φ.

2.236.3 ardorem simul et intensionem locis qui dolent infert et magnos dolores: inferit P1 v1 inferet M L2[7] (Gk II, 501, 22–3 καὶ τῷ φλέγειν ἅμα καὶ διατείνειν ἐπιφέρειν οἶδε μεγάλας ὀδύνας)

Here, β errs, as, although the structure of the Latin differs from that of the Greek, the *et* is required. Even if we reckon with an original version something like *ardore simul et intensione loci infert magnos dolores*,[8] β errs in the form of the main verb.

4.2.2. γ Errs

Other significant errors uniting M and P1 against the rest of the tradition, in passages for which u and v1 are not available, include the following:

1.85.2 ut legentes hunc librum non quaerant ex alio codice quae ad oculorum curationes sunt utilia: *om.* P1 M (Gk II, 3, 8–9 ὥστε τὸν ἐντυγχάνοντα τῷδε τῷ βιβλίῳ θεραπευτικῷ ὄντι(?) μὴ ζητεῖν ἐξ ἑτέρων ἀναλέγεσθαι περὶ(?) τῶν ἐν ὀφθαλμοῖς χρησίμων)

γ omits the words underlined.

2.7.2 flegmonem necesse est de his omnibus signis suspicari nos in pulmone esse factum: pleumone P1, pulmone M, flegmonem *cett. recte* (Gk II, 151, 5–6 φλεγμονὴν ἐξ ἀνάγκης ἐκ πάντων τούτων ὑποπτεύειν ἡμᾶς περὶ τὸν πνεύμονα γεγενῆσθαι προσήκει)

The original error here conceivably lies in γ using a phonetic spelling *fleumone(m)* for *flegmonem*,[9] *fleumone* being then corrected to a form of the word for 'lung', Greek in P1, Latin in M, in the latter perhaps in anticipation of the following *in pulmone*. Cf. 5.4 below and note ad loc.

2.7.3 si autem et . . . calor sentiatur multus in thorace, ita ut frigidum desiderent aerem: ita ut P3 m2 (*in marg. ad* et P3′) intus et M intus P1 id est ut AMu C G1 P2 L2 B ut O Ge φ et Ma P3′ D Ox (Gk II, 151, 8–9 εἰ δὲ καὶ . . . θέρμης αἴσθησις αὐτῷ γίνοιτο πολλὴ περὶ τὸν θώρακα, ὥστε ψυχρὸν ἐπιθυμεῖν ἀέρα ἀναπνεῖν)

M and P1 alone have *intus* for *ita ut*. It looks as if δ had *id est ut* (retained by η and θ′), and θ lost *id est*.

5 See Hofmann and Szantyr, 246 (including a reference to *pro quod=propterea quod* in Diosc. (Svennung, *Palladius*, 396f.) — cf. the reading of M here: does *pro hoc* recur in M? in other manuscripts?).

6 See Hofmann and Szantyr, 267 and, on the dubious instance at Scrib. Larg. 21, p. 22, 4–5, Langslow, *Medical Latin*, 52.

7 Given the numerous close links between G1 and L2, I would explain the *inferet* of L2 as reflecting *infer(unt) et*, the reading of G1 and B (presumably from θ′).

8 I owe this suggestion to Cloudy Fischer.

9 The cluster *gm* goes regularly to *um* in Late Latin (cf. e.g. *sagma* > *sauma* > French *somme* 'saddle').

2.9.2 Et spuunt nihil, neque soni aliquid aut ce*rcn*on patiuntur: sonum aliquem O Ma *fortasse recte*, sonum aliquid P1 sonum aliquod M aliquid P3′ (Gk II, 153, 2–4 καὶ οὔτε ἀναπτύουσιν οὐδὲν οὐδὲ ψόφον τινὰ οὐδὲ κέρχνον ὑπομένουσιν)

γ substitutes *sonum* for the probably original partitive genitive *soni*, which is preserved by δ. I presume that O and Ma 'correct' independently to *sonum aliquem* (though O might have found *sonum* in γ′: see 4.8.3 below).

4.2.3. δ Errs

1.19.2 Est autem quod defluit aut colericum aut flegmaticum interdum etiam et melancolicum: interdum etiam et γ C P3 φ aut δ (Gk I, 463, 4–5 ἔστι δὲ τὸ παραρρέον ὁτὲ μὲν χολῶδες ἢ φλεγματῶδες, ὁτὲ δὲ καὶ μελαγχολικόν)

δ substitutes a third *aut* for *interdum etiam et* (cf. ὁτὲ δὲ καὶ). Additional interest here lies in the distribution of the correct reading, in particular in the presence of C among the seven manuscripts which retain it. (On agreements of C with P3 and/or φ, see 4.7.5 below.)

1.87.1 magis capitalis incidenda est uena δ: incidenda est uena magis (magis *om.* M Ox P3′) capitalis γ Ox i. est m. c. u. D i. est m. u. c. P3 L2 m. i. est u. c. (capitis *ed.*) φ (Gk II, 5, 27 τέμνειν χρὴ τὴν φλέβα τὴν ὠμιαῖαν)

In view of the Greek, I here prefer the word-order of γ (and γ′, reflected in θ (D Ox P3 L2) and indirectly in φ). δ innovates by fronting *capitalis* in order to emphasize it, and Ma and Ge here follow θ′.

2.1.3 et quaequam (*quaedam*?) quidem earum ipsa loca patiuntur, alia etiam compatiuntur: quamquam A Mu C P2 L2 B (for further detail, see 5.4 and the app. crit. ad loc.) (Gk II, 147, 11–12 καὶ ὅτι αἱ μὲν αὐτῶν κατὰ πρωτοπάθειαν, αἱ δὲ κατὰ συμπάθειαν συνίστανται)

This is extremely messy (and there seems to be something missing in the Latin version), but η and θ′ appear to share the same erroneous deletion of *et* and the substitution of *quamquam* for *quaequam* (*quaedam*?) 'some of them'. This then would have already occurred in δ. The correct reading is preserved by γ, O and θ (O and θ presumably following γ′), although θ″, κ, κ′ and φ have each gone slightly their own way; see 5.4 below with app. crit. and note ad loc.

2.36.4–37.1 etiam lumbricorum signa sunt requirenda. +– –+ (37.1) Nam qui habent in stomacho mordicationem: Nam qui Ox u v1[10] in hanc qui P1 M hiis qui φ qui *cett.* (Gk II, 281, 3–5 καὶ τὰ τῶν ἑλμίνθων σημεῖα ζητεῖν· +–οὕτω γὰρ καὶ τὰ θηρία ταῦτα θανάτους αἰφνιδίους ἐργάζονται καὶ συγκοπὰς οὐδὲν ἧττον τῶν ὀλεθρίων χυμῶν.–+ (37.1) τοῖς οὖν ἔχουσι μοχθηροὺς καὶ δακνώδεις ἐν τῷ στόματι τῆς γαστρὸς χυμούς)

δ omits *Nam*. There is an obvious phonetic connection between *nam* and *in hanc*, the latter surely a corruption of the former in γ. *Nam* is quite appropriate here either as the first word of the lost sentence (for Greek γάρ, marked above) or as marking a move to a new subject (Greek τοῖς οὖν). Furthermore, the translator at this point begins every sentence with a particle. The presence of *Nam* in Ox may again reflect knowledge of γ′.[11]

[10] This is barely legible on the film of v1 but is confirmed by autopsy.

[11] *hiis* in φ is presumably an anticipation of 2.37.1 *eis*, unless it arose through a misreading of an abbreviation of *enim* as *h* (an idea I owe to Cloudy Fischer).

2.37.6 Nihil enim est aliud maius iuuamen P1 M P3 u v1: nullum *cett.* (Gk II, 281, 21–2 οὐδὲν γὰρ αὐτοῖς οὕτω συμβάλλεται)

It is probable that β (and hence γ′ reflected in P3?) preserves the original reading (cf. Greek οὐδὲν), δ showing a reinterpretation of *est* and presumably an attempt to improve the Latin.

2.37.10 malaxat et confortat P1 M P3′ u v1: malaxat autem et confortat *cett.* (Gk II, 283, 1 μαλάττει καὶ τονοῖ)

δ adds *autem*. β (including γ′, whence P3′) preserves the absence of particle in the Greek.

2.37.11 hoc enim medicamen ad haec optimum est: enim *om.* β P3′ (Gk II, 283, 1 τοῦτο τὸ βοήθημα κάλλιστόν ἐστιν)

δ adds *enim*. β (including γ′, whence P3′) preserves the absence of particle in the Greek.

2.37.14 quae proueniunt in stomacho simptomata P1 M u v1 (also G1 Ma P3′): quae proueniunt in stomacho cum simptomate *cett.* (Gk II, 283, 7–8 τῶν συμβαινόντων ἐν τῷ στόματι τῆς γαστρὸς συμπτωμάτων)

δ errs (with *cum simptomate* for *simptomata*) through dittography of *-co*, the last syllable of *stomacho*. θ″ (Ma P3′, followed here by G1 and L2) appears to have corrected the text; in the interests of parsimony (see 4.3.3, 4.7.2 below), I am reluctant to allow θ″ access to γ′. There is also the problem of where the corrector of P3 found the incorrect *cum*, if not in θ″ or γ′.

2.37.14 ex aegritudinibus diuersis augmentantibus humoribus: augmentantibus (aum- P1) P1 M u augmentatis *cett. etiam* v1 (*cf.* diuersorum augmentatione humorum θ″) (Gk II, 283, 9 διὰ ποσότητα πλεοναζόντων χυμῶν)

δ errs in corrupting *augmentantibus* to *augmentatis* (an easy corruption committed also by v1, although the converse — *augmentatis* > *augmentantis* > *augmentantibus* — is also thinkable, given confusion over the participle in Late Latin).[12]

2.158.1 Non scio si est alia peior passio ... non ob hoc solum quia ipsa per se ... occidere potest hominem sed quia ...: non enim P1 M nam ob D (Gk II, 187, 2–5 Οὐκ οἶδα πάθος, εἰ οὕτως ἄλλο χαλεπόν ἐστιν ...· οὐ γὰρ αὐτὸ καθ' αὑτὸ ... ἀναιρεῖν πέφυκεν, ἀλλὰ ...)

δ reflects an attempt to make sense of a nonsensical text preserved in β, where *non enim hoc solum* matches exactly Greek οὐ γὰρ αὐτὸ καθ' αὑτὸ, although neither of the Latin versions renders the Greek accurately. Note that, if we read *enim* instead of *ob*, *ipsa per se* seems to repeat *hoc solum*. One wonders whether one or the other entered the tradition as a gloss.

2.235.2 quia eius (i.e. *podagrae*) ignorantur natiuitates: ignoratur natiuitas M P3′ v1 ignorantis natiuitatis P1 natiuitatis ignorantia plurimis est po

There is nothing corresponding in the Greek at this point (II, 501, 12), but I incline to prefer the singular which β must have had (and γ′ reflected in P3′). The genitives in P1,

12 The presence of *aegritudinibus* may suggest that the translator read not ποσότητα but (the non-existent) νοσότητα, which would imply either that he was not concentrating or that Greek was not his first language: else he would have restored the opposition between quality and quantity (which he elsewhere correctly understands and translates). *Diuersus* usually (and frequently) stands for Greek διάφορος (e.g. 1.6=I, 447, 12; 1.6 *fin.*=Gk ms. Mf f. 4v; 1.21=I, 465, 17; 1.53=I, 509, 18). Here it matches nothing in the Greek: presumably the translator added it for clarity and naturalness. An alternative possibility (suggested to me by Michael Reeve) is that *diuersis* renders ποσότητα (although I am unable to find parallels for this).

although resembling a corruption of the plural, are easy slips given *-ti-* and *eius* just before.[13] (Note the transposition and the additional words in po.)

2.271.10 donec ... soluantur omnes carnes eius: omnes *om.* P1 M (Gk II, 575, 23–4 ἕως ἂν ἀναλυθῶσιν αἱ σάρκες αὐτῆς)

δ adds *omnes* absent from P1, M, and the Greek text.

2.271.12 coques autem oleum sicut dictum est (Gk II, 575, 27–8 ἕψε δὲ τὸ ἔλαιον, ὡς προγέγραπται)

δ omits *sicut dictum est* present in P1, M, and the Greek text.

4.2.4. β, γ and u v1

On the evidence at present available, it is not possible to establish beyond doubt the relations among the descendants of β. On the face of it, in 2.235–6 M and v1 agree very closely, often against P1, but P1 is nearly always in error and M and v1 probably merely transmit what was in β. In provisionally setting P1 and M against v1 and u, I have regard especially to the following shared errors.

2.36.3 ita ut interdum etiam aliqui mox derepente moriantur: iterum aut dementia aliquid M, iterum autem tumentia aliqui P1 (Gk II, 279, 22 ὥστε τινὰς παραυτίκα ἀπόλλυνται)

The nonsensical sequences in P1 and M are strikingly similar. u and v1 have the words underlined in common with the rest of the tradition.

2.37.2 in eius stomacho: in eo P1 M si in P3 φ (nothing corresponding in the Gk II, 281, 12ff.)

A small, phonetically-based error, but one shared only by P1 and M.

2.37.4 Ceterum autem oportet eis addere paulatim cibos qui tarde digeruntur: et rarum eis adhiuere paulatim M ceterarum autem oportit eis adibere paulatim P1 (Gk II, 281, 15–16 λοιπὸν δὲ δεῖ προστιθέναι κατὰ μέρος αὐτοῖς ὅσα δυσμετάβλητά εἰσι)

Both the corruption of the conjunction *ceterum* and the idiomatic but less appropriate choice of verb (*adhibere*) unite P1 and M in error. u and v1 both have *addere* with the rest of the tradition (although they follow β (including γ′, and hence Ox and P3) in placing it, probably rightly, before *paulatim*, as in the Greek); v1 has *Ceterum*, but u, like P1 and M, does not recognize the conjunction, and has *Ceteris*.

4.3. Daughters of δ

4.3.1. η Errs

The left-hand branch of the family deriving from δ — that is, those copies descending from what I am calling η — shows, at least in the chapters so far collated, apparently very few shared significant errors. Within η, there are problems in that C appears, at least in 1.85–7 and 2.1–11, to show contamination with a descendant of θ′, and in that in places O seems to share significant errors with β (presumably via θ or γ′).

[13] I owe this observation to Michael Reeve.

I begin, however, with the few innovations of η (in addition to those set out below, note 2.37.7 and 2.235.5 in 4.8.2 below).

1.19.7 Gustus igitur si amarus fuerit, cholericus est humor; salsus autem si fuerit, flegmaticus est; *acetosus autem*, melancholicus: salsedo autem A O Mu C | *acetosus autem*] aut η P1 acetosus Ox si (si autem Ge) acetosus *cett.* (Gk I, 463, 14–15 πικρότητος μὲν γὰρ αἰσθάνονται οἷς χολῶδές ἐστι τὸ αἴτιον· ἁλμυρᾶς δὲ ποιότητος, οἷς τὸ φλέγμα, ἰώδους δὲ, οἷς μελαγχολικός ἐστι χυμός)

This passage is surprisingly corrupt and messy (see my provisional text and notes ad loc.). What is clear is that *salsedo*, which A, O, Mu and C alone have, must have been an innovation in η for *salsus*. This passage may have been corrupt in δ (a possible trace of *acetosus* in the suffix of η's *salsedo*?) and heroically corrected by ε, all of whose descendants have *acetosus*.

2.1.2 aut alia aliqua qualitate assumpta (*abl. abs.*): sit (fit A′) qualitas (qualitas existens Mu′) assumpta A O Mu C qualitas assumpta (adsum ta P1) P1 M P2′ (*ante* qualitas *habet rasuram* (sit?) P2) (ab ...) qualitate assumptas φ qualitates assumptas (assupmtas Ma) *cett.* (Gk II, 147, 8–9 παντὸς τοῦ ἐπιρρέοντος χυμοῦ ἢ θερμὴν ἢ ψυχρὰν ἢ ἄλλην τινὰ ποιότητα προσειληφότος)

The innovation of η here consists in the insertion of *sit* to make a finite passive verb out of a failed attempt to translate the Greek genitive absolute (are there parallels for this?). It is important to note the detail that P2 appears to have corrected the text of η at this point, erasing a short word (*s/fit*?) before *qualitas*, adding *-s* to each word in the phrase *aliqua alia assumpta*, and changing *qualitas* to *qualitates*. This raises the possibility that P2 found the addition in δ (this is allowed for in the stemma, as there are other reasons to suppose that P2 had knowledge of δ: see 4.7.1 below), in which case it is even thinkable that *s/fit* was original and lost in β.

2.236.2 dolores facere +– in pedibus –+ solent nimios: inimicos A O Mu′ C (Gk II, 501, 20–1 ὀδύνην ἐργάζεσθαι πέφυκε σφοδράν)

inimicos is surely an error in η for *nimios*. Strikingly, it is corrected to *nimios* in Mu. I incline to think this a relatively easy correction, requiring in itself no assumption of an accessory model —for the possibility of contamination in Mu with reference to this very sentence see below under 'ε errs' (4.3.3).

4.3.2. η′ Errs (O Mu)

Apart from two possible links between A and Mu (see 4.8.4 below), the only clear relations between copies derived from η are between O and Mu, and these point to a lost daughter of η, η′. Evidence for η′ in the form of secondary readings exclusive to O and Mu is plentiful and scattered through all the chapters so far collated. Innovations of η′ include the following:

1.18.2 melanteria cum aceto acro inungues: *om.* O Mu (Gk I, 461, 21 Μελαντηρίαν μετ' ὄξους κατάχριε)

η′ omits *acro*, which, although it is not in the Greek, must have been in α.

1.19.3 subtilior apparet et subcolerico colore: et subcolerico apparet colore O Mu (Gk I, 463, 7–8 λεπτόν ἐστι τῇ συστάσει καὶ ὕπωχρον (ὑπόχολον Mf) τῇ χροιᾷ)

η′ moves the verb, with the result (if not the intention) of achieving a (for the Latin Alexander, characteristic) hyperbaton.

1.19.5 loca ex quibus fluit humor . . . ut nihil ex his defluat: humor fluit . . . defluat ex his O Mu (Gk I, 463, 10–11 οἱ τόποι ἐξ ὧν ἀπορρεῖ τὸ ὑγρὸν . . . ὡς μηδὲν ἐξ αὐτῶν ἀπορρεῖν)

η′ twice moves the verb so as to make it follow its subject, in contrast with the rest of the tradition and with the Greek.

1.85.1 et (scil. *modus*) qualiter conficiantur +– demonstratus est –+: demonstraturus O Mu′ -atus/a/um *cett.* (not in the Gk II, 3, 6)

The future participle makes no sense here, and in Mu has been corrected to *demonstratum*. This is not the only case in which the exclusive agreement is between O and Mu′ (Mu before correction): cf. 2.236.6 below.

1.85.7 sed adhuc etiam magis laeserunt (scil. *multi medici*): magis etiam O Mu magis M P2 B Ma ϕ (Gk II, 5, 4 ἔτι (ἔτι δὲ L) καὶ μεγάλως ἔβλαψαν)

In view of the common collocation *adhuc etiam* and the Greek at this point, *etiam magis* is probably right, and *magis etiam* a shared error.

1.86.2 rubra enim sunt omnia et sanguineo colore, et ipsa facies rubra: et *om.* O Mu (Gk II, 5, 20–1 ἐρυθρὰ γὰρ ἅπαντα καὶ αἱματώδη καὶ τὸ πρόσωπον ἐρυθρὸν)

η′ omits *et*, a small but important omission, exclusive to O and Mu.

1.86.2 et uene apparent [apertius et] plene: quia O quod Mu (Gk II, 5, 22 καὶ αἱ φλέβες εὐρύτεραι)

η′ makes a not-unintelligent, but clearly secondary, substitution of ‘because’ for ‘and’.

2.1.4 sine cognitione non possunt bene curari: *om.* O Mu (Gk II, 147, 15 ἄνευ διαγνώσεως οὐχ οἷόν τε θεραπεῦσαι καλῶς)

η′ omits *bene*.

2.10.1 Quando autem desubito qui laborant sentiunt coangustata praecordia se habere: coangustata A γ θ″ coangusta O Mu per-/prae- *cett.* (Gk II, 153, 8 Ὁπηνίκα δὲ ἀθρόως ὁ κάμνων αἴσθηται στενοχωρίας)

η′ writes by haplography the non-existent form *coangusta*. This was an easy mistake to make, but one confined among our eighteen witnesses to O and Mu. The translator uses *coangustare* and its participles quite frequently; *co-* is of course not an adjectival prefix.

2.37.5 Oportet autem his . . . suadere: *om.* O Mu (Gk II, 281, 20–1 δεῖ δὲ τούτοις . . . συμβουλεύειν)

η′ omits *his*.

2.37.6 Nihil enim est aliud maius iuuamen: iuuamen maius O Mu (nothing exactly corresponding in the Gk II, 281, 21–2 οὐδὲν γὰρ αὐτοῖς οὕτω συμβάλλεται)

η′ again reverses the order of a pair of words (cf. 1.85.7 above and 2.271.8 below).

2.236.6 Non enim solum oportet ut supercurrente materia reumatismi solent fieri sed et per simplicem solam qualitatem efficitur: *om.* O Mu′ (*add.* Mu m2) (Gk II, 503, 2–3 οὐ μόνον δὲ διὰ ἐπίρροιαν ὕλης οἱ ῥευματισμοὶ τοῖς ἄρθροις ἐπιγίνεσθαι πεφύκασιν, ἀλλὰ καὶ διὰ ψιλὴν ποιότητα μόνην)

η′ omits *et per* creating a nonsense. Mu′ attempts to restore sense by writing *efficit* for *efficitur*: a second hand then inserts *et per* and corrects *efficit* to *efficitur*. As in 1.85.1 above, the agreement is between O and Mu′.

2.236.6 ex calido, frigido, sicco et humido et duplicata distemperantia, id est aut calido et sicco aut calido et humido aut frigido et humido aut certe frigido et sicco: *alii alia*: ex calido et humido. Et duplicata distemperantia O Mu (Gk II, 503, 3–4 καὶ θερμὴν καὶ ψυχράν· ἔτι δὲ ξηρότης τε καὶ ὑγρότης)

Because of the high risk of a *saut du même au même*, the transmission of this passage is extremely messy (I seek a parallel for the Latin etiology, particularly given the contrast with the Greek). Given, however, the agreement of O and Mu, it is clear that η′ omitted the words *frigido sicco* in the list of the simple qualities.

2.236.7 Oportet ergo ... contemplari quales sunt causarum singularum qualitates uel quantitates: *om.* O Mu (not in the Gk II, 503, 5–6 δεῖ οὖν ... ὑποπτεύειν ἥτις ἀκριβῶς ἐστιν ἡ ποιητικὴ τοῦ πάθους αἰτία)

Although there is no corresponding word in the Greek, given the agreement of all the other Latin manuscripts, it is probable that *singularum* is original and lost already in η′.

2.236.7 et sic singularum causarum expedientem apponere curationem: purgationem O Mu (Gk II, 503, 6–7 καὶ τὴν ἁρμόττουσαν ἐπιφέρειν βοήθειαν)

η′ writes *purgationem* for *curationem*.

2.271.8 Mittens in caccabo olei communis sext. ii.: communis olei O Mu (Gk II, 575, 19 Βαλὼν εἰς κάκαβον ἐλαίου κοινοῦ ξε. β′)

Whatever the original case of the phrase underlined (the tradition offers accusative, ablative, and genitive), once again η′ reverses the order of two adjacent words (cf. 1.85.7 and 2.37.6 above).

4.3.3. ε Errs

The next important step in the history of this text was the recension reflected in ε, the common ancestor of eleven of the surviving copies as well as the early printing (*ed.*). Revisions affected minor changes in vocabulary and more significant changes in word-order. The fact that many of the descendants of ε are contaminated often makes it hard, sometimes impossible, to establish whether the corruption occurred already in ε or happened only later, in ε's daughter θ′, and passed by way of λ to Ma, D and Ge, appearing then in all the descendants of ε except Ox and P3, both of which are heavily contaminated with γ-readings. My reason for preferring the latter course (which of course reduces the features of ε, and adds to those of θ′) is that it allows γ-readings to enter the θ-family in a constrained fashion, through θ and P3 alone. Where θ agrees with γ, it is always possible to assume that θ has corrected the text inherited from ε with reference to γ′, and that the error was indeed in ε. It is interesting that the distribution of errors straightforwardly attributable to ε is complementary to that concerning θ′, and appears to increase sharply in the later chapters of Book 2 (there are hardly any compelling examples from Book 1 or the opening chapters of Book 2). If we assume a steady rate of error-commission by a given copyist, this could reflect a shift of source (or of main source, if two or more exemplars were available), such as, say, reduced use of γ′ by the maker of θ in the latter part of Book 2. There are too many ifs and buts here, of course, but the spread of errors through the text is an aspect that may repay further consideration at a later date. Be that as it may, this initial set of ε-errors is fairly strict and should be taken closely with those ascribed below to θ′ (4.4.1), some of which, as I say, may belong to ε. This initial list is reduced also in that it excludes those errors shared by (all or nearly all) the descendants of ε except P2: some of these, too, will have occurred in ε, but I present them among the principal cases of apparent contamination below (4.7.1) in order to illustrate the special position of P2.

1.18.t. Ad ulcera in capite spissa et rubra modica assimilantia titinulas, ex quibus tabes quaedam defluit: modica ulcera (modica sunt ulcera G1) G1 C L2 B Ma P3 D φ (Gk I, 461, 11–12 Πρὸς τὰ ἐν τῇ κεφαλῇ ἑλκύδρια πυκνὰ καὶ ἐρυθρὰ παραπλήσια θηλαῖς, ἀφ' ὧν ἰχῶρες ἀποτήκονται)

After the cautionary remarks in the last paragraph, this is a poor example to start with, as unfortunately, Ox, Ge and P2 omit *modica . . . defluit*. However, I tentatively ascribe to ε the insertion of a second *ulcera* (probably ending the title with *rubra* and beginning the chapter with *Modica*).

2.36.4 oportet non omnino existimare: non oportet omnino ε *praeter* P3 (Gk II, 281, 1–2 χρὴ μὴ πάντοτε νομίζειν)

A small normalization of the Latin, which nicely characterizes ε apart from P3 (which may follow γ′).

2.37.2 et panis in aqua frigida aut in calida aqua: in aqua frigida aut calida ε C (in aqua frigida infusus O in aqua frigida aut calida infusus D in aqua frigida infusus aut calida Ox in aqua calida aut frigida infusus P3)

Although there is some variation here, what is common to all the descendants of ε (and C) is the elimination of the repetition of *aqua*, which, in view of its distribution (η and β), is probably original. The distribution of *infusus* (O D Ox P3) makes me wonder whether it was in θ, in which case Ma and Ge must have preferred λ at this point.

2.158.3 +– quibus agnitis –+ sic curatio competens est adhibenda et differri non oportet: curatio competens sic est ε *praeter* D P3 (Gk II, 187, 6–7 καὶ οὕτω τὴν θεραπείαν ἐπιφέρειν καὶ μὴ ἀναβάλλεσθαι)

Given Greek καὶ οὕτω, and the fact that *sic* here surely means 'then, next', its position before *curatio* is probably to be preferred. If this is right, ε has here made a slight adjustment to the word-order (corrected by D and P3, the latter of which may have followed γ′).

2.235.3 Ego autem existimo ut quicumque eius bene potuerit natiuitates cognoscere uel diuersitates aut ipsas species quaecumque fiunt et qualiter contingunt bene et cito posse curare et facilius a medicis ab ipsis infirmitatibus liberari: fuerint G1 P2 L2 B D P3 *om.* Ox Ge (no direct correspondence in Gk II, 501, 12–14 ἐγὼ δέ φημι, ὡς, εἴγε διαγνωσθεῖεν καλῶς αἵ τε διαφοραὶ καὶ τὰ εἴδη αὐτῆς, ὅσα τε καὶ οἷα τυγχάνει, εὐθεράπευτος ἂν ῥᾳδίως ὑπὸ τῶν ἰατρῶν γενήσεται)

ε has *fuerint* for *fiunt*. κ′ omits the word. Ma and φ somehow have *fiunt*, probably independently, as these two forms are easily confused.

2.236.2 Etenim sanguis calidus supercurrens in articulorum cauitates, extenduntur et nerui quos sindismos uocant dolores facere +– in pedibus –+ solent nimios: concauitates extenditur θ′ (not C) θ″ κ φ *et* Mu! (Gk II, 501, 19–21 καὶ γὰρ αἷμα συρρεῦσαν ἐν τῇ τῶν ἄρθρων κοιλότητι θερμὸν καὶ διατεῖνον αὐτά τε καὶ τοὺς συνδέσμους ὀδύνην ἐργάζεσθαι πέφυκε σφοδράν)

Whatever the truth behind the Latin (where the construction seems to change after *cauitates*), ε apparently altered *cauitates* to *concauitates* and *extenduntur* to *extenditur*. It is striking that Mu here corrects *cauitates* to *concauitates* and *extenduntur* to *extenditur*. Is this independent, or is Mu contaminated? I have not allowed for the latter in the stemma, as this is the only potentially serious instance so far identified (but see 2.236.2 in 4.3.1 above).

2.236.6 Non enim solum oportet ut supercurrente materia reumatismi solent fieri sed et per simplicem solam qualitatem efficitur: oportet solum existimare Ma B existimare oportet P2 oportet existimare G1 D P3 φ | ut] a G1 P2 B Ma P3 φ | reumatismum solum fieri P2 solum reumatismum fieri G1 B Ma P3 φ (Gk II, 503, 2–3 οὐ μόνον δὲ διὰ ἐπίρροιαν ὕλης οἱ ῥευματισμοὶ τοῖς ἄρθροις ἐπιγίνεσθαι πεφύκασιν, ἀλλὰ καὶ διὰ ψιλὴν ποιότητα μόνην)

θ′ (but not C), θ″, D and φ, and therefore ε already, introduce *existimare*, and all but D also replace *ut* with the preposition *a* (governing *supercurrente materia*); only Ma and B retain *solum* early in the sentence. Before *fieri*, probably *solent* is original (Greek πεφύκασιν) but looked odd after *oportet ut*,[14] and was changed to *solum* and put before its noun (*reumatismum*) in ε (although P2 has the older word-order, perhaps by reference to δ).

κ has more or less the correct text, which poses a problem. Either θ corrects the text with reference to γ′, and makes it available to κ: this (unlike in 2.5.2 above, where P3 omits the relevant words) obliges me to suppose that P3 has the ε-error here from a third source (other than θ″ and γ′; cf. 2.37.14 above). Alternatively, κ had independent access to γ′: this is of course an easy solution, but one which, on grounds of parsimony, should be used only as a last resort. D and Ge (independently?) have *soleant* for *solent* after *oportet ut*, but D alone of the descendants of κ has the secondary *existimare*: did D here follow λ (as in 2.5.2 under 4.4.1 below)? or did κ′ (Ox Ge) omit *existimare* accidentally?[15]

All in all, this is a nice example of an unsuccessful attempt in the High Middle Ages to improve an obviously unacceptable text.

2.236.6 Ex quibus distemperationibus fiunt saepius reumatismi: distemperantiis O P2 B Ma D Ox Ge (nothing corresponding in Gk II, 503, 4–5 αἴτια γίνονται πολλάκις ῥευματισμῶν)

The distribution of *distemperantiis* is odd. Unless it is due just to sporadic and independent normalizations of *distemperatio* (*distemperantia* being the normal word), it was in ε, θ′/λ, θ (whence O) and κ, but corrected by θ″ (whence G1, P3 and φ).

2.271.6 Item aliud cerotum simile quod in statu passionis adhibeatur: Aliud quod ε Aliud. Aliud (*sic*) D Quod O Mu Ma Aliud cerotum quod C (Gk II, 575, 9 ἑτέρα κηρωτὴ ὁμοίως ἐν τῇ ἀκμῇ ἐπιτίθεσθαι δυναμένη)

γ and A are obviously right with *Item aliud cerotum simile quod*. ε has abbreviated this heading considerably, and is the source of the readings of D and Ma. The heading is abbreviated also (independently) in η′ (by mistake?) and in C (deliberately?).

2.271.7 Item aliud cerotum et ipsum mitigatiuum est: ipse γ, hoc ipsum ε (Gk II, 575, 12 Ἄλλη κηρωτὴ καὶ αὐτὴ παρηγορική)

The sequence *et hoc ipsum + another word* (…etiam P2 …enim Ma …autem B φ …antidotum P3) seems to be an innovation of ε. (Note that η (A O Mu; and incidentally L2) had *et ipsum enim*, so that probably the particle was introduced in δ. Save in Ma, *hoc* and *enim* are in complementary distribution, and *hoc* may have arisen from a misreading of the abbreviation of *enim* that resembles a small capital H.)

[14] *oportet ut* is wrong but evidently old and may reflect either δεῖ in the translator's Greek text (for δέ or διά, neither of which is translated in β or δ), or a corruption of *propter* (for διά).

[15] Note that κ′ lost *mediocriter* a few words earlier.

2.271.13 Sic enim facta coctio multum ualere potest: iuuare (Ch) G1 P2 L2 B Ma P3 φ *om.* Ox Ge (Gk II, 575, 30 οὕτω γὰρ ποιῶν ἐπιτεύξῃ)

Again (as in 2.158.6 under 'θ′ errs' below), κ (though here we have only D!) disagrees with ε. It is at least thinkable that *facta coctio* (not in the Greek) was added as an explanatory gloss, and that the alternation *ualere/iuuare* arose in the same way, which obviously reduces its value for present purposes. (In any case, what is (Ch) doing agreeing with ε?!)

2.271.13 Sufficiat haec de anodinis et paragoricis cataplasmatibus dixisse: podagricis ε (but not C) (Gk II, 575, 29–30 τοσαῦτα περὶ τῶν ἀνωδύνων καὶ παρηγορικῶν ἐπιπλασμάτων μοι λέλεκται)

Although *paragoricus* was fairly common and might have been left alone, this is a perfectly intelligent substitution at the end of the chapters on gout, which nicely characterizes all copies descending from ε, and shows that ε did not refer to the Greek text.

3.59 [*post uerba* nullo modo in aere tardandus est infirmus, *hoc est post finem cap. 59 ed.*:] In uisceribus autem oleo infundendum est magis et exeunte de balneo depones in frigidam piscinam non tantum aquam frigidam habentem sed lactaneam. Inuolutus ergo sabanis non satis remoretur in eis. Volens autem ... Quod si sitem habet infirmus et in sabanis adhuc positus accipiat tunc magis traditur nutrimentum per totum corpus: *haec uerba habent soli* γ (P1 M) Mu ba[16] (Gk I, 363, 16–26)

As this omission is in P2 and in all the manuscripts deriving from θ, including φ, it must have been in ε. Of the copies deriving from η, Mu has the missing lines, C omits them, and – alas! – we do not have this chapter in A, O, or (Ch). As there are other reasons for believing C to be contaminated, it is simpler to assume for the moment that C followed his θ′-source at this point (B stops before this chapter, but G1 and L2 have it and omit the lines), rather than that the omission was already in δ and that Mu recovered the material from an accessory model: while I think that O must have known θ (and conceivably γ′), it seems that where O agrees with θ (or γ′) it disagrees with Mu, so that I am reluctant to ascribe knowledge of θ or γ′ to η′.

4.4. Descendants of ε

4.4.1. θ′ Errs

θ′ is one of two lost daughters of ε, and heads a family which is hard to characterize, because virtually every member appears to have an accessory model. I regard θ′ as representing innovations common to (at most) G1, P2, L2 and B, some of which are followed by MaDGe (see 4.4.2 below), and some by C (which I see as essentially a daughter of η, but for which a descendant of θ′ close to G1 was apparently an accessory model). Of the main members of this group, G1 and L2 are sometimes strikingly close to P3; P2 also had an accessory model in a higher descendant of δ; and there are one or two hints that even B may have had relations outside θ′ (on all these, see 4.7 below).

[16] That ba has the missing lines provides another instance of an excerpting manuscript — in this case, a relatively late one (early thirteenth century) — with a source relatively high in the stemma. I have yet to determine the genetic affiliations of the exemplar of ba.

The following list of features of θ′ may include errors that occurred already in ε (see the introductory paragraphs to 4.3.3 above and 4.4.2 below).

1.19.1 ex quibus fluit humor similis quod icor Gracci uocant: similis γ A C Ox P3′ *s. s.* Ma *om.* ε η′ (Gk I, 463, 3 ἐξ ὧν ἔξεισιν ὑγρὸν ἰχῶρι παραπλήσιον)

θ′ (and independently η′) omits *similis*. Its presence in η (A C), γ (P1 M) and the Greek (παραπλήσιον) guarantee that it is original. Ox, P3′ and the corrector of Ma will have inherited it from θ (and it could have been in γ′).

1.19.2 cognosci ergo oportet: uero G1 P2 L2 B Ma Ge autem D C (Gk I, 463, 5 διαγινώσκειν οὖν χρὴ)

θ′ replaces *ergo* (οὖν) with *uero* (further altered to *autem* by D and C). Ox and P3′ (one of them here followed by ϕ) will have inherited *ergo* from θ (and it could have been in γ′).

1.85.11 et si unus ex ipsis est qui molestatur humor aut duo commixti: mixti G1 C P2 B Ma Ge (Gk II, 5, 13–14 καὶ πότερον εἷς ἐστιν ὁ λυπῶν χυμὸς ἢ δύο συμπεπλεγμένοι)

θ′ (including C but not L2), Ma and Ge substitute *mixti* for *commixti* which matches the Greek and obviously fits better. Ma and Ge follow θ′, while θ″ and κ (including D) follow θ.

1.87.2 Si autem colericus acer humor cum sanguine appareat mixtus: mixtus appareat G1 C P2 B Ma Ge (Gk II, 5, 28–7, 1 εἰ δὲ καὶ χολώδεις καὶ δριμεῖς χυμοὶ σὺν τῷ αἵματι φαίνοιντο)

θ′ (including C but not L2), Ma and Ge transpose *appareat* and *mixtus*.

1.88.2 Superinunctiones autem et inquimatismata +– sequenti sermone sunt ordinanda –+: superunctiones ε *praeter* Ox P3 (Gk II, 7, 19 ἐπιχρίσμασι δὲ καὶ ἐγχυματισμοῖς τοῖσδε)

Admittedly a small discrepancy, but one that neatly characterizes the descendants of ε except, as often, Ox and P3, whose readings derive from θ (and could have been in γ′).

2.1.1 initium habet (scil. *tussis*) modo a calida distemperantia, est autem quando a frigida: est autem quando γ η θ″, quandoque G1 C P2 L2 B, modo κ ϕ (Gk II, 147, 5–6 ποτὲ μὲν γὰρ ἄρχεται ἀπὸ θερμῆς δυσκρασίας, ἔσθ' ὅτε δὲ καὶ ἀπὸ ψυχρᾶς)

θ′ (followed by C) replaces *est autem quando* (for Greek ἔσθ' ὅτε δέ) with *quandoque*.[17]

2.2.5 Sic enim erit cognoscenda calida distemperantia a praedictis signis: erit cognoscentia P2 B G1 L2 Ge cognoscetur C erit agnoscenda D Ma P3 (Gk II, 147, 24–5 οὕτω γὰρ ἔστι τὴν διὰ θερμὴν δυσκρασίαν βῆχα ἀπὸ τῶν παρόντων σημείων διαγινώσκειν)

θ′ (G1 P2 L2 B) and λ (followed by Ge) replace *cognoscenda* with *cognoscentia*.

2.2.6 Nihil igitur minus et a praecedenti qualitate calidi aeris: contingit tussis ex P2 D Ge contingit tussis Ma fit ex G1 L2 contingit tussis et fit ex B (Gk II, 147, 25–6 οὐδὲν δὲ ἧττον καὶ ἀπὸ τῶν προηγησαμένων ἐξ ἐγκαύσεως)

G1, P2, L2, B, Ma, D and Ge have additions in common (B apparently with a combination of G1 and P2). This is ε minus P3, Ox and ϕ, and the addition is probably best understood as an innovation of θ′, with the readings of P3 and Ox deriving from θ.

[17] B actually has *quandoque autem*, which could be seen as a blend of two models(?).

2.4.2 materiale*s* autem [si accesserit tussis] amitrotera*s*, et non oportet <t>alia iterum dicere: (Gk II, 149, 12–14 διαφέρουσι δὲ τοῦ μᾶλλον τὰς δραστικὰς ἔχειν ἐναργέστατα σημεῖα, τὰς δὲ ὑλικὰς ἀμυδρότερα καὶ οὐ χρὴ ταὐτὰ (ταῦτα? *Fischer*) πάλιν λέγειν)

The Latin tradition offers various explanatory notes to Greek ἀμυδρότερα, among which P2 and B alone have *leuior ad curandum*, and G1 alone the very similar *leuis ad curandum.*[18] The Greek text was evidently totally misunderstood at this point.

2.5.2 Vnde et ex quibus transmittitur locis, haec omnia utique contemplari oportet: Vnde et *ras.* P2 *om.* G1 L2 B D (Vnde ... locis *om.* θ″) (Gk II, 149, 16–17 ὅθεν δὲ καὶ ἐξ ὁποίων ἐπιπέμπονται μορίων, κἀνταῦθα διορίζεσθαι δεῖ καὶ προσέχειν)

G1, P2, L2, B and D omit *Vnde et* (θ″ omits *Vnde et ex quibus transmitttur locis*). The error must therefore have been in θ′. D, unless erring independently, has the error from λ. θ will have inherited the missing words from ε (or found them in γ′), and made them available to Ox, Ge, and φ. (If the erasure in P2 was of *Vnde et*, these words were presumably from δ: see 4.7 below).

2.36.2 maxime his qui nimis sensibilem habent stomachum, ita ut interdum etiam aliqui mox derepente moriantur: nimis sensibilem η (*praeter* C) u v1 nimis sunt debelem P1 nimis debilem M P3 sensibilem nimis θ′ debilem nimis φ debilem uel sensibilem (uel s. *s. s.*) nimis Ge sensibilem L2 (Gk II, 279, 21 ἐὰν οὖν εὑρεθῶσί τινες ἔχοντες τῆς γαστρὸς αἰσθητικὸν τὸ στόμα, παραυτίκα ἀπόλλυνται)

Whatever lies behind *nimis* (not in the Greek),[19] *sensibilem* is to be preferred (for αἰσθητικὸν) and *debilem* is to be seen as a corruption of it (possibly via *sunt debilem*, as in P1). The other corruption evident here is the 'normalizing' of the order adjective + *nimis* in keeping with the habits of the translator (*sensibilem nimis*, *debilem nimis*). *sensibilem nimis* is in θ′ (G1 P2 B and C) and possibly θ (Ma D Ge), in which case the reordering could have occurred already in ε. Ma, D and Ge, however, could as well reflect λ, in which case *nimis sensibilem* may have survived for Ox to find in θ. Here again it looks as if the most likely model of φ is Ge.

2.37.5 Oportet autem his cum requieuerit +– aut lenimentum acceperit –+ passio suadere semper ut citius cibos accipiant: his aut cum Ma L2 his autem cum G1 D his ut cum B his cum aut P2 φ his qui cum M v1 his qui Ox cum η′ (*cf.* his et cum passio uel quieuerit P3) (Gk II, 281, 20–1 δεῖ δὲ τούτοις καὶ μετὰ τὸ παύσασθαι τῆς ἐπιχεούσης διαθέσεως ἀεὶ ταχύτερον συμβουλεύειν ἐσθίειν)

This is messy, but what all the copies deriving from ε (except Ox) have in common is the insertion of a word for 'either' before *requieuerint.* Originally, there was probably a word corresponding to Greek καὶ, which may be reflected in *et* in P3 (and possibly in *qui* in M, v1 and Ox), and which, as it was not convincing Latin, was either dropped (in η) or changed to *aut* (in ε). P3 may have found *et* in one source and *aut* in another and revised the sentence to incorporate both, but Ox is surely following θ (following γ′), and I hence ascribe the insertion of 'either' to θ′ rather than to ε.

[18] cf. *leuior facilior ad curandum* Ma *.i. leuis* P3 m3(?) *.i. facilis ad cognoscendum* Ox φ.

[19] Possibly *inuenti s(unt)*: cf. Greek εὑρεθῶσι?

2.37.7 For the text and variants, see 4.8.2 below.
Here θ′ (followed by λ and hence Ma D Ge) makes another change in the word-order, moving the subordinate verb (*ut assumant*) next to the main verb *suadendum est* (which was certainly in δ); note also *in aqua calida aut frigida* (ε except P3) and *panem in aqua calida aut frigida infusum* (ε except Ox and P3).

2.158.6 Diabrosin dicunt quando uena, amisso nutrimento, caro desuper ipsam extenuatur: uene Ox Ge | carnis G1 P2 L2 B P3 Ma | extenuat γ fit extenuata η κ (!) (not in the Greek text)

The Latin presumably means: 'They call *diabrosis* the case when the vein, because its nourishment has ceased, the flesh over it is extenuated' (with *uena* nominative and change of construction). The nominative *uena* could explain the substitution of *carnis* for *caro*. It is possible that this substitution occurred in ε, and was preserved in θ′ and θ″, and that κ here made an independent correction back to *caro* (which κ′ then better accommodated by changing *uena* to *uene*).[20] The remarkable presence in η and κ of *fit extenuata* for *extenuatur*, however, is not so easily explained. Independent innovation is unlikely, and there is no trace of the periphrastic passive in γ at this point. The only possible explanation is that δ and possibly ε and θ had *fit extenuata*, that *extenuatur* is an innovation of θ′ followed by λ and Ma, and that P3 also had access to a descendant of θ′. (For another possible disagreement between κ and ε, see 2.271.13 under 4.3.3 above.)

4.4.2. λ Errs (MaDGe)

Further significance attaches to θ′ in that its lost daughter λ was known to Ma (a daughter of θ″) and to D and Ge (daughters of κ). This is the most economical explanation I can think of for cases where one or more of MaDGe (whom I have come to regard as a friend!) disagree with the other descendants of θ, in particular with Ox and P3 (see 4.4.3). I have as yet identified only one significant innovation which would distinguish λ, the accessory model of MaDGe, from θ′ (note also, however, 2.9.2 under 4.4.3). I represent λ as a daughter of θ′, as in this way some of the errors I for a long time ascribed to ε (including 1.19.1, 1.19.2, 1.88.2, 2.2.6) could in fact be errors of θ′. This may seem pedantic, but it allows direct knowledge of γ′ to be restricted to θ (and P3) among the descendants of ε, which considerably simplifies the stemma (see 4.7.2).

2.7.3 Si autem et sitis sit nimia, et frequenter ad haec signa et calor sentiatur multus in thorace: et frequenter] frequenter et (etiam D) O D Ox P3 | *post* frequenter] expirent (expirent *s. s.* Ma) Ma Ge etiam expirent D respirent et φ | ad haec signa *om.* P3′ Ma D Ge | calor multus sentitur P3 Ma φ (Gk II, 151, 6 εἰ δὲ καὶ δίψη σφοδρᾷ συνέχοιτο πρὸς τοῖς σημείοις τούτοις καὶ θέρμης αἴσθησις αὐτῷ γίνοιτο πολλὴ περὶ τὸν θώρακα)

θ transposes *et* and *frequenter*, but is followed only by O, Ox and P3 (and in part by D), as MaDGe (λ, which may be the third source of P3) omits *ad haec signa*,[21] and adds *exspirent* (*respirent* φ[22]) after *frequenter*. The Latin appears to be a translation of διψῇ

[20] Or, less probably, κ followed γ′ (*caro* γ), but I am trying to restrict knowledge of γ′ to θ and P3.
[21] P3 m3 adds *ad hec signa* in the margin with an indication that it belongs after *Si autem*.
[22] φ could have got *respirent* from Ge (see 4.6 below).

σφόδρα συνεχῶς τε.[23] θ″ (Ma, P3 and hence φ) eliminates the hyperbaton (and the subjunctive) in *calor sentiatur multus*.

4.4.3. θ Errs

θ is the other daughter of ε, and the mother of θ″ and κ (important, if indirect, sources of φ). Some errors in θ are also in O. Earlier I thought these must reflect independent use of γ′ by O and θ″ and κ. I now think O might have known not (or not only) γ′ but θ, and that θ knew γ′. (For some slight hints that O had direct knowledge of γ′, see 4.8.3 below.)[24]

The number of innovations attributable to θ has increased considerably following the reconstruction of λ and the recognition that agreements between Ox and P3 may reflect θ, whether or not they are shared with γ.

1.19.8 Minus autem frigidus melancolicus inest humor: Si autem minus Ox P3 | *om.* Ox P3 φ (Gk I, 463, 17–18 ἧττον δὲ ψυχρὰ ἐφ' ὧν μελαγχολῶδες)

θ, here the common source of Ox and P3 alone, starts a new sentence with *si autem minus*. Ox and P3 also omit the final *inest humor*, and in this are followed by φ.

1.85.1 Iam enim in aliis tribus libris a me scripta sunt de oculorum passionibus qualiter oporteat cognosci in eis consistentes passiones, et causas eorum et curationes: scriptis oculorum passiones et causas earum qualiter oportet cognoscere et earum curationes Ox P3 (Gk II, 3, 2–3 Ἤδη μὲν οὖν ἐν ἄλλοις τρισὶ βιβλίοις ἀναγέγραπταί μοι περὶ τῶν ἐν ὀφθαλμοῖς παθῶν)

θ, here the common source of Ox and P3, has substantially recast this opening sentence in a sort of tidying-up operation, making *scriptis* adjectival, and *oculorum passiones* the direct object of the following indirect question, omitting *in eis consistentes passiones*, and putting *et causas earum* before the indirect question.

1.85.11 Aut enim ex sanguine nigro aut coleribus aut flegmate aut melancholia est quod fluit: aut ex Ox P3′ L2 φ (Gk II, 5, 12–13 ἤτοι γὰρ αἷμα μᾶλλον ἢ χολὴ ἢ φλέγμα ἢ μελαγχολικὸς χυμός ἐστι τὸ ἐπιρρεῦσαν)

θ, here the common source of Ox and P3′ (here followed by L2 and φ), omits *enim*. (P3, Ma, D and Ge could then have found *enim* in λ.)

1.85.11 et si unus ex ipsis est qui molestatur humor aut duo commixti: et si unus M et unus P1 Ox P3′ et aut unus η (A O Mu C) P3 aut unus D G1 aut et unus P2 aut etiam unus Ma L2 B φ an et unus Ge (Gk II, 5, 13–14 καὶ πότερον εἷς ἐστιν ὁ λυπῶν χυμὸς ἢ δύο συμπεπλεγμένοι)

Ox and P3′ (and P1) omit *si* (πότερον)(?). I take it that *si* is the original, automatic and nonsensical translation of Greek πότερον, variously corrected in the tradition.

2.1.3 Scire autem oportet et hoc quomodo differunt abinuicem tussiculae secundum causas singulas sed quoniam et secundum loca: et G1 P3 Ma′ D Ox Ge sed et φ (Gk II, 147, 9–10 εἰδέναι δὲ δεῖ καὶ τοῦτο, ὡς οὐ διαφέρουσιν ἀλλήλων αἱ βῆχες κατὰ τὴν αἰτίαν μόνην, ἀλλὰ καὶ κατὰ τοὺς τόπους)

[23] This suggestion was inspired by Cloudy Fischer.

[24] In view of the ages of the relevant manuscripts, it is worth bearing in mind the possibility that O was the source, rather than the recipient, of some of these shared readings. I am grateful to Michael Reeve for this observation.

θ omitted *sed quoniam*, perhaps deliberately in order to improve the Latin; *sed quoniam* was in γ and δ, and the corrector of Ma will have found it in θ′. The Greek text has just ἀλλὰ,[25] but ὅτι may have followed in the translator's Greek text. On the agreement of G1 with P3 and Ma′, see 4.7.3. Note that θ″ and φ have *quoniam* for *propterea/propter quod* in the next sentence, 2.1.4.

2.3.2 Et laeduntur ex frigidis et iuuantur ex calefactionibus, et acitonicum magis quam amaritudinem habere se sentiunt: se sentiunt habere P3 Ma Ox G2 (Gk II, 149, 4–6 καὶ βλάπτονται μὲν ὑπὸ τῶν ψυχόντων, ὀνίνανται δὲ ὑπὸ τῶν θερμαινόντων, καὶ ὀξίδος μᾶλλον ἢ πικρίας, ὡς ἐπὶ τὸ πολὺ, αἰσθάνονται)

θ, here the common source of θ″ and Ox, transposes *habere* and *se sentiunt* (unless the transpositions were made independently).

2.3.3 Et praecessit eos magis frigdor quam calor, et balneo non in tempore competenti et potionibus et cibis usi sunt frigidis: competenti tempore P3′ Ma Ox φ (Gk II, 149, 6–8 καὶ προηγεῖται μᾶλλον τούτοις ψῦξις ἢ ἔγκαυσις καὶ λουτρῶν ἀκαίρων καὶ πομάτων καὶ ἐδεσμάτων ψυχρῶν χρῆσις)

θ, here the common source of θ″ and Ox, transposes *tempore* and *competenti*.

2.7.4 Si autem et colericum sputant nec nimis grauiter angustiam sentiunt +– se habere praecordiae loca –+ sed magis calida esse: in praecordie loca M P2 praecordie loca P1A Mu C circa praecordiorum loca θ″ κ O in praecordiorum locis G1 L2 B Ge φ | sed magis] magis θ″ κ O φ (Gk II, 151, 10–11 εἰ δὲ χολῶδες ἀναπτύοιτο, μὴ πάνυ δὲ βάρους ἢ στενοχωρίας συναίσθησις γίνοιτο ἀλλὰ μᾶλλον θέρμης)

θ, followed by θ″, κ and O, inserts *circa*,[26] and omits *sed* (as does φ).

2.8.2 supercurrens <pus?> ex subitaneis mutatis euersionibus et sonos aurium cum obclusione saepius patiuntur: ex *om.* γ O P3 Ma D Ox | subitaneas mutatas euersiones (*plus minus*) γ O P3 Ma D (Ox has ablative) (Gk II, 151, 18–19 περιρρέοντος αὐτοῦ ἐν ταῖς ἀθρόαις μεταστροφαῖς καὶ ψοφοῦντος ἀκούειν πολλάκις)

The Latin text is uncertain here, but there is a clear division in the tradition between θ and γ (and O) without *ex* and with the accusative, and δ (seen in η and θ′ – A Mu C G1 P2 L2 B – and λ followed by Ge) with *ex* + ablative.

2.8.3 manifeste confidendum est quia pus est quod in thorace continetur: est quod *om.* O P3′ Ma D Ox | non continetur O P3′ Ma (Gk II, 151, 22–3 δῆλον ὅτι ὁμολογούμενον πῦόν ἐστι τὸ περιεχόμενον ἐν τῷ θώρακι)

θ (whence θ″ and κ and O) omitted *est quod*; θ probably also added *non* before *continetur*, but this was corrected by κ and belatedly in P3 (with dots under *non*, and *est quod* added by m2 in the margin). Again, Ge follows λ.

2.9.1 Quodsi fyma meditauerit fieri in pulmone: editauerit et fuerit M medetauerit fierit P1 fuerit (*post* pulmone O P3 Ma) O P3 Ma D Ox euenerit fieri *cett.* (Gk II, 151, 26 Εἴπερ εἴη φῦμα [μὴ] μελετηθὲν ἐν τῷ πνεύμονι)

O agrees with both θ″ and κ (although Ge follows λ and preserves *euenerit fieri*) in replacing whichever main verb phrase was in this clause with a simple *fuerit*, and with

[25] cf. just *sed* in φ, a possible hint (although a very slight one) that (a) a Greek text was consulted, or (b) φ had a third Latin source, in addition to Ox and P3 (possibly B: see 4.8.9).

[26] Alternatively, *in* is original and lost independently in P1 and η, rather than introduced independently in M and P2: do we then have *in* + accusative of place where? Note that ε replaced *precordie* with *precordiorum*. Again φ requires a source other than Ox and P3, which here could be Ge or B.

θ″ in moving it to the end of the clause, after *in pulmone*. Given that *euenerit fieri* — which is at least intelligible — was already in δ, it is probable that the more radical solution of O, θ″ and κ is owed to θ (possibly from γ′) and possible that it arose through the omission, whether accidental or deliberate, of the first of two future perfect verbs in a sequence something like that preserved in M (*editauerit et fuerit*).

2.9.2 Neque enim contingere poterit nisi ex indigesto et necdum permixto *fymate*: enim hoc P3 Ma D Ge | poterit Ma poterat P1 potest *cett.*; *post* potest *add.* patienti O P3 Ma D Ox ϕ (*praeter ed.*) (Gk II, 153, 3–4 οὔτε γὰρ συμβῆναι δυνήσεται ἔτι ἀπέπτου καὶ μηδέπω ἀποβεβλημένου τοῦ φλέγματος)

θ inserts *patienti*, which is copied by O and survives in θ″ and κ and hence ϕ (though Ge follows λ). The distribution of *hoc* after *enim* makes it look like an innovation of λ (in which case λ could be the third source of P3).

2.10.1 Quando autem desubito qui laborant sentiunt coangustata praecordia se habere et absque febribus molestari et siti multa: absque aliquibus febribus κ P3 (a quibus febribus P3′) aliquibus febribus O Ma (Gk II, 153, 8–9 Ὁπηνίκα δὲ ἀθρόως ὁ κάμνων αἴσθηται στενοχωρίας ἐκτὸς ὀχλήσεως πυρετοῦ καὶ δίψης πολλῆς)

θ substitutes *aliquibus* for *absque*. O, θ″ and κ alone have *aliquibus*, either instead of or in addition to *absque*. The source of *aliquibus* is surely the correct *absque* itself. O and θ″ (note P3′ *a quibus*) reflect uncritical copying of θ; κ and P3 have reinserted *absque* from an accessory model, but without eliminating *aliquibus*.

2.10.1 sed habet etiam quendam raucorem cum tusse: et (*om.* Ma) acrorem *add.* θ″ κ ϕ (*om.* L) (Gk II, 153, 9 ἔχῃ δέ τινα κέρχνον μετὰ βηχός)

θ adds *et acrorem* (or perhaps just *acrorem*, as in Ma) in the first instance probably as a gloss on *raucorem*.

2.10.1 qui ibidem fluunt de capite aut ex alio aliquo membro: altero aliquo O aliquo altero M P3 Ma D aliquo alio Ox L2 (Gk II, 153, 11–12 τὸ περιεχόμενον ἐν τῷ πνεύμονι καὶ συρρεῦσαν ἐκ τῆς κεφαλῆς ἢ ἐξ ἄλλου τινὸς μορίου)

θ (perhaps following γ′: cf. M) substitutes *altero* for *alio*, and is then followed by O, θ″ and κ (but Ox, Ge and L2 hold themselves aloof, or make independent corrections: Ge could have followed λ, and L2 could have followed G1).

2.11.3 Iste uir per multum tempus molestiam sustinens de tusse: per multa tempora O per multo tempore M per multum tempore P1 multo tempore κ (Gk II, 153, 22–3 οὗτος ὁ ἀνὴρ πολὺν χρόνον ὀχληθεὶς ὑπὸ τῆς βηχός)

θ (perhaps following γ′: cf. M) substitutes the ablative for the accusative, and is then followed by O and κ but corrected by θ″.

2.11.6 Redeamus igitur et de curis aliqua breuiter dicere non omittamus: cura M O P3′ Ma curas P1 (not in Gk II, 155, 22)

θ (perhaps following γ′: cf. M) substitutes the singular for the plural, and is then followed by O and θ″ but corrected by κ. (*cura* M and *curas* P1 can of course reflect a single form, as word-final *-s* was not pronounced in some varieties of Latin. Equally, they may reflect a 'vulgar' accusative after *de*.)

2.36.3 lumbrici saepius superiora petentes ex inferioribus partibus ad stomachum necesse est ut faciant cardiacam passionem: stomachi θ″ κ stomacho ϕ (Gk II, 279, 23–5 πολλάκις δὲ καὶ ἕλμινθες ἐκ τῶν κάτω μερῶν ἀναδραμόντες ἐπὶ τὸ στόμα τῆς γαστρὸς ἐργάζονται καρδιακὰς διαθέσεις) θ presumably saw no sense in *ad stomachum* and so replaced it with *stomachi* (construing it, erroneously, with *ex inferioribus partibus*).

4.4.4. θ″ Errs

There are numerous significant secondary readings common to P3 and Ma, which oblige us to reconstruct yet another lost copy as the immediate common ancestor of P3 and Ma (θ″ in the stemma). θ″ represents an in many places substantial revision of the inherited text, as is clear especially from the longer extracts set out below.

2.1.1 [sed] quoniam initium habet (scil. *tussis*) modo a calida distemperantia: quoniam P3 Ma (Gk II, 147, 5–6 ποτὲ μὲν γὰρ ἄρχεται ἀπὸ θερμῆς δυσκρασίας)

θ″ deletes *sed*. Given the evidence of the manuscripts, *sed* must have been in the Latin version,[27] but we are much better off without it, as the maker of θ″ saw.

2.1.1 initium habet (scil. *tussis*) modo a calida distemperantia, est autem quando a frigida: ex (*bis*) P3 Ma (Gk II, 147, 5–6 ποτὲ μὲν γὰρ ἄρχεται ἀπὸ θερμῆς δυσκρασίας, ἔσθ' ὅτε δὲ καὶ ἀπὸ ψυχρᾶς)

θ″ twice substitutes *ex* for *a* (ἀπό).

2.1.2 et secundum humorum superfluentium <qualitates> similiter exist*it* (scil. *tussis*): humorum superfluentium γ humores superfluentes P3 Ma, humorum superfluitates *cett.* (Gk II, 147, 7–8 καὶ καθ' ὕλην ἐπίρρυτον ὡσαύτως συνίσταται)

As if with knowledge of both variants, θ″ retains the adjectival participle of γ′ but corrects it to an accusative after *secundum*.

2.3.1 Tussiunt etiam plurimi ex frigida distemperantia: Si autem tussis ex frigida distemperantia ... fit P3 Ma (Gk II, 149, 2 ὅσοι δὲ βήσσουσι διὰ ψυχρὰν δυσκρασίαν)

θ″ completely rewrites this sentence, making it a conditional clause dependent on the statement of symptoms which follows.

2.5.2 Vnde et ex quibus transmittitur locis, haec omnia utique contemplari oportet: *om.* P3 Ma (Gk II, 149, 16–17 ὅθεν δὲ καὶ ἐξ ὁποίων ἐπιπέμπονται μορίων, κἀνταῦθα διορίζεσθαι δεῖ καὶ προσέχειν)

θ″ omits the opening of this sentence, if not by accident then on the grounds that this question was mentioned in the previous sentence.

2.7.2 si nihil dignum sputent uix respirantes, flegmonem necesse est de his omnibus signis suspicari nos in pulmone esse factum: uix digne respirantes P3 Ma φ[28] (Gk II, 149, 5–6 εἰ καὶ μηδὲν ἄξιον ἀναπτύεται δυσπνοούντων αὐτῶν, φλεγμονὴν ἐξ ἀνάγκης ἐκ πάντων τούτων ὑποπτεύειν ἡμᾶς περὶ τὸν πνεύμονα γεγενῆσθαι προσήκει)

θ″ erroneously repeats (a form of) *dignum* with *respirantes*.

2.7.3 et adhuc magis existimari oportet ignitum esse flegmonem in pulmone: *om.* P3 Ma (Gk II, 151 ἔτι καὶ μᾶλλον ὑπονοεῖν δεῖ ζέουσαν εἶναι τὴν φλεγμονὴν περὶ τὸν πνεύμονα)

θ″ omits *et adhuc magis*.

[27] Puschmann reports L ἄλλοτε in place of ποτὲ, and I wonder whether the translator's Greek text might not have had ἀλλ' ὅτι, whence *sed quoniam*.

[28] φ erroneously eliminates the first *dignum*.

2.11.6–8 +– de curis aliqua breuiter dicere non omittamus –+. Ad autem facile inueniend*um*, per partes ad tussem adiutoria et expedientia et a multis probata scribam. Vnde in sequenti generaliter curas et ipsas differentias uobis exponam, ut non alibi indigentes adiutoria requiratis:

P3 de curis (*corr. ex* cura m2) aliqua (*corr. ex* aliqual *pro* aliquid) breuiter dicere non obmittamus <*add.* m2 *in marg.*: Ad hec enim facile inuenienda sunt per partes ad tussem adiutoria expedientia et a multis probata> ut non alibi adiutoria requirantur unde in consequenti generaliter curas <scribam *add. in marg.* m3> et ipsarum differentias uobis exponam <ut non alibi indigentes adiutoria requiratis *add. in marg.* m2>.

P3′ de cura aliquid breuiter dicere non obmittamus ut non alibi adiutoria requirantur unde in consequenti generaliter curas et ipsarum differentias uobis exponam.

Ma de cura aliquid breuiter dicere non omittamus ut non alibi adiutoria requirantur unde in consequenti generaliter curas et ipsas differentias uobis exponam.

(Gk II, 155, 22–8 πρὸς δὲ τὸ εὐχερῶς εὑρίσκειν τὰς κατὰ μέρος ὕλας τῶν βηχικῶν βοηθημάτων καὶ ἁρμόζειν δύνασθαι +–πρὸς τὴν ὑπὸ τῆς διαγνώσεως ὑπαγορευομένην διάθεσιν–+, ἀκόλουθον ἐνόμισα +–μετὰ τὰς διαγνώσεις καὶ τὴν καθόλου ἀγωγὴν καὶ τὰς διαφορὰς –+ ὑμῖν ἐκθέσθαι τῶν βοηθημάτων μετὰ τῆς ἀκριβοῦς αὐτῶν συσταθμίας, ὥστε μὴ παρ' ἑτέρου δεῖσθαι μανθάνειν, +–ἀλλ' ἐντεῦθεν ἀναλέγεσθαι τὸ ζητούμενον–+)

θ″ significantly revised the end of this chapter, as we see by comparing Ma with the original text of P3 (P3′ above). Note: *cura* for *curis*; *aliquid* for *aliqua*; the omission of a sentence after *non obmittamus*(!); the transposition of the last two clauses (*unde* ... and *ut non* ...); *in consequenti* for *in sequenti*;[29] the omission of *indigentes*. P3′ and Ma are almost identical, and very different from any other surviving copy (including P1 and M, so that it is not likely that γ′ was the model for the revision).[30]

2.36.2 Contingit autem his quibus pessimi et uenenosi cum mordicatione stomachi ibidem colliguntur humores: ibidem colliguntur humores cum mordicatione P3′ Ma stomachi *add. in marg.* P3 m4 (Gk II, 279, 19–21 συμβαίνει δὲ τοῦτο, εἰ μοχθηροὶ καὶ δακνώδεις καὶ ἰώδεις ἀθροισθῶσιν ἢ συρρεύσωσιν ἐν τῷ στόματι τῆς γαστρὸς χυμοί)

θ″ reversed the order of the two three-word phrases (*cum mordicatione stomachi* and *ibidem colliguntur humores*) and omitted what was then the last word, *stomachi*.

2.37.4 Ceterum autem oportet eis addere paulatim cibos qui tarde digeruntur: Oportet autem eis dare cibos paulatim P3 Ma (P3 notes the variant *addere*, which *cett.* have except P1 M *adhibere*) (Gk II, 281, 15–16 λοιπὸν δὲ δεῖ προστιθέναι κατὰ μέρος αὐτοῖς, ὅσα δυσμετάβλητά εἰσι)

θ″ must have: (a) omitted *ceterum* and fronted *oportet*; (b) substituted *dare* for *addere*; (c) transposed *paulatim* and *cibos*.

[29] I write these as two words for the purpose of showing how the variant arose.

[30] The text against which P3 was corrected was close to κ′ or φ, which alone have *scribam* before *curas*, and of our surviving copies closest to Ge (note *ad hec enim facile*, and *ipsarum differentias*).

2.37.12 scio autem quia et anacardia antidotum ad tales passiones benefacit et pigra datum iuuat sed nullum sic sicut glicea adiuuat (Gk II, 283, 2–5 οἶδα δὲ, ὅτι καὶ ἡ δι' ἀνακαρδίων πρὸς τὰ τοιαῦτα ποιεῖ καὶ ἡ πικρὰ, ἀλλ' οὐδὲν οὕτως (?) ὡς τὸ βοήθημα τοῦτο)

Ma Scio autem quia et antidotum hoc in plurimis aliis passionibus iuuat et pigra datum et
P3 [S. a. q. *add. ante* et pigra] plurimis aliis passionibus iuuat et pigra datum et
Ma anacardion iuuat sed non sicut glicea.
P3 anacardi<n>on iuuat sed non sicut glicea.

θ″ has revised this sentence in several important respects, and P3 and Ma reflect knowledge of the same, radically-altered model. Notice: (a) the order and placement of *anacardia* and *pigra*; (b) *plurimis aliis passionibus* for *ad tales passiones*; (c) the sequence of verbs *iuuat – iuuat – NOTHING* for *benefacit – iuuat – adiuuat*; (d) *non* for *nullum*. Each of these features is exclusive to, and identical in, P3 and Ma.

2.82 – 86 – 83 – 87 *order of chapters*

θ″ transposes chs 83 (*De lacte dando*) and 86 (*De cibo dissintericorum*) of Book 2 (chs 84 and 85 being inventions of φ: see 4.5).

4.4.5. κ Errs

When D and Ge are not following λ, they appear to follow another daughter of θ, κ, which is also the source of Ox. The evidence for κ is, I confess, rather thin, mainly no doubt because D and Ge are contaminated, but it is still more than adequate to require the reconstruction of a further lost copy. (In addition to the passages set out below, note 2.158.6 in 4.4.1 and 2.271.13 under 4.3.3 above.)

1.87.3 mitigat et digerit satis igneos oculorum flegmones: totum igneum D Ox totos igneos L2 | flegmonem D Ox (*uerba* satis *et* oculorum *om.* Ox) (Gk II, 7, 7 πραΰνει καὶ συμπέττει τὰς πάνυ ζεούσας τῶν ὀφθαλμῶν φλεγμονὰς)

κ replaces *satis igneos ... flegmones* with *totum igneum ... flegmonem*. The fact that D has both *satis* and *totum* (and L2, *satis totos*), while Ox has just *totum*, perhaps suggests that *totum* had been added to κ (or earlier) in such a way that it could be, but need not be, read as a gloss or correction. I cannot explain the near-agreement of L2, which diminishes the probative power of this example for the establishment of κ.

1.87.4 postquam autem repressum fuerit reuma, cum melilota crocus et glaucion ... superponantur: tunc D Ox (Gk II, 7, 10–11 τὸ αὐτὸ δὲ ποιοῦσι καὶ οἱ φοίνικες μετὰ τοῦ ἐπέχειν τὸν ἐπιφερόμενον ῥευματισμὸν μετὰ τῶν μελιλώτων (τοῦ –ου?) καὶ κρόκου καὶ γλαυκίων (–ου? *Fischer*))[31]

κ interprets *cum* as the conjunction, and substitutes *tunc* in order to have a main clause after the subordinate *postquam*-clause.

2.9.1 Quod si fyma meditauerit fieri in pulmone: fuerit D Ox (Gk II, 151, 26 Εἴπερ εἴη φῦμα [μὴ] μελετηθὲν ἐν τῷ πνεύμονι)

(On this passage, see above, 4.4.3.) θ (whether or not following γ′) substitutes *fuerit* for the main verb phrase and puts it at the end of the clause (*in pulmone fuerit* in θ″ and O). κ moves *fuerit* away from the end of the clause, perhaps to prevent its juxtaposition with *erit*, which begins the next clause (*erit omnino difficultas spirandi*).

[31] There are surely things wrong with the Greek text at this point, including ἑπτά probably for ἑφθά, participle of ἕψω. I am indebted to Cloudy Fischer for helpful discussion of these points.

2.11.6 Redeamus igitur et de cura aliqua breuiter dicere non omittamus: Redeamus ad tussem D Ox (not in Gk II, 155, 22)

κ inserts *ad tussem* in this resumptive sentence which takes us back from the case-report of the man who coughed up a stone to remedies for the treatment of coughing.

2.236.2 extenduntur et nerui quos sindismos uocant dolores facere in pedibus solent nimios: neruis D Ox Ge | solet Ox Ge P3 *ex corr.* (Gk II, 501, 20–1 καὶ διατεῖνον αὐτά τε καὶ τοὺς συνδέσμους ὀδύνην ἐργάζεσθαι πέφυκε σφοδράν)

Whatever the Latin was at this point, D, Ox and Ge all replace *nerui* (subject of *solent*?) with *neruis* (presumably dative of disadvantage after *sanguis* ... *dolores facere* ... *solet*). The change of *solent* to *solet*, more or less required by *neruis*, is made by Ox and Ge (κ′), for some reason not by D. (The corrector of P3 must have taken *et nerui* with *extenduntur*.)

2.271.1 Haec ergo per os sunt danda quae mitigare possunt dolores: per os sunt danda γ η G1 P3] sunt danda θ′ danda sunt D Ox danda L2 (Gk II, 573, 25 Ταῦτα μὲν οὖν παρηγορεῖν οἶδε διδόμενα διὰ στόματος)

The abbreviated writing of *p(er) os sunt* led to the phrase being read as *possunt* and corrected to *sunt*.[32] κ transposes *sunt danda*.

2.271.9 turpidinem piscem maritimum uiuum: turpitudinem de D Ox Ge B (Gk II, 575, 20 τουρπαίνης θαλασσίας ζώσης)

The writing of *turpitudo* for *turpido* looks like an error in κ, although it is shared also with B. The preposition *de*, also in L2 and Ma, and before the *turp*. word in G1 and P3, presumably reflects *id est*, which is in ϕ, and which was probably already in ε (note that P2 has a small erasure after *turpidine*, made perhaps after consultation of δ: on P2 and δ, see 4.7.1).

4.4.6. κ′ Errs (Ox and Ge)

As we have seen, λ was one of the models of Ge, which as a result in places (e.g. 1.85ff.) agrees with Ma in particular. In most of the passages collated from Book 2, however, Ge agrees closely with Ox, often very strikingly. Since Ge shares errors with D and Ox, and thus appears to be a descendant of κ, these agreements with Ox are ascribed provisionally to a lost descendant of κ, κ′ in the stemma. An alternative account would be to take them as features of κ, and assume that D uses another source in these places. (In addition to the passages set out here, note also 1.19.6 under 4.7.1 below.)

2.10.4 Sunt autem et alia de quibus in sequenti dicturi sumus, ubi de ulceratione et ruptione uenarum et diabroseos cogemur scribere: dicemus Ox Ge ϕ | dicturi sumus Ox Ge ϕ, dicturi sumus (sumus uel G1) cogimur scribere G1 P3 (Gk II, 153, 16–18 εἰσὶ δὲ καὶ ἄλλα, περὶ ὧν ὕστερον λεχθήσεται, ἔνθα καὶ περὶ ἑλκώσεως καὶ ῥήξεως καὶ διαβρώσεως ἀναγκαζόμεθα γράφειν)

[32] The fact that G1 and P3 have the correct reading makes it likely that θ had *possunt* (perhaps from γ′), which was wrongly changed by κ but correctly restored by the immediate common ancestor of G1 and P3 (while MaGe took *sunt danda* from λ).

It looks as if the common source of Ox, Ge and P3′ (θ? with Ma D following λ?) erroneously repeats *dicturi sumus* from the previous clause in place of *cogimur scribere*. κ′, here followed by φ, achieves variation by replacing the first *dicturi sumus* with the synthetic future *dicemus*. P3 is able to improve this by adding *cogimur scribere* from a second source (not θ″, if θ was the source of the error in the first place, but λ?). Note the agreement in error of G1 with P3 (see 4.7.3).[33]

2.235.2–5 ideo nullo modo ab artificibus medicinae sanari potest quia eius ignoratur natiuitas. (3) ego autem existimo ut quicumque bene potuerit natiuitatem cognoscere uel ... species quaecumque fiunt ... bene et cito posse curare et facilius a medicis ... liberari (4) et sic postea curationes ipsas exponemus. (5) Credo enim quia si ea quae scripta tradimus diligentius attendantur [naturam uniuscuiusque] [uoluerit operari], multos poterit liberare: nullo modo ideo Ox Ge | eius *om.* Ox Ge | fiunt *om.* Ox Ge | a medicis et facile Ox Ge | ipsas *om.* Ox Ge | quia *om.* Ox Ge | naturam uniuscuiusque *om.* Ox Ge

I deliberately run several sentences together in order to show a series of agreements between Ox and Ge in rearrangements of, and omissions from the inherited text. Note also that towards the end of the passage from 2.236.2 quoted in 4.4.5 above, Ox and Ge alone have *solet in pedibus*; in 2.236.4 Ox and Ge alone have *ledens eodem modo* (*eodem modo ledens* cett.); in 2.236.5 Ox and Ge alone omit *mediocris/mediocriter* before *commotio*; in 2.236.6 Ox and Ge alone have *solam simplicem* (*simplicem solam* cett.), and they alone omit *aut calido et humido* from the list of types of *duplicata distemperantia*.

In 2.271 there are similar exclusive agreements between Ox and Ge, although less numerous. They alone have 2.271.5 *infundes in aquam* (for *in aqua(m) infundes*); they alone omit all of 2.271.12, and they alone insert *autem* after 2.271.13 *Sufficiat* (*Sufficiant* κ φ ?O).

4.5. THE φ-RECENSION (G2 *ed.* L1)

The φ-recension was the latest and the most thorough-going. There are innovations exclusive to G2, L1 and *ed.* in almost every section of every chapter collated. Many are quite minor, but a good number involve important changes affecting vocabulary, word-order, and syntax, as well as insertions of new material, some of these extensive.

That G2, L1 and *ed.* are very closely related is immediately apparent from collation of even a short section of text. Provisionally, I represent L1 and *ed.* as in effect daughters of G2 because, while *ed.* and L1 each has many errors exclusive to itself (see section 4.9 below), I have yet to find places where G2 errs significantly and independently of *ed.* and L1. Lost copy φ survives from the time when I regarded G2, L1 and *ed.* as sisters. If G2 is correctly represented as the ancestor of L1 and *ed.*, φ may be otiose. For the moment, I retain it as a convenient shorthand reference to this family.

In the following paragraphs, I first of all list innovations more or less peculiar to φ, and then (4.6) consider the sources of φ, of which there are at least two.

[33] Although in this particular case the agreement could be independent, in that the error could be essentially dittographic (the repetition of *dicturi sumus*) and corrected by each copyist taking another look at the exemplar. I owe this observation to Michael Reeve.

1.85.10 [*ante* Prouidendum est autem unde prorumpat quod supercurrit:] Quandoque enim contingit passio quia uitium est in qualitate humoris sola .i. quando est humor maliciosus sed non multus quandoque e conuerso quandoque utroque modo: *haec verba habent soli* G2 *ed.* L1 (not in the Gk II, 5, 9)

ϕ inserts a long sentence of explanation not in the Greek original nor anywhere else in the Latin tradition.

2.36.2 Contingit autem his quibus pessimi et uenenosi cum mordicatione stomachi ibidem colliguntur humores: generantur ϕ (Gk II, 279, 19–21 συμβαίνει δὲ τοῦτο, εἰ μοχθηροὶ καὶ δακνώδεις καὶ ἰώδεις ἀθροισθῶσιν ἢ συρρεύσωσιν ἐν τῷ στόματι τῆς γαστρὸς χυμοί)

ϕ substitutes the banal *generantur* for the more accurate *colliguntur* (ἀθροισθῶσιν).

2.36.3 lumbrici saepius superiora petentes ex inferioribus partibus ad stomachum necesse est ut faciant cardiacam passionem: superiora sepius ϕ superiora G1 C (Gk II, 279, 23–5 πολλάκις δὲ καὶ ἕλμινθες ἐκ τῶν κάτω μερῶν ἀναδραμόντες ἐπὶ τὸ στόμα τῆς γαστρὸς ἐργάζονται καρδιακὰς διαθέσεις)

ϕ transposes *saepius* and *superiora*.

2.36.3 ex inferioribus partibus ad stomachum: stomacho ϕ, stomachi θ″ κ (Gk II, 279, 24 ἐπὶ τὸ στόμα τῆς γαστρός)

(For a fuller text, see 4.4.3) ϕ 'improves' what is seen as a faulty construction *facere passionem ad* + accusative by substituting the dative for *ad* + accusative.

2.37.1 Nam qui habent in stomacho mordicationem de malignis humoribus et propterea sincopos patiuntur [Cap. 37. Curatio cardiace] inprimis oportet eis cibos offerri: (Gk II, 281, 5–7 τοῖς οὖν ἔχουσι μοχθηροὺς καὶ δακνώδεις ἐν τῷ στόματι τῆς γαστρὸς χυμοὺς καὶ διὰ τοῦτο συγκοπῆναι κινδυνεύουσιν ἁρμόζει πρῶτον αὐτοῖς ἁπάντων ἐκεῖνα τῶν ἐδεσμάτων προσφέρειν)

ϕ disastrously misplaces the title of what then becomes ch. 37 of Book 2 in the middle of the first sentence![34]

2.75=2.84–5

ϕ erroneously repeats ch. 2.75 (*De potionibus et cathaplasmatibus ad epaticam dissinteriam*) in the intrusive chapters (which occur only in ϕ) 2.84 (*De potionibus ad epaticam dissinteriam*) and 2.85 (*De embroca et cathaplasmate ad calidam epatis distemperantiam*).

2.158.7 Anastomosin autem dicunt cum ora uenarum uirtute amissa apertiora effecta et laxiora sanguinem refundunt intrinsecus et sic aut uomitur aut per uentrem deducitur in secessus: extrinsecus G2 *ed.* exterius L1 (not in Gk II, 187, 11)

ϕ substitutes *extrinsecus* for *intrinsecus*; the latter is probably correct, as this is surely a reference to internal bleeding (although it is possible that the writer had in mind blood getting *out of* the vein[35]).

2.235.5 multos poterit liberare, et non solum eos quibus mox ab initio curationem adhibet curationem: exhibet ϕ (Gk II, 501, 16–17 ὠφελήσει πολλοὺς οὐ μόνον τοὺς ἀρχὴν ἔχοντας εἰς τὸ πάθος)

[34] B, L2 and D have this title a little later (before 2.37.2 *Infrigidant igitur*), G1 and P3 (rightly) a little earlier, before 2.37.1 *Nam qui habent in stomacho* . . ., where, according to Puschmann, p. 281 n. 1, the Greek manuscripts have the title Περὶ καρδιαλγίας; P3 has *Curatio cardiacorum*, of which there is perhaps a reflection in Ma's otherwise inexplicable *quorum*, for *qui*. P3 also has *Curatio cardiacorum* where ϕ has it, and in red, but it is here deleted in black. In the same place, Ge has *Cura* in red.

[35] I owe this observation to Cloudy Fischer.

φ substitutes *exhibet* for *adhibet*.

2.236.t. [*ante* Multa igitur sunt uitia:] Cap. 236 De causis podagre: *haec verba habent soli* G2 *ed.* L1 (not in Gk II, 501, 18)

φ inserts a chapter-break and a title occurring nowhere else in the Latin tradition nor in the Greek original.

2.236.6 Non enim solum oportet ut supercurrente materia reumatismi solent fieri sed et per simplicem solam qualitatem efficitur: *om.* φ (Gk II, 503, 2–3 οὐ μόνον δὲ διὰ ἐπίρροιαν ὕλης οἱ ῥευματισμοὶ τοῖς ἄρθροις ἐπιγίνεσθαι πεφύκασιν, ἀλλὰ καὶ διὰ ψιλὴν ποιότητα μόνην)

φ omits *solam*.

4.6. THE SOURCES OF φ

φ appears to represent a recension which employed more than one exemplar of the text. One exemplar must have derived from κ, and must have been particularly close to Ox and Ge. Another source of φ must have been close to θ″, and especially to P3. (There are possibly one or two hints that B was a third source of φ: I list them in 4.8.9 below, but remain to be convinced that they merit even a dotted line on the stemma.) It is noteworthy that, while φ has many γ-errors and many good γ-readings, it never agrees alone with γ, but nearly always with Ox and/or P3 as well.

4.6.1. φ AND κ (OR κ′)

2.1.1 quoniam initium habet (scil. *tussis*) modo a calida distemperantia, est autem quando a frigida aut humida aut etiam sicca: modo a (modo de D) D Ox Ge φ (Gk II, 147, 5–6 ποτὲ μὲν γὰρ ἄρχεται ἀπὸ θερμῆς δυσκρασίας, ἔσθ' ὅτε δὲ καὶ ἀπὸ ψυχρᾶς ἢ ξηρᾶς ἢ ὑγρᾶς)

κ and φ match the Latin form of the second alternative to that of the first (*modo a* X, *modo a* Y).

2.1.4 de qua re oportet nos accedere cum omni studio: nos oportet Ox φ | attendere Ox φ accendere D (Gk II, 147, 12–13 δεῖ καὶ ἡμᾶς ἐλθεῖν μετὰ πάσης σπουδῆς)

Ox and φ transpose *nos* and *oportet*, and substitute *attendere* for *accedere* (Greek ἐλθεῖν). *attendere* may be a correction (by Ox followed by φ?) of *accendere* (in D and perhaps in κ).

2.1.4 oportet nos accedere cum omni studio ad cognoscendam uniuscuiusque ueritatem: uarietatem Mu C ε *praeter* B, tussis uarietatem Ox φ (nothing corresponding in the Gk II, 147, 13–14[36])

Ox and φ insert *tussis* before *uarietatem*, the latter a corruption of *ueritatem* (in view of its distribution, a polygenetic corruption, I think — but that may be cowardice on my part).

2.2.1 Quod si de calida distemperantia pura uel simplici generata fuerit tussis: sola Ox φ (Gk II, 147, 17 ψιλῆς τοίνυν οὔσης τῆς θερμῆς δυσκρασίας)

Ox and φ substitute *sola* for *pura*.

[36] However, Cloudy Fischer suggests that Latin *uniuscuiusque* may somehow reflect a part of Greek ὁποῖος for ποιούσης.

2.2.1 For the text and variants, see 4.7.3 below.

For *sentiunt enim merito*, the reading of Ox *et in inicio sentiunt* is strikingly similar to *et merito sentiunt* in φ. I would suggest that Ox and φ found *et merito sentiunt* in their common source, and that Ox then attempted to make some sense of the phrase.

2.3.1 Tussiunt etiam plurimi ex frigida distemperantia: quam plurimi Ox C φ (Gk II, 149, 2 ὅσοι δὲ βήσσουσι διὰ ψυχρὰν δυσκρασίαν)

Ox and φ (and presumably independently C) replace *plurimi* with *quam plurimi*, a common phrase in our translation.

2.3.4 Sic enim ex frigida distemperantia cognoscitur generata tussis: tussis generata cognoscitur Ox Ge tussis esse generata cognoscitur φ (Gk II, 149, 8–9 οὕτω μὲν αἱ διὰ ψυχρὰν αἰτίαν ἢ θερμὴν διαγινώσκονται βῆχες)

κ′ (Ox and Ge) transposes *cognoscitur generata tussis*, and φ takes this new word-order and inserts *esse*, thus making a nominative + infinitive construction.

2.4.2–5.1 materiales autem [si accesserit tussis] amitroteras, et non oportet <t>alia iterum dicere. ... (5. 1) Supercurrente igitur materia efficitur tussis: tussis efficitur Ox φ (Gk II, 149, 12–14 διαφέρουσι δὲ τοῦ μᾶλλον τὰς δραστικὰς ἔχειν ἐναργέστατα σημεῖα, τὰς δὲ ὑλικὰς ἀμυδρότερα. καὶ οὐ χρὴ ταὐτὰ πάλιν λέγειν)

The Latin tradition offers various explanatory notes to Greek ἀμυδρότερα, among which Ox and φ alone have *facilis ad cognoscendum*. Ox and φ also transpose *efficitur* and *tussis*.

2.5.2 et attendere seu de capite fluit qui mouet tussem, siue ex altero membro: qui γ η P3′ humor qui P3 (*add.* m2) Ge φ quod G1 P2 L2 B Ma D Ox (Gk II, 149, 17–18 καὶ προσέχειν εἴτε ἐκ τῆς κεφαλῆς ἐπιρρεῖ τὸ κινοῦν τὴν βῆχα εἴτε καὶ ἐξ ἑτέρων)

Ge, φ and the first corrector of P3 alone insert *humor*, necessary to make sense of *qui*. The Greek text would speak for the indeterminate neuter pronoun. (Neater Latin would be <*id*> *quod*, avoiding the possibility of taking *quod* with *capite*.[37]) This and the next passage pose a problem for the stemma, requiring one of two additional hypotheses for which I have little, if any, independent evidence: *either* these innovations are of λ, Ma and D here follow θ″ and κ, respectively, and (additional hypothesis 1) P3 knew λ; *or* they are of θ, Ma and D here follow λ, and (additional hypothesis 2) Ox had an accessory source. I am at present at a loss.

2.5.3 Etenim pulmo suscipit primum, est autem quando et thorax et latera uel praecordia et alia altera patiuntur membra: thorax suscipit Ge φ (Gk II, 149, 19–20 καὶ γὰρ ὁ πνεύμων ἀδικεῖται πολλάκις· πρῶτος γάρ ἐστιν, εἶτα ὁ θώραξ ἢ πλευρὸν ἢ τὸ διάφραγμα ἢ ἄλλο τι μόριον)

Ge and φ alone repeat the first main verb (*suscipit*) in the second clause. This and the next passage would seem to confirm the proximity of Ge to the κ-source of φ (but see the comment at the end of the preceding passage).

2.7.t.–2.7.1 Signa si de capite in pulmonem fluat (7.1) Quod si in pulmonem fluat: fluat humor P3 Ge φ | Quod si amplius Ge φ (nothing corresponding at Gk II, 151, 1 Φλεγμονῆς ἐν τῷ πνεύμονι σημείωσις)

Ge, φ and P3 alone insert *humor* (as in 2.5.2 above). Ge and φ alone add *amplius*.

[37] I owe this suggestion to Cloudy Fischer.

4.6.2. ϕ AND θ'', ESPECIALLY P3

2.1.4 Propter quod non una est causa tussis sed uaria: quoniam G1 P3 Ma ϕ (Gk II, 147, 12 ἐπεὶ οὖν οὐ μίαν αἰτίαν ἡ βὴξ, ἀλλὰ ποικίλην κέκτηται)

θ'' (and in this case G1) and ϕ replace *propter quod* with *quoniam.*

2.5.1 et exinde nascentiam tussis habet: tussis nascitur P3 Ma ϕ (Gk II, 149, 16 αἱ βῆχες ... τὴν γένεσιν ἔχουσιν)

θ'' and ϕ replace *nascentiam tussis habet* with the simpler *tussis nascitur.*

2.5.5 et omnino nihil praetermitti debet de tusse: praetermittendum est P3 Ma praetermittendum ϕ (Gk II, 149, 22 ὡς πανταχόθεν ἀπαράλειπτον εἶναι τὸν περὶ τῆς βηχὸς λόγον)

θ'' and ϕ replace *praetermitti debet* with *praetermittendum (est).*

2.7.3 Si autem et sitis sit nimia, et frequenter ad haec signa et calor sentiatur multus in thorace: calor multus sentitur P3 Ma ϕ (Gk II, 151, 6 εἰ δὲ καὶ δίψη σφοδρᾷ συνέχοιτο πρὸς τοῖς σημείοις τούτοις καὶ θέρμης αἴσθησις αὐτῷ γίνοιτο πολλὴ περὶ τὸν θώρακα)

θ'' and ϕ eliminate the hyperbaton (and the subjunctive) in *calor sentiatur multus.* (On this passage, see also 4.4.3 above.)

2.37.2 si is qui patitur sit temperantia satis calida, et in eius stomacho contineantur humores mordicantes et acres nimis: si in stomacho P3 ϕ (Gk II, 281, 12–14 εἴπερ οἱ πάσχοντες ἦσαν τῇ κράσει θερμοὶ πάνυ καὶ οἱ περιεχόμενοι χυμοὶ δακνώδεις καὶ δριμεῖς ἄγαν)

P3 and ϕ alone omit *eius* and make a second conditional clause.

2.271.12 coques autem oleum sicut dictum est in hospitio pede plano mense Martio quinta feria: die iouis γ, feria quinta P3 ϕ (Gk II, 575, 27–8 ἕψε δὲ τὸ ἔλαιον, ὡς προγέγραπται, ἐν οἰκήματι κατωγαίῳ μηνὶ μαρτίῳ πέμπτῃ)

P3 and ϕ alone transpose *quinta* and *feria.*

4.7. THE PRINCIPAL CASES OF APPARENT CONTAMINATION

The tradition of the Latin Alexander is enormously complicated by contamination. In my judgement, (apart from the recension represented by ϕ, at the very end of the manuscript tradition of the text) two of the daughters of η (O and C) and all but one (B) of the descendants of ε made more or less extensive use of an accessory model (the most extensive contamination being apparent in, from left to right, C, P2, G1 and P3). Of the ε-family, P2 appears to have known a copy close to δ, while at a lower level G1, a daughter of θ', shares errors on the one hand with C (daughter of η), and on the other hand with daughters of θ'', P3 in particular, and lower still L2 may be represented as following now G1 and now P3.

These individual cases apart, the single most important aspect of the contamination of this tradition lies in the presence of readings characteristic of γ (or β) in O on the one hand and in nearly all of the descendants of θ on the other. On the stemma I have represented all of these cases of contamination as due to the accessory use of a lost daughter of γ, γ', probably a sister of M, but the truth may of course have been much more complicated.

The contaminations, perhaps inevitably, have seriously delayed the present account of the relations between the manuscripts, and even now I can neither pretend to have identified every case of contamination, nor be sure that I have nowhere called polygenesis contamination. For now, I present the clearest instances illustrating the main lines of contamination in turn. I hope and trust that, as work on the edition proceeds, collation of further passages will bring further clarification of the uncertainties that I have tried to signal in my notes on the passages discussed in this chapter, and in the remaining problems noted in 4.8 below.

4.7.1. P2 AND δ

To begin with ε, we find a number of significant secondary readings shared by a group comprising all (or nearly all) the descendants of ε except P2. At an earlier stage of this project, I considered the possibility that not P2 but θ′ was contaminated, i.e. that P2 was a second source of θ′, intermediate between ε and θ′, with a sister (then called ζ) the immediate ancestor of θ′ and θ. Since, however, P2 agrees with δ rather than with ε when not agreeing with θ′, I think we must take it that P2 had an accessory model in a descendant of δ higher than ε, which we may as well call δ.

1.19.6 Ceterum autem et quae praecesserunt causae, seu temperantia aegrotantis: considerande sunt cause G1 C L2 B P3 D φ cause sunt considerande Ma (considerande sunt *habet* P2 *in marg.*) cause attendere oportet (a. o. *s. s.* Ge) Ox Ge | distemperantia ε *praeter* P2 P3 Ox′ Ge (Gk I, 463, 12–13 λοιπὸν δὲ καὶ τὰ προηγησάμενα αἴτια, ἥ τε κρᾶσις τοῦ πάσχοντος)

ε inserts *considerandae sunt* (altered to *attendere oportet* by κ′ (Ox Ge)) in order to make a complete sentence, but γ and η have the same verbless sentence as the Greek, which must be original. ε or θ′ also changes *temperantia* to *distemperantia* (γ′ showing the correct reading to θ and hence P3 and Ox′). In both cases, P2 agrees with, and is presumably following, δ.

1.19.8 sed et tactu cognoscere poteris: cognosci potest G1 L2 B Ma D Ge (Gk I, 463, 16 ἀπὸ τῆς ἁφῆς δὲ διαγινώσκειν ἐστί σοι δυνατόν)

θ′ (except P2) and λ (followed by Ma D Ge) change *cognoscere poteris* to *cognosci potest*. P2 follows δ, and Ox and P3 (and hence φ) follow θ.

1.85.9 Fit [et]enim plenitudo materiae supercurrens ut solum ex hoc uideas fieri dolorem et qualitate, saepius autem ex utrisque fit, ex qualitate scilicet et ex quantitate: *post* supercurrens *habent verba* dolorem efficit G1 B D dolorem facit C uel ita Ma Ge | *post* qualitate *habent* dolores efficiunt Ma dolorem efficit Ge | ut solum ex *om.* G1 C D (Gk II, 5, 7–9 καὶ πλῆθος ὕλης ἐπιρρέον μόνον οἶδε ποιεῖν ὀδύνην καὶ ποιότης, πολλάκις δὲ καὶ τὸ συναμφότερον, καὶ ποιότης ἅμα καὶ ποσότης)

After *supercurrens*, θ′ (G1 and B, here followed by C) and D have ‘causes pain’, Ma and Ge have *uel ita* here and ‘cause(s) pain’ later, after *qualitate* (and φ in fact adds a longer explanatory note after *quantitate*). Presumably, Ma D Ge here follow λ, P2 here follows δ, P3 and Ox follow θ (and L2 follows P3?).

1.87.3 Lac mulieris cum oui uitello et oleo roseo superpositum +– –+ mitigat: uitello cocto (coctum P3 cocta D) θ′ C θ″ κ (Gk II, 7, 6 Γάλα γυναικὸς μετὰ κρόκων ᾠῶν καὶ ῥοδίνου διατιθέμενον +–θαυμαστῶς–+ πραΰνει)

ε inserts *cocto* (although curiously it is added in P3 Ma Ge, and is not in L2 or φ), but P2 follows δ.

1.87.4 A*d* autem <eum> cui cum nimio flegmone uel tumore ingenti +– dolor fuerit ortus –+ bene facit crocus: Quando autem cum nimio G1 C P3 Ma Ge Ox Quando autem cum non nimio L2 B φ At autem cui cum (cum om. O) nimio A O Mu At autem cui non nimio P2 Quod si cui cum nimio D aut (aut om. M) qui cum nimio P1 M (Gk II, 7, 8–9 πρὸς δὲ τὰς μεγίστας φλεγμονὰς καὶ ἐν ὄγκῳ μείζονι ποιεῖ καὶ ὁ κρόκος)

ε replaces *At* with *Quando* and loses the relative pronoun, while P2 follows δ. After *At autem*, *cui cum* is probably right (as this sequence is also in γ), although *cui* lacks an antecedent.[38] (For further details, see my provisional text in 4.10.3 and notes ad loc.)

2.10.1 s*ed* habent etiam quendam raucorem cum tusse, interea et proiciunt humores: interius ε (*cum* O C) *praeter* P2 (Gk II, 153, 9–10 ἔχῃ δέ τινα κέρχνον μετὰ βηχὸς, ἔσθ' ὅτε δὲ καὶ ἀναγωγὴν ὑγροῦ)

ε erroneously substitutes *interius* for *interea*, but P2 follows δ. While *interius* makes perfectly good sense, *interea* 'sometimes' (cf. 5.4, note ad loc.) is clearly demanded by the Greek (ἔσθ' ὅτε).

2.37.1 oportet eis cibos offerri qui et refrigerandi habeant aliquid et confortare possint: uirtutem ε *praeter* P2 (Gk II, 281, 7–8 ἁρμόζει πρῶτον αὐτοῖς ἁπάντων ἐκεῖνα τῶν ἐδεσμάτων προσφέρειν, ὅσα μετὰ τοῦ ψύχειν ἔτι (ἔχει τι M) καὶ ῥωννύειν δύναται)

With *habeant aliquid* cf. the reading of Greek ms. M ἔχει τι,[39] although Latin *et* ... *et* nicely translates Greek μετὰ ... ἔτι καί. The substitution of *uirtutem* for *aliquid* makes the text clearer and no less idiomatic. Once introduced, *uirtutem* was not likely to be corrected, and hence neatly characterizes ε, although again P2 follows δ.

2.37.4 quaecumque ... uincere possunt malos qui continentur humores: malos humores qui continentur ε *praeter* P2 Ox (Gk II, 281, 19–20 ὅσα δύνανται ... νικᾶν τὴν κρατοῦσαν κακοχυμίαν)

The hyperbaton is so much a feature of the translator's style that we can be confident that ε or θ′ has here normalized. P2 either reintroduced the hyperbaton himself, or took it from δ.[40]

2.37.7 aut mela aut citri deforis mundaturam: citri β P2 citrie η P2′ citr(i)um *cett.* | mundaturam (mundati ad P1) β η mundatum ε mundati P2 (Gk II, 281, 24 ἢ μῆλον ἢ κίτρον ἐκτὸς τοῦ λέπους αὐτοῦ)

The reinterpretation (thanks to the writing of *-tur-* as *t̃*) of the last word as a past participle in agreement with *citr(i)um* — 'peeled on the outside' rather than 'without its peel' — may have occurred already in ε, but the readings of ε and P2 are nicely distinguished, and I take it from the presence of *citrie* in P2′ and η that δ had *citrie*, and that P2 knew δ. (I am not inclined to associate the readings of P1 and P2: P1's *mundati ad* is probably a graphic corruption of *mundat(ur)a(m)* + anticipation of the *d* of *dieta*.)

2.37.11 non solum cardialgias sanat (scil. *glicia remedium*) ... sed et alia plurima: alia multa θ′ *praeter* P2 Ox P3 (Gk II, 283, 2–3 οὐ μόνον γὰρ ἰᾶται καρδιαλγίαν, ἀλλὰ καὶ ... ἄλλα πλεῖστα)

[38] Where does the negative come from in P2, B, L2 and φ? I can see that *cum* could be read as *cui n(on)*, so perhaps it reflects a dittography of *cum* which is then dealt with in various ways.

[39] For this use of *aliquid*, cf. 1.63, 139, 142, 146, *et passim*.

[40] As the stemma stands, either Ox reintroduced it himself, or the innovation was in θ′ (and P3 had access to it, say via λ), and Ox inherited the correct text via θ.

Given the Greek πλεῖστα and the distribution of the Latin variants, it is reasonable to suppose that θ' has normalized *plurima* to *multa*, while P2 has followed δ. Ox (and P3) would then have the correct reading from θ. (P3 is rather creative at this point but reflects a model containing *plurima* rather than *multa*: *sed et plurimis aliis passionibus iuuat.*)

2.236.6 non enim solum oportet, *etc.*: for the text and variants, see above under 'ε errs'. P2 alone of the descendants of ε has *existimare oportet* (*oportet existimare* ε) and *reumatismum solum* (*solum reumatismum* ε). P2's word-order may be due to reference to δ (which had *solum oportet* and *reumatismi solent*).

2.236.6 et per simplicem solam qualitatem efficitur (scil. *reumatismus*) id est per distemperantias ipsarum (scil. *qualitatum*): distemperantias ipsas (distemperantiam ipsam L2) ε *praeter* G1 P2 (nothing corresponding in the Gk II, 503, 3–4)

ε changes *ipsarum* to *ipsas*, but P2 follows δ. As *qualitas* does not appear in the plural, it was all too easy to make *ipsarum* agree with the adjacent *distemperantias* (as L2 also does, making the phrase singular). Once the change was made, there was no reason to undo it, and so G1's *ipsarum* is not easy to explain: it may reflect another agreement between G1 and P3, where *ipsas* is a correction, presumably of *ipsarum*.

4.7.2. θ, P3 AND γ'

In a striking number of instances, there is agreement in error between at least one of the descendants of γ and at least one of the descendants of θ, above all Ox and/or P3, but in fact D, Ge and Ma (Ma more rarely) are also implicated. The question arises, how many members of the θ-family knew γ' directly? In principle, we could be generous, moderate, or parsimonious. In generous mood, we could allow all of them — the five surviving copies and the two lost copies θ'' and κ — as well as θ itself direct access to γ'. This is of course the easiest solution, but also the least satisfactory, not only because it makes the stemma virtually unreadable, but more importantly because it is historically implausible and moreover ignores certain clear patterns of agreement. A choice between the moderate and the parsimonious availability of γ' is, however, less obvious. For a long time I adopted the moderate approach: I observed that D quite often shared γ-errors alongside Ox and P3, Ge less often, and Ma more rarely still, and consequently allowed θ, κ, Ox and P3 each the possibility of following γ' independently. From the first, however, I was acutely aware of the complexity and apparent chaos that even this compromise brought to the stemma, and dissatisfied by an approach that was in reality arbitrary and only apparently principled. The reconstruction of λ as the accessory model of Ma, D, and Ge brought at last a realistic chance of making a parsimonious approach work, and it is this that I seek to represent — I hope consistently — in the present work. Given that Ma, D and Ge can reasonably be held to derive non-γ-readings from λ, daughter of θ', that there is some reason to think that P3 had a non-γ-source other than θ'', and that Ox is not obviously contaminated (while P3 very evidently is), I think we may account for all significant agreements between γ- and θ-family manuscripts by allowing θ itself and P3 alone among its descendants direct access to γ'.[41]

[41] Note also good readings by contamination, e.g. of P3 in 2.37.6, 10, 11 under 4.2.3 above.

1.85.1 qualiter oporteat cognosci in eis consistentes passiones, et causas eorum et curationes et diuersitates colliriorum, et modus qualiter oporteat adhiberi: modo nos qualiter M modum nos qualiter P1 modum qualiter nos Ox P3′ (nothing corresponding in Gk II, 3, 3–5 πῶς διαγινώσκειν χρὴ τὰ ἐν αὐτοῖς συνιστάμενα πάθη καὶ τὰς αἰτίας τούτων καὶ τὰς θεραπείας καὶ περὶ διαφόρων κολλουρίων καὶ τοῦ τρόπου τῆς χρήσεως αὐτῶν)

γ and γ′, and hence θ, Ox and P3′, inserted *nos* with *oporte(a)t adhibere.*

[1.85.4 Incipiamus ergo [nunc] iam dicere: iam γ Ox P3, iam nunc G1 C L2 ϕ (Gk II, 3, 8–9 ἀρξώμεθα οὖν ἤδη τοῦ λόγου)

γ and γ′, and hence θ, Ox and P3, may here preserve a correct reading: *nunc* looks like a gloss on *iam.*]

1.85.6 Quando ergo dolores nimii et intolerabiles occupauerint oculos: dolor nimius ... -is M D Ox P3 doloris nimio ... -is P1 (Gk II, 3, 11–5, 1 εἰ οὖν ὀδύναι σφοδραὶ καὶ ἀκαρτέρητοι περιέχουσι τοὺς ὀφθαλμοὺς)

γ and γ′, and hence θ, κ (D and Ox) and P3, substitute singular *dolor nimius* for plural *dolores nimii.*

1.85.6 non, sicut multi faciunt, narcoticis confectis praesumendum est uti colliriis: praesumant γ Ox praesumendum P3′ (Gk II, 5, 2–3 μὴ ὡς πολλοὶ τοῖς ναρκωτικοῖς σκευαζομένοις θαρρήσῃς κολλουρίοις)

γ and Ox (presumably via θ) have *praesumant* for *praesumendum est*; or can this be by chance?

1.85.10 Prouidendum est autem unde prorumpat quod supercurrit ... et qualis utique superfluitas est: qualis γ Ox P3 (Gk II, 5, 9–11 θεωρεῖται δὲ καὶ πόθεν ὁρμᾶται τὸ ἐπιρρεῦσαν ... καὶ οἷον ἄρα τὸ ἐπιρρέον ἐστίν)

γ and γ′, and hence θ, Ox and P3, omit *et.*

1.86.1 Si ergo sanguineus fuerit humor qui ...: humor fuerit M D Ox P3 humor P3′ (Gk II, 5, 19 Εἰ μὲν οὖν αἱματικὸς εἴη χυμὸς)

M and γ′, and hence θ, κ (D and Ox) and P3,[42] transpose *fuerit* and *humor* (εἴη χυμὸς).

1.86.2 Rubra enim sunt omnia et sanguineo colore et ipsa facies rubra et in tumore magno sunt posita: nimio M D Ox P3 L2 ϕ omnia C (Gk II, 5, 20–1 ἐρυθρὰ γὰρ ἅπαντα καὶ αἱματώδη καὶ τὸ πρόσωπον ἐρυθρὸν καὶ ἐν ὄγκῳ μείζονι)

M and γ′, and hence θ, κ (D and Ox) and P3 (and L2), substitute *nimio* for *magno*; *nimio* is perfectly idiomatic, but, in view of Greek μείζονι, surely secondary. If this is right, we have here an agreement in error setting M and γ′ against P1 (which has *magna*).

1.86.2 et pigritia in omnibus consuetis actionibus accidit: omnis consuetas accionis P1 omnes consuetas actiones M omni consueta accione D Ox omnibus consueta accione P3 (Gk II, 5, 22–3 καὶ ὄκνος περὶ τὰς συνήθεις ἐνεργείας)

κ (D and Ox) and P3 agree in error in substituting singular *consueta actione* for plural *consuetis actionibus*, and I wonder whether this was inspired by (or represents a correction of) the accusative plural **consuetas actiones* in γ′ via θ (cf. the evidence for γ provided by P1 and M) — especially if γ′ had lost one or two final esses; the accusative plural could perfectly well have been in the original.

1.86.3 Et si in his neque mordicans lacrima neque acris uideatur: uel acris (agris P1 acres M) uidetur γ Ox P3 (Gk II, 5, 23–4 εἰ δὲ πρὸς τούτοις μηδὲ τὸ δάκρυον δακνῶδες καὶ δριμὺ φαίνοιτο)

[42] But note that P3′ omits *fuerit*, and has just *sanguineus humor qui.*

In view of the Greek text, γ and γ′, and hence θ, Ox and P3, probably here preserve the original reading — though parallels must be sought for *neque … neque* and *neque … uel*.

1.87.1 Si enim sanguineus esse tibi manifestus fuerit flegmon: *om.* M Ox P3′ (not in Gk II, 5, 27 Εἰ μὲν οὖν αἱματικόν σοι φανείη τὸ τὴν φλεγμονὴν ἐργασάμενον αἴτιον)

M and γ′, and hence θ, Ox and P3′, omit *esse*. Again, M and γ′ would agree in error against P1.

1.87.1 incidenda est uena (magis) capitalis γ D Ox P3

γ and γ′, and hence θ, κ (D and Ox) and P3, preserve the correct word-order in this phrase. (On this passage, see above under 'δ errs'.)

1.87.2 Si autem colericus et acer humor cum sanguine appareat mixtus: enim M D Ox P3 (Gk II, 5, 28–7, 1 εἰ δὲ καὶ χολώδεις καὶ δριμεῖς χυμοὶ)

M and γ′, and hence θ, κ (D and Ox) and P3, substitute *enim* for *autem* (most probably repeating *enim* from 1.87.1 *Si enim sanguineus …*). Again, M and γ′ would agree in error against P1.

1.87.3 Extrinsecus autem superponenda sunt adiutoria haec: igitur γ D Ox P3 φ (nothing corresponding in Gk II, 7, 5 Περὶ τῶν ἔξωθεν ἐπιτιθεμένων βοηθημάτων)

γ and γ′, and hence θ, κ (D and Ox) and P3, substitute *igitur* for *autem*.

1.87.4 Similiter autem et dactili faciunt — postquam autem repressum fuerit reuma: postea repressa P1, postquam repressa M, postea cum repressa P3 (no exact correspondence in Gk II, 7, 10–11 τὸ αὐτὸ δὲ ποιοῦσι καὶ οἱ φοίνικες μετὰ τοῦ ἐπέχειν τὸν ἐπιφερόμενον ῥευματισμόν)

Rightly or wrongly, γ and γ′, and hence probably θ and P3, agree in omitting *autem* and in treating *reuma* as feminine. (The Latin version incorrectly takes Greek μετά + genitive as meaning 'after'.)

1.87.4 crocus et glaucion et ouorum uitella cocta et oleum roseum permixta superponantur: superimposita γ et superimposita (superposita Ox) mitigant dolores Ox P3 L2 φ mitigant D (nothing corresponding in Gk II, 7, 11–12 μετὰ … κρόκου καὶ γλαυκίων καὶ πυρρῶν ᾠῶν ἑπτὰ ἐκζεστῶν καὶ ῥοδίνου)

γ and γ′, and hence θ, Ox and P3 (and L2), substitute *superimposita* for *superponantur*. θ, κ (D and Ox) and P3 (and L2) also reflect the supplying of a new main verb phrase, *mitigant dolores*, as the second participle would require: there is no hint of this in γ.

1.88.1 Cataplasmata igitur extrinsecus ad flegmonem talia qualia diximus sunt utenda: que γ P3 (not in Gk II, 7, 18–19)

γ and γ′, and hence P3, have *que* for *qualia* (*que* may very well be right).

2.36.2 For the text and variants, see 4.4.1 above.

P1, M and P3 alone have *nimis debilem* for *nimis sensibilem*, and presumably P3 here follows γ′.[43]

2.37.2 si is qui patitur sit temperantia satis calida, et in eius stomacho contineantur humores mordicantes et acres nimis: distemperantia P3 D Ox Ge φ | acrissimi M acerrimi P3 φ (Gk II, 281, 12–14 εἴπερ οἱ πάσχοντες ἦσαν τῇ κράσει θερμοὶ πάνυ καὶ οἱ περιεχόμενοι χυμοὶ δακνώδεις και δριμεῖς ἄγαν)

[43] Note that u and v1 here preserve the correct reading *nimis sensibilem*, which further supports the placing of γ′ closer to γ than to u and v1, or even the idea that u, v1 and α all derive from α′ (see 4.8.1).

In the second case, the common source of P3 and φ surely had access to a copy in which *acres nimis* had been changed into a superlative form, perhaps in the first instance a barbarous one such as that in M. In the first case, *distemperantia* (for *temperantia*) was surely in θ and corrected by Ma alone of the descendants of θ, possibly by reference to λ.

2.158.3 sic curatio competens est adhibenda et differri non oportet: dilatare γ P3 (Gk II, 187, 6–7 καὶ οὕτω τὴν θεραπείαν ἐπιφέρειν καὶ μὴ ἀναβάλλεσθαι)

P1, M and P3 alone have *dilatare* for *differri*, and presumably P3 here follows γ′.

4.7.3. G1 and θ″, especially P3

A few significant innovations are exclusive to G1, P3 and Ma, and imply an accessory use by G1 of a daughter of θ″ (close to P3 in particular, see below). I have represented this with a dotted line on the stemma.

2.2.1 Quod si de calida distemperantia pura uel simplici generata fuerit tussis – sentiunt enim merito calorem quasi per aliquas qualitates taliter tussientes et respirantes – desiderium habent frigidi aeris: sentiunt enim merito γ η sentiunt et merito B P2 L2 et merito sentiunt φ merito sentiunt et Ge merito sentiunt G1 P3 Ma | quem super P1 quas per M quia per G1 P3′ Ma (*dots under* quia P3 m2) (Gk II, 147, 17–19 Ψιλῆς τοίνυν οὔσης τῆς θερμῆς δυσκρασίας αἰσθάνονται μὲν ἴσως διά τινος ποιότητος τοιαύτης, οἷον δυσκρασίας θερμῆς, βήσσοντες καὶ ἀναπνεῖν ἐπιθυμοῦσι ψυχρὸν ἀέρα)

Although things are messy at this point and the Latin text (not to mention the Greek!) is far from clear (see 5.4 below and the notes ad loc.), we see that G1, P3 and Ma agree within the space of a few words in omitting *et* (or *enim*) and in substituting *quia* for *quasi*.

2.37.2 et panis in aqua frigida aut in calida aqua: in aqua calida aut (uel G1) frigida G1 P3 Ma (Gk II, 281, 12 καὶ ἄρτος εἰς ὕδωρ ψυχρὸν καὶ εὔκρατον)

While the Greek and the rest of the Latin tradition have ‘cold or hot’, G1, P3 and Ma (and I presume θ″) have ‘hot or cold’. (On this passage, see also 4.3.3 above.)

G1 never agrees with Ma against P3, and that G1’s accessory model was especially close to P3 is suggested by the following agreements. Individually, I acknowledge, many of these are very slight, but taken together they are not negligible, and one in particular — 2.271.4 — is surely decisive. Note that in 1.19.3, 2.271.2–4, and 2.271.5, G1 and P3 agree also with a descendant of γ. (Cf. 2.271.1 under 4.4.5 above, and note ad loc.)

1.19.2 Est autem quod defluit aut colericum ...: qui defluit humor G1 P3 (Gk I, 463, 4 ἔστι δὲ τὸ παραρρέον ὁτὲ μὲν χολῶδες ...)

1.19.3 et subcolerico colore: cum colerico M G1 P3 (Gk I, 463, 7–8 καὶ ὕπωχρον (ὑπόχολον Mf) τῇ χροιᾷ)

2.37.t. on the (correct) placement by G1 and P3 (perhaps by θ″) of an additional title (Curatio cardiace G1 Curatio cardiacorum P3) misplaced elsewhere in the tradition, see under 4.5 above.

2.158.7 et sic aut uomitur aut per uentrem deducitur (scil. *sanguis*) in secessus: per uomitum G1 per uomitur P3 (not in the Gk II, 187, 11)

G1 and P3 alone have *per*. This could admittedly be a good correction, made independently by each, of the transmitted version, but it is certainly secondary: for *per uomitum aut per uentrem*, cf. e.g. 2.24 *ad fin.*, 2.54 *ad init.*

2.236.4 et flegma eodem modo laedens dolores fortissimos facit: fortissimos dolores G1 C P3 L2 (Gk II, 501, 23–4 ἔτι δὲ φλέγμα χωρῆσαν εἰς τοὺς εἰρημένους τόπους ὀδύνης ἰσχυροτέρας αἴτιον γίνεται)

The Greek word-order suggests that *dolores fortissimos* is original, but *fortissimos dolores* is better Latin. Was the improvement made independently by θ″ (whence G1, P3 and L2?) and C, or is this another agreement linking C with manuscripts outside η (see below)? Or was it just an accident? To what extent is the Greek word-order noun-adjective retained in the Latin translation?

2.236.6 et per simplicem solam qualitatem efficitur (scil. *reumatismus*): perficitur G1 P3 L2 (nothing corresponding in Gk II, 503, 3)

G1 and P3 have the certainly erroneous *perficitur* for *efficitur*. The *per-* was perhaps suggested by the preposition a few words earlier, in which case this could again involve independent error. This is perhaps supported by the fact that the error is shared also with L2; on the other hand, there are other places where L2 agrees in significant error with G1 and P3 (note especially the next three passages).

2.271.2 et hi in accessione dolores ferre non possunt: hi cum G1 P3′ L2 | accessionibus G1 P3 L2 (not in Gk II, 575, 2)

G1 and P3 and L2 alone have *accessio* in the plural, and they alone provide a logical link by means of the conjunction *cum* between this sentence and the next (which announces some pain-killing remedies).

2.271.2–4 cerotaria anodina quae mox sine dolore faciant. (3.) Ordinamus cerotum quod dum in statu accessionis fuerit superpositum mox sine dolore locus efficitur. (4.) +– Recipit autem haec.–+ Croco opio ÷ iiii.: cerotaria anodina que mox sine dolore faciant ordinamus. Quorum unum recipit opii croci G1 P3 L2 (Gk II, 575, 4–5 Κηρωτὴ ἐν τῇ ἀκμῇ τῶν παροξυσμῶν ἐπιτιθεμένη, ἀνωδύνους ποιοῦσα. +– –+ Κρόκου, ὀποῦ μήκωνος, ἀνὰ οὐγγ. δ′)

This is a very striking set of exclusive agreements between G1 and P3 and L2. Notice (a) *quorum unum* for *cerotum quod dum*; (b) the lacuna (*in statu* ... *efficitur*); (c) the asyndeton after *recipit*; (d) the order of the first two ingredients of the recipe.[44]

2.271.5 Crocum et opium infundes in uino, panem uero in aqua infundes: uero γ G1 P3 L2] *om. cett.* | infundes] *om.* G1 P3 L2 C (Gk II, 575, 6–7 τὸν κρόκον καὶ τὸν ὀπὸν ἀπόβρεχε ἐν οἴνῳ, τὸν δὲ ἄρτον ὕδατι)

Again, G1 and P3 and L2 are very close, and again a descendant of β is probably involved.

4.7.4. C and θ′, especially G1

C shares important η errors such as 2.236.2 *inimicos* (for *nimios*, see 4.3.1), and important correct η readings, such as 2.271.4 *paragoricis* (*podagricis* ε, see 4.3.3),

[44] Note that the fourth feature, (d), is also in M, which also omits *que mox sine dolore faciant* ... *recipit autem hec*. Note also that *que mox sine dolore faciant ordinamus* is an addition in P3. It is likely that the source of G1, P3 and L2 here was an exemplar very like M (γ′), and that *quorum unum recipit* was an improvised filling of what was obviously a lacuna between *cerotaria anodina* and *opii croci*. An accessory model then gave P3 *que mox sine dolore faciant ordinamus* and (probably) a nonsensical *autem* added after *recipit* (although of course some changes/innovations could have been made without reference to another model!).

(and at e.g. 2.236.7 — although this is a very messy passage — C agrees perfectly with A), and therefore, if the agreements with θ′ are significant, they presumably arise through contamination. In addition to the passages presented under 4.4.1 above, I note the following agreements in error with G1 in particular.

1.85.t. De oculorum passionibus: passionibus oculorum G1 C (Gk II, 3, 1 Περὶ θεραπείας ὀφθαλμῶν)

The ancestor of G1, here followed by C, transposes *oculorum* and *passionibus*.

1.85.4 Incipiamus ergo [nunc] iam dicere: iam nunc C G1 L2 φ, nunc iam *plerique* (Gk II, 3, 8–9 ἀρξώμεθα οὖν ἤδη τοῦ λόγου)

G1 and C (and L2 and φ) agree in putting *nunc*, which may have begun as a gloss (it is not in γ or Ox or P3), after *iam*, rather than before it as in the other descendants of δ.

2.5.1 et quod spuitur plenitudo: quod γ η P3′ eo quod P2 ex eo quod *cett. etiam* C (Gk II, 149, 14–15 αὐτῷ τῷ ἀναπτύεσθαι πλῆθος)

C shares in the elaboration of *quod* to *ex eo quod*, an innovation probably of ε (note the further slight discrepancy between P2 and ε (cf. 4.7.1 above): did δ have *eo quod*?).

2.36.4 lumbrici saepius superiora petentes ex inferioribus partibus: *om.* G1 C (Gk II, 279, 23–4 πολλάκις δὲ καὶ ἕλμινθες ἐκ τῶν κάτω μερῶν ἀναδραμόντες)

The ancestor of G1, here followed by C, omits *saepius*.

2.236.2 Etenim sanguis calidus supercurrens in articulorum cauitates: *om.* G1 C (Gk II, 501, 19 καὶ γὰρ αἷμα συρρεῦσαν ἐν τῇ τῶν ἄρθρων κοιλότητι θερμὸν)

The ancestor of G1, here followed by C, omits *calidus*.

2.271.9 coques lignis de uitibus, id est sarmentis, donec bulliat: *om.* G1 C L2 (Gk II, 575, 19–20 ἕψε ξύλοις ἀμπελίνοις, ἕως οὗ βράσῃ σφοδρῶς)

The ancestor of G1 and L2, here followed by C, omits *id est sarmentis*.

4.7.5. C AND P3 (AND/OR φ)

Nearly all of the aberrant readings in C can be explained in terms of contamination with θ′. Some, however, including some striking ones, unite C in error with P3 and φ, or with φ alone.

1.17 *ad fin.*[45] Item aliud ad eas quae in capite scabias sunt. Rutam et stipteria teres cum melle, et ungues caput; antea tamen rades. Si autem recesserit a capite cutis, oliuae folia cocta [trita?] cum melle cataplasmabis: Item ... quae] Item C Iterum φ | in capite scabias sunt] ueteres autem scabies capitis illinies C ueteres scabies capitis sic curabis φ in capite scabies ueteres (ueteres *s. s.*) sunt P3 | Si autem recesserit a capite cutis] si autem cutis recesserit a capite cortice C P3 φ | oliuae folia cocta [trita?] cum melle] cortice oliue et foliis coctis et (et *s. s.* P3) tritis cum melle C P3 φ (Gk I, 461, 7–10 Πρὸς τὰ ἐν τῇ κεφαλῇ ψωρώδη καὶ ἰχωρώδη. Πήγανον καὶ στυπτηρίαν λεάνας μετὰ μέλιτος χρῖε τὴν κεφαλὴν προξυρῶν· ἐὰν δ’ ἀφιστῆται τῆς κεφαλῆς τὸ δέρμα, ἐλαίας φύλλα ἑφθὰ μετὰ μέλιτος κατάπλαττε)

This short recipe (omitted by *ed.*) throws up several significant agreements involving C, P3 and φ. C and φ alone abbreviate the beginning of the recipe, replacing the introductory relative clause with a main-verb instruction, and C and φ together with a

[45] I have yet to subdivide 1.17, as I have collated only the recipe omitted by *ed.* See 4.10.1.

corrector of P3 insert *ueteres* before *scabies*. They also agree (together with D, Ox and Ge) in a dittography of *cutis*, whereby the second occurrence is reinterpreted as a form of *cortex* and as referring to the skin of the olives. Finally, they agree in resolving the asyndeton *cocta trita* by inserting *et* between the two participles. (For further details of this revealing passage — bearing also on other branches of the tradition — see 4.10.1.)

1.18.t. ex quibus tabes quaedam defluit: uelut quedam tabes C φ (Gk I, 461, 12 ἀφ' ὧν ἰχῶρες ἀποτήκονται)

C and φ alone insert *uelut* and transpose *tabes quaedam*. This surely cannot be due to independent innovation.

1.19.2 cognosci ergo oportet passionis ipsius proprietatem: cognoscere (agn- M P3) γ C P3 φ | ipsam passionem et C P3 φ ipsius passionis M (Gk I, 463, 5–6 διαγινώσκειν οὖν χρὴ τὸ κυρίως αἴτιον)

C, P3 and φ have the active infinitive (in common with γ and the Greek) and a reworking of *passionis ipsius* (conceivably based on γ′: cf. the word-order of M).

4.8. Remaining Problems

Given the complexity of this tradition, and the inevitably provisional nature of some of the relations argued for in this chapter, it may be useful to rehearse briefly some of the outstanding problems and questions, the loose ends which I am as yet unable to tie up. This I do in chronological order, by the age of the principal manuscript(s) concerned, beginning with the oldest.

4.8.1. γ, u, v1 and α: Two Problems

With regard to β, γ and δ, it is important to note two potential problems with the stemma as at present proposed.

In the first place, there are two passages in which we have to reckon with the possibility that u and v1 alone preserve the correct reading. In this case, either γ and δ have erred independently, or the error was in α and the common ancestor of u and v1 descends not from α but from a very similar copy (α′). In the latter case, in sections 4.2 and 4.8.2 we are reconstructing not β and γ vs δ, but α vs α′: agreements in error between γ and u and v1 presumably reflect errors in α′ corrected not in α but in δ; correct readings shared by γ and u and v1 allow us to suppose error in δ, as before. (On the implications for the top of the stemma, cf. the remarks in 3.2.5 and 4.1.2 above.)

Here are the two passages in question.

2.36.3 cardiacas passiones Ox P3′ u v1: cardiacam passionem *cett.* (Gk II, 279, 25 καρδιακὰς διαθέσεις)

In view of the plural in the Greek, u and v1 may be right (Ox and P3 getting the correct reading from γ′). (This is, admittedly, a small matter, but the pattern of agreements appears not haphazard.)

2.36.3 ita ut aliqui statim a lumbricorum mordicatione pereant P3 u v1: statim a mord. lumbr. φ statim in malo (mala D Ox C B malo a Ma Ge) lumbr. mord. *cett.* (Gk II, 279, 25–281, 1 ὥστε τινὰς παραυτίκα ὑφ' ἑλμίνθων δακνομένους ἀπόλλυσθαι)

Here again u and v1 may have the correct reading (which was preserved also in γ′, the descendant of β known to P3, which in turn transmitted it to φ, which normalized the word-order) as there is nothing in the Greek to warrant the words *in malo*. It is striking that the three unwanted syllables more or less exactly repeat three syllables in the sequence *statimalumbricorum. Are we to reckon with some sort of dittography, perhaps caused by double reading/hearing of syllables in *scriptio continua*?[46] The converse — haplography of e.g. *statĩĩ malulũ bricorũ — is also conceivable, but raises further problems, including the question of the meaning of *in malo lumbricorum*.[47] We are not helped by the fact that the Latin Alexander appears not otherwise to use *perire*!

Secondly, while setting up γ vs v1 and u as I do in the stemma, I must acknowledge and here highlight a possibly significant agreement (in error?) of M and v1:

2.235.3 Ego autem existimo ut . . . bene et cito possit curari et facilius a medicis ab ipsis infirmitatibus liberare: et cito] citto P1 credo M v1 *om. Pod.* | possit P1 M P3 posunt Ox posse *cett.* (Gk II, 501, 12–14 ἐγὼ δέ φημι ὡς . . . εὐθεράπευτος ἂν ῥᾳδίως ὑπὸ τῶν ἰατρῶν γενήσεται)

M and v1 alone have *credo* for *cito*. On the other hand, of the copies deriving from β, only v1 changes *possit* (required after *existimo ut*) to *posse* (required with *credo*), and P1 agrees with M and v1 in omitting *et* (required by the substitution of *credo* for *cito*), so that the error may have occurred in β (*bene credo possit*) and have been faithfully copied in M, partly corrected in P1 (*bene citto possit*), and properly incorporated by means of a further change in v1 (*bene credo posse*) (cf. my provisional text in 4.10.6 and notes ad loc.).

4.8.2. Who Errs, β or δ?

For the record, I add a further set of passages in which the manuscripts show a clear β vs δ division but where I am not yet able to say with confidence which side of the tradition is in error. At some future date, some at least of these passages will serve for further definition of β and δ.

2.1.4 Propter quod non una est causa tussis sed uaria: propter quod γ O D, propterea A Mu C Ox Ge P2 L2 B, quoniam G1 Ma P3 φ (Gk II, 147, 12 ἐπεὶ οὖν οὐ μίαν αἰτίαν ἡ βὴξ, ἀλλὰ ποικίλην κέκτηται)

η and θ′ (and perhaps θ whence κ′), and therefore δ already, have *propterea*, β has *propter quod*. The latter is much more common than the former in A's version of Books 1 and 2, but I cannot at this point decide between the two. θ″ (here preferred by G1) evidently innovates with *quoniam*. O may have found *propter quod* in γ′.[48]

2.36.4 oportet non omnino existimandum: existimandum M u v1 existimandis P1 estimandum Ox existimari P3 existimare *cett.* (Gk II, 281, 1–2 χρὴ μὴ πάντοτε νομίζειν)

Either δ has normalized an original gerundive, or β has vulgarized an original infinitive.[49] The (near-)agreement of Ox with β may reflect use of γ′ by the maker of Ox.

[46] I owe this suggestion to Cloudy Fischer.

[47] Might *malum lumbricorum* have been a phrasal term of the type *passio lumbricorum* (Langslow, *Medical Latin*, 223, with references)? Are there parallels in the Latin Alexander?

[48] D may be ignored, as he is indulging in free composition at this point, writing between *quod* and *non* the words *per partes agnoscenda sunt quia*.

[49] For *oportet* with the gerundive see Hofmann and Szantyr, 374 with literature.

2.37.7 his ergo hora tertia panem infusum in calida aqua [ut] adsumant aut in aqua frigida infusum P1 v1: sumant M P3 in calida ... infusum *om.* u
his ergo hora tertia suadendum (suad. est C) panem infusum ... ut assumant (assumere O[50]) ... infusum A O Mu C
his ergo hora tertia suadendum est ut assumant (accipiant B) panem ... infusum *cett. praeter* Ox P3 (Gk II, 281, 22–3 ἀλλὰ περὶ ὥραν τρίτην ἢ τετάρτην ἄρτον εἰς εὔκρατον λαμβάνειν ἢ εἰς ὕδωρ ψυχρὸν)

The difficulty here centres on *suadendum est*, which was certainly present in δ. We may suppose either:
(a) β (including γ′ reflected in P3) errs in losing *suadendum est*; P1 and v1 blindly preserve the tell-tale *ut* before *assumant*, but M and γ′ (cf. P3) drop the *ut* and change *assumant* to *sumant*; η (A O Mu C) preserves the correct reading (probably minus *est*, which is only in C) from δ, while ε normalizes the elaborate word-order and structure (which is in keeping with the Greek and probably original); or
(b) the jussive subjunctive (*assumant*) is original, and *suadendum est* is part of an attempt by δ to restore sense to a garbled text.
In favour of (a) is the otherwise inexplicable *ut* before *assumant* in P1 and v1, but I leave both possibilities open for now. In either case, the Latin version, unlike the Greek, obviously began a new sentence here, with *His ergo*.

2.235.2 Relinquitur eius aliquid in ipsis locis, et ideo nullo modo ab artificibus medicine sanari potest: potuerunt P1 v1 poterunt M po poterit P3 (Gk II, 501, 11–12 ὑπόληψιν δὲ ἐκ τούτου τὸ πάθος ἀνιαρὰν ἐκτήσατο, καὶ μηδὲ ὅλως ὑπὸ τέχνης ἰατρικῆς ἰαθῆναί ποτε δυνηθῆναι)

The Greek means, 'as a result, the disease [gout] acquired the unholy reputation that it had never actually been susceptible of being completely cured by the art of medicine', and the Latin seems to be a bad mistranslation, which starts by misconstruing ὑπόληψιν as a part of ὑπολείπω. Given the confusion, it would be hazardous to favour any particular tense of *posse*. We can, however, be confident that δ had *potest*, while β (including γ′ reflected in P3) had the future or the perfect.

2.235.5 Credo enim quia si ea que scripta tradimus diligentius attendantur [naturam uniuscuiusque] multos poterit liberare: attendantur po] attendendo α | *ante* multos *habent* quicumque (quisquis Ma quis P3 L2 *om.* η) uoluerit operari *omnes praeter* P1 M v1 po (Gk II, 501, 15–16 ἐλπιζέτω γὰρ ὅτι τοῖς γεγραμμένοις ἐάν τις ἀκριβῶς προσέχοι, ὠφελήσει πολλούς)

Provisionally (and tentatively), I take it that, given that there is nothing corresponding in the Greek, and that it adds nothing to the sense, the words *uoluerit operari* were inserted by δ rather than lost by β. The line would be that, following the corruption of *attendantur* into *attendendo*, it became apparent to the maker of δ, but not to the maker of β, that the *si*-clause had no finite verb, and *uoluerit operari* was added.

An intelligible alternative would be the text of η: *Credo enim si* (*si quis* η′) *ea quae scripta tradimus, diligentius attendendo naturam uniuscuiusque, uoluerit operari, multos poterit liberare* 'For I believe that if anyone wishes to apply the things which we are transmitting in writing, while/by paying careful heed to the nature of each

[50] cf. Greek λαμβάνειν!

individual (case/patient), he will be able to cure many people'. On this account, β omits *uoluerit operari*. In the text of A of Book 1, I have counted forty-two instances of ablative gerund + main verb.

In either case, I think it more probable that the indefinite pronoun as subject of *uoluerit* (*quicunque* repeated from 2.235.3) was added by ε rather than lost by η; δ might have understood the subject as unspecified 'he', the doctor. (See my provisional text in 4.10.6 and the notes ad loc.).

2.236.5 sed et grauitate sua facta sentitur <non> mediocris commotio: mediocris effecta M v1 po mediocriter effecta P1 mediocriter *cett. om.* Ox Ge (Gk II, 503, 1–2 ἀλλὰ καὶ τῷ βάρους ἐπιτελεῖν αἴσθησιν οὐ μετρίους ἐργάζεται τοὺς παροξυσμούς)

(On the omission of the negative in all the Latin manuscripts, see under α above.) Here one can argue either:

(a) the translation is poor, and on a meaningless, word-for-word basis *facta* for ἐπιτελεῖν and *effecta* for ἐργάζεται in β is clearly closer to the Greek and therefore likely to be right: δ's deletion of *effecta* would then have been prompted by the thought that it merely repeated *facta*; or

(b) β and po understood *facta* to go with *grauitate*, felt the need for another participle with *sentitur commotio*, and added *effecta*.

A possible argument in favour of (b) is that ἐργάζομαι appears to be rendered rarely or never by *efficio*,[51] but regularly and frequently by *facio*.[52] If this is right, *effecta* is more likely to be secondary than the original equivalent of ἐργάζεται.

2.271.7 Opium soluens cum lacte muliebri addes olei rosei ÷ vi. cera ÷ vi. et sic miscebis cerotum et uteris: addes *om.* P1 M | miscis P1 M misces P3 (Gk II, 575, 13–17 Ὀπίου δραχ. δʹ ἐν ἄλλῳ ηʹ κηρωτῆς ῥοδίνου λιτρ. αʹ. λείου γυναικείῳ γάλακτι τὸ ὄπιον καὶ οὕτω μίσγε τὴν κηρωτὴν ἐν τῇ θυΐᾳ καὶ χρῶ ὡς πάνυ καλλίστῃ.)

The Latin text is abbreviated and seems to be corrupt (e.g. there is no indication of the quantity of *opium* to be used). Either β lost *addes*, or, more probably, δ added it in an effort to make sense of the recipe. And, whichever the original form of the instruction to mix, there is a clear distinction between δ and β (with γ′ reflected in P3).

4.8.3. O AND γ′?

Nearly all of the aberrant readings in O can be explained through contamination with θ; remarkably, eight of the innovations with which I characterize θ above are shared by O (see 4.4.3 above). Two innovations in O, however, seem to unite O alone in error with γ, and therefore to suggest that O had direct knowledge of γ′. I remain very tentative on this relation, which I do not represent on the stemma, as the evidence is as yet slight, but here for the record are the passages in question (note also 2.1.4 under 4.8.2 above).

[51] Possibly at 1.35=I, 487, 11 (a mistranslation).

[52] Note e.g. 2.184=II, 473, 5; 2.236.2=II, 501, 21; and especially 2.200, where in the space of two lines *factus*=II, 495, 2 ἐργάζομαι, but *effectus*=γινόμενος (as often: cf. e.g. 1.29, 1.34, 2.40, 2.41, 2.59).

2.2.3 Quod si haec fuerint passi et sola distemperantia fuerit: fuerint passi et *recte* δ (A Mu P2) fuerit passus et P1 M O passio ex ε C (Gk II, 147, 21 εἰ μὲν οὖν οὕτως εἴη μόνη ψιλὴ ποιότης)

ε (θ and θ′, the latter followed by C [but P2 follows δ]) lost *fuerint* and then replaced *passi et* with *passio ex*. O here agrees in error with γ, and conceivably reflects γ′, although the substitution of singular for plural could be polygenetic.

2.3.1 Tussiunt etiam plurimi ex frigida distemperantia: Tussent P1 Tussem M Tusse O Si autem tussis ... fit P3 Ma | plurima O (Gk II, 149, 2 ὅσοι δὲ βήσσουσι διὰ ψυχρὰν δυσκρασίαν)

γ and O (conceivably reflecting γ′) appear to share the replacement of the verb *tussiunt* by the noun *tusse(m)*, although O alone tries to make the syntax work (with the ablative absolute *Tusse ... plurima ... existente*). The three variants, *tussent, tussem* and *tusse* (but is the first a possible form?) would have been pronounced very much alike. (On this passage, see also 4.4.4 above.)

4.8.4. η: A and Mu (?)

As for the relations between the copies descended from η, it is beyond doubt that O and Mu derive from a lost descendant of η (η′: see 4.3.2 above). The only other striking agreements in error within η would link A and Mu, but I have found to date only two such errors, and I think both of them, while prima facie quite telling, could have been made independently. Nevertheless, I am keeping an open mind on this point. The two shared errors in question are:

2.1.1 initium habet (scil. *tussis*) modo a calida distemperantia est autem quando a calida distemperantia est quoque quando a frigida (the dittography is only in A and Mu: A appears to have marked the error with ″ after the second *distemperantia*; Mu does not mark it)

2.6.1 per uuam (gulam Mu) intra arteriam: in tracheam arteriam *cett.* (Gk II, 149, 25–6 κατὰ τὴν σταφυλὴν ἢ τὴν τραχεῖαν ἀρτηρίαν).

4.8.5. Contamination of Mu?

In only one passage (2.236.2, discussed under 4.3.1 and 4.3.3 above) have we seen grounds for suspecting that Mu had more than one model at any point. Further slight circumstantial evidence may be sought in the fact that some of the errors that Mu shares with O (reflecting error in η′: see 4.3.2 above) have been corrected in Mu, though it is not clear that the corrections must derive from another copy.

4.8.6. Contamination of Ox?

In such a contaminated tradition, it is something of a relief to be able to treat any manuscript as derived from a single source. Remarkably, of the surviving descendants of θ, only Ox is so far not demonstrably contaminated. One could take the view that Ox's purity has been bought at a high price: θ must be regarded as heavily contaminated with readings from γ′, and some or all of Ma, D and Ge as copying λ whenever they disagree with Ox (or Ox and P3), so that Ox can take all of its inherited readings from θ via κ. For the material so far collated, this seems to work well enough, but it bears repeating that we have noted difficulties with at least three passages in passing (see the next paragraph), and that further collation may yield patterns of agreement which require Ox (or κ′ or κ) to have an alternative means of access to γ′ or ε or both.

4.8.7. A third source of P3?

As for Ox, so for P3, limiting direct knowledge of γ′ to θ and P3 itself has permitted a straightforward account of nearly all patterns of agreement so far encountered. In a few passages, however, it has seemed desirable to give P3 access to an ε or θ′ reading which neither γ′ nor θ″ could make available. This often goes hand in hand with a complementary need to make a reading available to κ,[53] which is why I list the relevant passages together. The simplest solution would be to allow P3 a third source in λ. I list the passages where either this or contamination of Ox was mooted, in case there are more to be found:

1.85.11 the recovery of *enim* (under 4.4.3 above).
2.5.2 and 2.7.t.–2.7.1 the two additions of *humor* (under 4.6.1 above).
2.10.4 the recovery of *cogimur scribere* (under 4.4.6 above).
2.37.4 the elimination of the hyperbaton (under 4.7.1 above).
2.158.6 access to *extenuatur* (under 4.4.1 above).

4.8.8. Contamination of B?

Like Ox among the descendants of θ, B is alone among the daughters of θ′ in having yielded so far no palpable evidence of contamination, and even B has shown one or two possible traces of the use of a second model, which I list here, in case there are more to be found:

2.1.1 B's *quandoque autem* appears to combine *quandoque* θ′ with *est autem quando* γ η ε (under 4.4.1 above).
2.2.6 B's *contingit tussis et fit ex* appears to combine *contingit tussis* P2 Ma D Ge with *fit ex* G1 L2 (under 4.4.1 above).

4.8.9. B as a source of φ?

There are a few places where φ shows innovations which are neither in P3 nor in κ′ (Ox and Ge) but which are attested elsewhere in the tradition, notably in B, and the question arises whether φ had a third source in B or a close congener. The agreements I have noted so far do not, I think, merit a line on the stemma, but I report them as a starting-point, in case there are more to be found.

1.87.4 A*d* autem <eum> cui cum nimio flegmone uel tumore ingenti +– dolor fuerit ortus –+ bene facit crocus: Quando autem cum non nimio L2 B φ (Gk II, 7, 8–9 πρὸς δὲ τὰς μεγίστας φλεγμονὰς καὶ ἐν ὄγκῳ μείζονι ποιεῖ καὶ ὁ κρόκος)

[53] Note especially 2.158.6 *fit extenuata* in, of all places, η and κ (discussed under 4.4.1 above).

(For further details, see under 4.7.1 above.) The tradition is confused at this point. L2, B and φ alone have *Quando autem cum non nimio*.

2.1.3 Scire autem oportet et hoc quomodo differunt abinuicem tussiculae secundum causas singulas sed quoniam et secundum loca: et G1 P3 Ma′ D Ox Ge sed et φ (Gk II, 147, 9–10 εἰδέναι δὲ δεῖ καὶ τοῦτο, ὡς οὐ διαφέρουσιν ἀλλήλων αἱ βῆχες κατὰ τὴν αἰτίαν μόνην, ἀλλὰ καὶ κατὰ τοὺς τόπους)

For discussion of this passage see 4.4.3 above. Note that if *sed* in φ is not by conjecture, the only descendants of ε with *sed quoniam et* at this point are P2, L2 and B.

2.3.t. De tusse quae ex frigida distemperantia fit: si ... oritur B φ (Gk II, 149, 1 Περὶ βηχὸς διὰ ψυχρὰν δυσκρασίαν γινομένης)

B and φ alone substitute *si ... oritur* for *quae ... fit*.

2.7.1 et lingua aspera et mela rubra: mela P1 A] mala *cett.* maxilla *s. s.* B φ (Gk II, 151, 3 γλῶττα τραχεῖα καὶ μῆλα ἐρυθρά)

B and φ alone gloss the erroneous *mala* with *maxilla*.

2.236.3 colericus humor saepius supercurrens super neruos aut inter ipsos residens: *om.* B φ (Gk II, 501, 21 χολὴ πολλάκις ἐπιρρυεῖσα μεταξὺ τῶν νεύρων)

B and φ alone omit the preposition *super*, presumably in order to avoid repeating the preverb of *supercurrens*.

4.9. The Nature of the Text in Single Manuscripts and Individual Secondary Readings

Finally, I give a brief general impression of the nature and quality of each manuscript copy, and some illustration of significant secondary readings occurring in single manuscripts. These affect all the witnesses including the excerpts (u and v1) and the early printing (*ed.*), with the possible exception of G2, which is why G2 alone of the surviving copies is represented in the stemma as a sole source for later copies. For ease of reference, the manuscripts are arranged in alphabetical order by siglum, and in each case I give much briefer context than hitherto. (On spellings in the manuscripts, see 5.2 below.)

A

Consistent and reliable use of *e* caudata; very occasionally hypercorrect use of *ae*, e.g. 1.19.1 *ipsae* for *ipsa*; alone of the competently written manuscripts spells *abundans* without initial *h*-. Very accurate copying, very correct Latin, very little interference:

1.19.2 *om.* aut flegmaticum interdum etiam et melancholicum (Gk I, 463, 4–5)
1.86.3 *flegmonem facit* for *facit flegmonem* (but also in C, and possibly already in η)
2.7.4 *om.* grauiter (Gk II, 151, 10 πάνυ)
2.10.t. *-que* for *et*
2.37.6 *adiumentum*: iuuamentum *ed.*, iuuamen *cett.* (no direct match Gk II, 281, 21–2)
2.158.3 *om.* aegritudinum (Gk II, 187, 8 νοσημάτων)

B

Much use of abbreviations. Pretty accurate copying, with little interference:

1.19.1 *Greci ycora* for *ycora Greci*
1.19.8 *si <tibi> locus appareat*

1.85.5 *om.* nimio (Gk II, 3, 11 σφοδρά)
2.37.7 *accipiant*: sumant M P3 accipiant Ox[54] assumant *cett.* (Gk II, 281, 23 λαμβάνειν)

C

Much use of abbreviations. Good copying, with little interference, including the occasional particle:

1.19.3 *si h(ab)undet h(umor)* for *abundans humor*
1.19.7 *fit* for *fuerit*
1.19.7 *aut melancolicus est* for *est aut melancolicus* of η
1.19.8 *si autem frigidior melancolicus* (points under) *flegmaticus est [h(umor)]*
2.7.3 *extrinsecus*: intrinsecus *cett. recte* (not in Gk II, 151, 8–9)
2.36.3 *mouentes*: appetentes β, petentes *cett.* (Gk II, 279, 24 ἀναδραμόντες)
2.271.9 *om.* secundam aut tertiam (Gk II, 575, 21–2 δεύτερον ἢ τρίτον)

D

Generally good copying and a good knowledge of Latin, but quite a bit of inventive interference:

1.85.1 *add.* a me [plurima] scripta sunt: *non habent cett.* (not in Gk II, 3, 2)
1.85.2 *hunc librum [curationum]*
1.85.8 *non enim una est [in hac passione] qualitas cause* for *non enim est una qualitas cause*
2.37.13 *add.* de acredine humorum [in stomacho existentium] cum mordicatione: *non habent cett.* (not in Gk II, 283, 6–7)

ed.

Essentially the text of φ with numerous errors, though (often, at least) with *mihi*, *nihil* for *michi*, *nichil* in G2 and L1:

1.18.t. *scrissa* for *scissa*
1.19.5 *melancolicum* for *modicum*
1.19.8 *est humor* for *inest humor*
1.85.2 *que [horum] ad oculorum curationem*
1.85.9 *fieri dolores et aliquando ex qualitate qualitas sepius* for *fieri dolores et qualitates sepius* in φ
1.87.1 *capitis*: capitalis *cett.* (Gk II, 5, 28 ὠμιαῖαν (φλέβα))
2.81 *om.* cum insomnietate to end of chapter
2.235.6 *agendo*: attendendo *cett.* (Gk II, 501, 16 προσέχοι)
2.236.2 *add.* in articulis [seu articulorum] concauitates: *non habent cett.* (Gk II, 501, 19 ἐν τῇ τῶν ἄρθρων κοιλότητι)
2.271.11 *mollificatiuum*: mollissimum *cett.* (Gk II, 575, 27 ἁπαλωτάτην)

[54] But B and Ox are otherwise very different here.

G1

Much use of abbreviations. Good copying, though with a little modification:

1.85.1 *scripta sunt a me* for *a me scripta sunt*
1.85.1 *monstratus* for *demonstratus*
1.85.9 *dolorem efficit et qualitates doloris* for *fieri dolorem et qualitates*
1.85.11 *aut ex uentositate <spiritus>*
1.87.3 *uitello oui* and 1.87.4 *uitella ouorum* for *oui uitello, ouorum uitella*
1.88.1 *.i. infusiones* written above *talia*
2.7.2 *suspicari flegmonem*: *cett.* have *flegmonem* at the start of the clause (as does Gk II, 151, 5)
2.8.t. *humorum*: humor *cett.* (no title in Gk II, 151, 12)
2.8.2 *om.* mutatis (?cf. Gk II, 151, 19 μεταστροφαῖς)
2.11.3 *om.* non poterat fortiter extussire (Gk II, 153, 23–4 οὐκ ἠδυνήθη τοῦ βήσσειν ἰσχυρῶς ἀπαλλαγῆναι)
2.11.7 *adiutoria ad tussem*: ad tussem adiutoria *cett.* (Gk II, 155, 23 τῶν βηχικῶν βοηθημάτων)

G2

A very good copy of ϕ, much preferable to *ed.* and L1. At 1.85.9 *dolores et qualitas* does not make sense, as *dolores* is accusative, so that *qualitas* is probably an instance of a very rare error in G2 (although the Greek has ποιότης here!).

L1

The text of ϕ with numerous errors of all sorts:

1.19.5 dittography of *cuti*
1.19.7–8 omission of *si salsus ... inest humor*, in consequence of a big *saut du même au même*
1.85.2 *unde nunc bene <hic> michi* (text of ϕ)
1.85.2 *careant*: querant *cett.* (Gk II, 3, 8 ζητεῖν)
1.85.8 *antecedentes*: attenden(te)s *cett.* (Gk II, 5, 5 ἀποβλέποντα)
1.85.10 dittography of *et qualis*
1.85.11 *aut colerico* for *aut coleribus*
1.87.2 *apparuerit maxime* for *appareat mixtus*
1.88.t. omission of the last four words
2.37.2 *add.* [assumptus seu] acceptus: *non habent cett.*[55] (nothing corresponding in Gk II, 281, 10)
2.235.1 *om.* <Podagre> passiones: *habent cett.* (Gk II, 501, 8 τὸ τῆς ποδάγρας πάθος)
2.235.5 *om.* uerum etiam diuturnas iam existentes> podagras: *habent cett.* (Gk II, 501, 17–18)
2.236.6 *frequenter*: sepius *cett.* (Gk II, 503, 5 πολλάκις)
2.271.7 *om.* rosei

[55] Note, however, the reading *asseptus* in D, a blend of the two variants?

L2

Some abbreviations. Good copying with some intelligent corrections, the occasional transposition and omission:

1.19.8 *potest cognosci*: cognosci potest θ' MaDGe cognoscere poteris *cett.* (Gk I, 463, 16 διαγινώσκειν ἐστί σοι δυνατόν)

1.85.4 *incipiamus ergo iam nunc <dicere>*

1.85.6 *oculorum occupauerint* for *occupauerint oculos*

1.85.10 *aut ... aut ... aut ... uel ... aut* for *utrum ... aut ... aut ... aut ...aut*

1.87.3 *herbe uiole* for *uiole herbe*

1.87.4 *fuerit repressum* for *repressum fuerit*

2.2.6 *nihil enim minus*: nihil igitur minus *cett.* (Gk II, 147, 23 οὐδὲν δὲ ἧττον)

2.5.2 *itaque*: utique *cett.* (a mistranslation of the first syllable of Gk II, 149, 16 κἀνταῦθα)

M

An erratic copy, sometimes good, sometimes with crass errors betraying a basic ignorance of Latin, and omissions not always with the excuse of a *saut du même au même*:

1.18.t. *ex quibus si talis quidem defluit humor for ex quibus tabes quedam defluit*

1.19.4 *non fuerit [fuerit] suptilis est pignosus et glutinosus for non fuerit subtilis sed pinguis et glutinosus*

1.19.6 *que solent accesserint case sue* for *que precesserunt causae, seu*

1.19.7 *sic amarus fuerit coricus est humor* for *Gustus igitur si amarus fuerit, colericus est humor*

1.19.7 omission of *salsus autem ... melancolicus*

1.19.8 *si uissicula* for *si tibi locus*

1.19.8 ends with the first instance of *humor*, omitting the last eleven words

1.85.1 *om.* passionibus <qualiter oporteat ... consistent*ibus* passion*ibus*>[56] et causam: *habent plerique* (Gk II, 3, 3–4)

1.85.2 *conscribam quid*: constricteque *cett.* (Gk II, 3, 6 συντόμως)

2.36.2–3 *om.* <stomachi ... et do>minantur: *habent cett.* (Gk II, 279, 19–20)

2.36.4 *operibus*: humoribus *cett.* (Gk II, 281, 2 χυμῶν)

2.158.6 *descendat*: desudat *cett.* (this section not in Gk)

Ma

A very good copy, with some careful corrections and only very occasional omissions or transpositions:

1.19.4 *flegmaticus humor <salsus> augmentatus*

1.19.8 *si autem flegmaticus frigidior <est>* for *si autem frigidior, flegmaticus est*

1.87.5 *cum sapa* correctly, corrected from *cum supradictis*(!)

2.36.4 *uentosis*: uenenosis *cett.* (Gk II, 281, 2 μοχθηρῶν)

[56] I have made the last two words dative-ablative plural, as in P1, as this would explain M's omission as another *saut du même au même*.

2.37.10–11 *om.* <malaxat . . . ad hec> optimum est <et non solum> (Gk II, 283, 1–2)
2.158.6 *mundatur*: nudatur *uel* nudata *cett.* (this section not in Gk)

Mu

A very good copy, with some use of abbreviations, although with many endings unclear because of the state of the manuscript. Little, if any, interference: unlike the corrector of A, did not mark the dittography in η at 2.1.1, but corrected the *demonstraturus* of η′ to *demonstratus* at 1.85.1; 1.19.5 *orum* for *horum*. Note above all the loss of a folio between fol. 40vb (2.147 *De potionibus ad splenem*) and 41ra (2.161 *Signa anastomoseos*).

O

A very good copy, with problems caused by the small size of the hand and damage to the manuscript. Some use of abbreviations, including non-standard ones, e.g. *mŏs* for 1.85.1 *modus*. Occasional omissions and transpositions:

1.19.1 *capitis cute* for *cute capitis*
1.19.2 *cognosci ergo <oportet>*
1.85.2 *de his debeam* for *debeam de his*
1.85.8 *qualitatem cause; <et . . . cause;> sed multe*, a *saut du même au même* (Gk II, 5, 5–6)
1.86.3 *om.* existima <qui fluit et facit flegmonem> (Gk II, 5, 24–5)
1.88.2 *super inunctiones* written as two words
2.37.7 *om.* mela aut (Gk II, 281, 24 μῆλον ἢ)
2.158.2 *que res*: querela (nothing corresponding in Gk II, 187, 6)
2.236.3 *neruos*: ipsos *cett.* (nothing corresponding in Gk II, 501, 21)

Ox

A messy copy, with numerous interventions, some quite intelligent, others apparently arbitrary:

1.18.1 *[ana ÷ ii] delauabis*
1.18.2 *acri* for *acro*
1.19.1 *similis [illi] quod ycor Greci uocant*
1.19.3 *colericus igitur humor si h(ab)undat* for *colericus igitur abundans humor*
1.19.7 *Igitur si amarus fuerit gustus* for *Gustus igitur si amarus fuerit*
1.85.t. *De [diuersis] oculorum passionibus*
1.85.9 *fieri dolores et sepius ex qualitate, sepius autem* for *fieri dolorem et qualitates, sepius autem*
1.85.12 *faciunt <dolorem uel tumorem>*
1.87.3 *iuuant* for *mitigat*
2.8.3 *om.* manifestum <spuentes . . . manifeste considerandum> est: *habent cett.* (Gk II, 151, 21–2)
2.36.4 *add.* [mordicationes et] subitaneas sincopas: *non habent cett.* (not in Gk II, 281, 2)
2.271.8 *om.* Item aliud cerotum ad podagram . . . et sic miscebis cerotum et uteris. (Gk II, 575, 12–17)

P1

Very occasional probable traces of an uncial exemplar: *sineolas* (for *singulas*); more frequent signs of careless reading of minuscule: *mundati ad* for *mundatura(m)*, *supra* for *rubra* (on the spelling, see 5.2). The endings are all over the place, betraying a basic ignorance of Latin. Omissions, additions and other changes are also common:

1.19.1 *tabum* for *tabem*
1.19.5 *si autem nihil <horum> fuerit*
1.19.5 *et sup(er)emittis cutem et constrictio* for *et supereminentia cuti et constricta*
1.19.6 *causes eu* for *cause seu*
1.19.8 omission of *sed ... qualis sit*
1.19.8 *calidior enim si [fueri]tibi locus apareat*
1.85.8 *unaq:q: causa adtendens currare < > sed multias et uarias s(unt)*
1.85.12 *contingit enim haec et bonum solum* for *contingit enim et unum solum*
1.86.1 *enim* for *ergo*
1.86.2 *supra* for *rubra*
1.87.2 *p:quod* for *postquam*
2.158.7 *relatiores*: relaxatioris M, laxiora *cett.* (this section not in Gk)
2.235.4 *cognita enim*: cognitiones *cett.* (Gk II, 501, 15 διαγνώσεις)
2.235.5 *habet*: adhibet *plerique recte* (nothing corresponding in Gk II, 501, 17)[57]
2.235.5 *inexistentis*: iam existentes *cett.* (nothing corresponding in Gk II, 501, 17–18)
2.271.5 *om.* donec ... ceram (Gk II, 575, 7–8)

P2

Some use of abbreviations. A very good copy, showing very good knowledge of Latin, and evidence of careful correction, with only occasional error:

1.19.7 *si acetosus, melancǫlicus, si salsus salsum flecma habundat*, a good reconstruction of this corrupt passage
1.19.8 *sed et tactu [melius] cognoscere poteris*
1.85.10 *unde autem est* (est *add.*) corrected to *autem est unde*
1.86.1 *flegmonem [tibi] fecerit, erit tibi*
1.87.3 *igneos oculorum [dolorum] flegmones*
2.37.4 *om.* uincere (Gk II, 281, 20 νικᾶν)[58]
2.37.5 *om.* ut <citius> cibos accipiant: *habent cett.* (Gk II, 281, 21 ταχύτερον)

P3

Apparently complete chaos because of all the different correctors' hands and the infinite number of marginalia, but the quality of the copying, the correcting, and the philology is of the highest order throughout:

1.19.5 (in agreement with *locus*, the reading of γ for *loca*) *supereminens cutem et constrictus sic ut nichil ex hoc* (hoc *corr. ex* his)

[57] 2.235.6 non solum eos quibus mox ab initio curationem adhibet (scil. *medicus*): cf. Gk II, 501, 17 οὐ μόνον τοὺς ἀρχὴν ἔχοντας εἰς τὸ πάθος — but it is unlikely that *habet* in P1 is related to Greek ἔχοντας.
[58] P2 inserts *in stomaco uincere* in smaller letters at line-end after *humores*.

1.85.4 *solent contingere* for *contingere solent*
1.85.7 *ledunt* for *leserunt* (*lesit* γ)
1.85.8 *attendendo* for *attendens*
1.85.13 *ad unam "ergo" quanque earum*, and 1.87.5 *"fuerit" coctum* carefully corrected
1.86.3 *existimabis* for *existima* (*-ant* γ)
1.88.t. *humore sanguineo* for *sanguineo humore*
2.6.t. *de capite ... humores*: ex capite ... humor *cett.* (Gk sg. II, 149, 24 ἐκ τῆς κεφαλῆς ἐπιρρεῖ)
2.37.6 *om.* accepti (nothing corresponding in Gk II, 281, 22)
2.37.9 *quod ita conficitur*: cuius confectio recipit haec *cett.* (Gk II, 281, 26 οὗπερ ἡ σκευασία ἔχει οὕτως)
2.271.2 *debilitatem*: imbecillitatem *cett.* (Gk II, 573, 26 τὸ ... πεπονθέναι)

u

2.36.4 *lumborum*: lumbricorum *cett.* (Gk II, 281, 1 ἑλμίνθων)
2.37.7 *om.* in calida ... frigida infusum (Gk II, 281, 23 ἄρτον εἰς εὔκρατον λαμβάνειν ἢ εἰς ὕδωρ ψυχρὸν)
2.37.9 *aloe epantite ... feniculi radices cortices ... mel*: feniculi radicum cortice ... aloe epatite ... melle attico (Gk II, 281, 28–30 μαράθρου ... ἀλόης ... μέλιτος Ἀττικοῦ)
2.37.11 *reumachus*: stomachus *cett.* (not in Gk II, 283, 3)
2.37.13 *om.* sufficiant haec ... de acredine (Gk II, 283, 5–7 τοσαῦτα περὶ τῆς καρδιακῆς διαθέσεως εἰρήσθω τῆς γινομένης ἐπὶ δήξει τῶν δακνόντων καὶ μοχθηρῶν χυμῶν)
2.37.14 *om.* last word *humoribus* (Gk II, 283, 9 χυμῶν)

v1

2.36.2 *moribus*: uenenosis humoribus, *vel sim. cett.* (Gk II, 279, 23 χυμῶν)[59]
2.37.5 *causa*: cibos *cett.* (nothing corresponding in the Gk II, 281, 20–1)
2.37.7 *add.* mala [non satis dulcia]: *non habent cett.* (Gk II, 281, 24 μῆλον)
2.37.12 *dianacardion*: anacardion/-ium/-ia *cett.* (cf. Gk II, 283, 4 ἡ δι' ἀνακαρδίων)[60]
2.236.3 *om.* diximus: *habent cett.* (not in Gk II, 501, 20)
2.236.7 *om.* oportet ergo ... quales sunt causarum: *habent cett.* (Gk II, 503, 5–7 δεῖ οὖν ἀκριβῶς, ὡς ἔφαμεν, ὑποπτεύειν, ἥτις ἀκριβῶς ἐστιν ἡ ποιητικὴ τοῦ πάθους αἰτία, καὶ τὴν ἁρμόττουσαν ἐπιφέρειν βοήθειαν)

4.10. A Provisional Text of the Chapters Collated and Referred to in Chapter 4

The stemma explained and defended in the present chapter was reconstructed principally on the basis of collation and close consideration of the manuscript versions of, in all, twenty-two chapters selected from Books 1 and 2 of the Latin Alexander.

59 Could *uenenosis* be secondary, an addition in α, v1 reflecting α′? 'Poisonous' is not in the Greek.
60 Another correct reading preserved in v1 alone!

Eleven of these — the first eleven chapters of Book 2, on coughing — have been worked up into a sample fragment, as it were, of the proposed edition, and are presented in Chapter 5. The other eleven chapters are presented here in a more rudimentary form, partly in order to facilitate the putting into context of the many individual passages discussed in the foregoing account of the relations between the manuscripts (in 4.1–4.9), and partly in the hope of stimulating from interested readers further comment on the business of reconstructing the Latin Alexander.

The Latin text presented here in these 'appendices' to Chapter 4 is, I stress, provisional. My original intention was to give just the corrected text of ms. A. In coming to views on 'right' and 'wrong' readings in certain key passages in the process of collating and relating the manuscripts, I made (I hope) progress towards reconstructing the text of the archetype for longer extracts, and it is the interim results of this work that I present: here and there, however, bias may remain towards readings of δ, η and A in particular when these disagree with β.

While some passages are relatively straightforward, others are extremely confused either in the archetype or in the tradition or in both. What I print here in such cases is uncertain in the extreme, pending further work on other portions of the text — if, indeed, this will throw new light on the problems so far encountered. To take a more positive view, publishing these extracts in this rather raw and preliminary form will illustrate the nature and extent of the difficulties to be faced in reconstructing this text.

For the first passage only (4.10.1), which is much the shortest in terms of the amount of Latin text involved (a single recipe from 1.17), I offer, in addition to my provisional Latin text and Puschmann's Greek text, a transcription of each manuscript version (which may be useful also for giving a ready impression of the orthography of each witness, to supplement 4.9 above and 5.2 below), as well as a commentary in the main text on the reconstruction of the text and its transmission. For the other pieces (4.10.2–4.10.7), I present only a provisional Latin text, Puschmann's Greek text, and a few brief notes on text-critical and linguistic points.

4.10.1. Book I.17

This short passage (a recipe omitted from the early printing, *ed.*) neatly illustrates many of the relationships between the surviving witnesses, and the puzzling position of ms. C in particular (cf. 4.7.4 and 4.7.5 above).

Below, after Puschmann's Greek text (with some variants from ms. Mf), I offer my provisional text of the Latin version, with a select apparatus criticus and comments on each point. (For ease of reference, in such a short but confused extract, I append a transcription of each Latin manuscript version, in alphabetical order by siglum.) With regard to the form of the translator's Greek text at this point, it is worth noting that the Latin version sides with Puschmann's text and against ms. Mf on three or four points in as many lines (no indication of quantity after Πήγανον; presence of καὶ στυπτηρίαν; absence of τὰς τρίχας; preposition with μέλι). This is a salutary reminder that it will not do simply to equate the translator's exemplar with Zipser's α or a close congener of Mf (cf. the comparisons offered in 2.4.1 above).

(I, 461, 7–10) Πρὸς τὰ ἐν τῇ κεφαλῇ ψωρώδη καὶ ἰχωρώδη. Πήγανον (-ος *cum mensura* Mf) καὶ στυπτηρίαν (καὶ στ. *om.* Mf) λεάνας μετὰ μέλιτος χρῖε τὴν κεφαλὴν προξυρῶν (προξυρίσας τὰς τρίχας Mf)· ἐὰν δ' ἀφιστῆται τῆς κεφαλῆς τὸ δέρμα, ἐλαίας φύλλα ἑφθὰ μετὰ μέλιτος κατάπλαττε (μέλιτι καταπλάσσε Mf).

[Item aliud?] ad eas quae in capite scabias sunt. Rutam et stipteria teres cum melle, et unges caput; antea tamen rades. Si autem recesserit a capite cutis, oliuae folia cocta [trita?] cum melle cataplasmabis.

Item aliud ad P1M A P3] Item aliud OMu Item ad G1P2L2B Ma DOxGe (Item C Iterum G2 L1) | **eas quae** G1P2L2B Ma DOxGe] ea P1M eos quibus P3 quibus OMu *om.* A C φ

NB initium cap. in A C P3 φ:
Item aliud ad scabeas in capite A
Item ueteres autem scabies capitis illinies ut sunt C
Item aliud ad eos quibus in capite scabies ueteres (ueteres *s. s.*) sunt P3
Iterum ueteres scabies capitis sic curabis φ

Item aliud is not in the Greek, and Ox may alone have the right text. If Ox is right, however, it is probably by accident, for, given the agreement of A and γ, we must suppose that *Item aliud* was in α. As to the form of the pronoun, it may be no accident that *ea* in γ preserves the gender of the Greek (at least this is a possibility worth bearing in mind). If the neuter form is old, then ε made the easy correction to the feminine (*eas*). P3 and independently η′ alter the wording slightly to make the heading refer to the patients rather than the disease. The variety of versions of this simple heading (note also A and C) may indicate damage or corruption at any rate in η (contrast A and η); cf. the next paragraph. In the attachment of *ueteres* to *scabies*, we see the first of several agreements between C, P3 and φ, as in 1.18–19.

in cap. scab. sunt P1M OMu P3′] in capite sunt scab. G1P2L2B Ma DOxGe scab. in capite A ueteres autem scab. capitis C ueteres scab. capitis φ ueteres *add. super* sunt P3

The Greek word-order is reflected in γ, η′ and P3 (presumably from γ′), and I take this to be original in the Latin, too. Something has probably gone wrong with the end of the heading after *in capite* (cf. Greek ψωρώδη καὶ ἰχωρώδη). Latin *scab-* presumably reflects Greek ψωρ-. If the Greek text is like that used by our translator(s), we should have expected Latin *scabiosa* <*et icorosa*>. It is conceivable that *et icorosa* lies behind the curious addition of *ueteres* in C, P3 and φ. An alternative, perhaps more likely, explanation is that it is a corrupt form of the word *uteris* in the previous sentence ('Vteris autem illo magis ad humidas et impetiginosas'): C, P3, G2 and L1 all have *uteris* correctly at this point, but it is striking that *ueteris* for *uteris* is here attested both in the *Liber passionalis* (**s**, p. 309, where it is corrected from *Vteris*!) and in the oldest manuscript of the *Tereoperica* (Par. lat. 11219, f. 49ra *ueteris*).

unges *scripsi*] unguis M OMu unges C φ inunguis P1 P3 inlines A illinies *cett. NB* illinies … unges] Item ueteres autem scabies capitis illinies ut sunt ruta et stipt(er)ea teres cum mell(e) et unges caput C

I would defend a form of *ung(u)o* on the grounds that it is attested on both sides of the stemma (in descendants of γ and of η), while *illino* is attested only in descendants of δ (A, C and ε). The fact that C has both verbs, about a line apart (with *illinies* coming a line too early), suggests that *illinies* was written as an alternative over *unges* in C's exemplar but read with the preceding line by the copyist of C.

si autem rec. a cap. cutis (cortix *pro* cutis M) P1 MAOMu Ox] si autem cutis a cap. rec. G1P2B Ma D si autem cutis a cap. rec. cortice Ge si autem cutis rec. a cap. cortice C P3 φ.

Again, I follow the word-order attested in γ and η and in the Greek. I take it that ε 'improved' the order by putting the subject first and the verb last. The curious *cortice* (in C P3 DOxGe and ϕ; cf. *corticibus* in D and Ox) must surely reflect the corruption of *cutis* in γ′ (*cotis* → *cortis* → *cortix*/*cortex*; cf. *cortix* in M), interpreted as referring to the skins of the prescribed olives, and incorporated and adapted to the recipe by a majority of the descendants of ε. Note again the agreement of C P3 ϕ.

oliuae fol. coct. [trit.?] cum mel. P1M AOMu] oliue fol. coct. cum mel. trit. G1P2B Ma D (coct. et corticibus cum . . . D) cortice oliue et fol. coct. cum mel. trit. Ge cort. oliue et fol. coct. et trit. cum mel. C P3 ϕ (oliue cortice et fol. coct. trit. cum mel. Ox′: et corticibus *add. supra post* fol. [cf. D!])

It seems that *trita* was, if not original (it is not in the Greek), added very early to the Latin version, in asyndeton with *cocta*. A perceived harshness in the asyndeton was eased in ε by moving *trita* to the end of the phrase, in C, P3 and ϕ by inserting *et* between *cocta* and *trita*. The assumption into the tradition of olive-*skins* (*cortice*, *corticibus*: see above), in addition to leaves, required the addition of another *et*.

The manuscript versions, in alphabetical order by siglum (with *Lib. pass.* and *Ter.* at the end):

A 4vb Item aliud ad scabeas in capite Rutam et stipteria teres cum melle; et inlines caput. Antea tamen rades. Si autem recesserit a capite cutis; oliuę foliis coctis tritis cum melle cata plasmabis.

B 145r Item ad eas que in capite sunt scabies. rutam teres et stipteram alumen (alumen *s. s.*) cum melle et illinies caput ante autem rades. Si autem cutis a capite recesserit oliue foliis coctis cum melle tritis cathaplasmabis.

C 7v Item ueteres autem scabies capitis illinies ut sunt ruta et stipt(er)ea teres cum mell(e) et unges caput an(te)a t(ame)n radas. Si autem cutis recesserit a capite cortice oliue et foliis coctis et tritis cum mell(e) cathaplasmabis.

D 4vb Item ad eas que in capite sunt scabies. rutam stiptеream teres cum melle et illinies capud antea tamen rades. Si autem cutis a capite recesserit oliue foliis coctis et corticibus cum melle tritis cataplasmabis.

ed. *om.*

Ge 148v Item ad eas que in capite sunt scabies. rutam et stiptеream teres cum melle et illinies capud. ante tamen rades. Si autem cutis a capite recesserit cortice oliue et foliis coctis cum melle tritis cathaplasmabis.

G1 5r *et* **L2** 6vb Item ad eas que in capite sunt scabies rutam et stipt(er)eam t(er)es cum melle et illinies caput antea t(ame)n rades. Si autem cutis a (autem nondum a L2) capite recesserit oliue foliis coctis cum melle tritis (tritis *s. s.* G1) cataplasmabis (catha- L2).

G2 15r *et* **L1** 13v Iterum ueteres scabies capitis sic curabis. rutam et stiptеream teres cum melle et unges caput. antea tamen radas. Si autem cutis recesserit a capite cortice oliue et foliis coctis et tritis cum melle cataplasmabis (catha- L1).

Ma 6v Item ad eas que in capite sunt scabias (sic *uel* fit). rutam et stiptеream teres cum melle et illinies caput. Antea tamen rades. Si autem cutis a capite recesserit oliue foliis coctis cum melle tritis cataplasmabis.

M 288b Item aliud ad ea que in capite scabia sunt. Ruta et stiptiria teris cum mel et unguis caput antea tamen radis. Si autem recesserit a capite cortix oliue folia cocta trita cum mel catapl(asm)as.

Mu 2vb *et* **O** 5ab Item aliud quibus in capite scabies sunt. rutam et stipt(er)iam t(er)is cum melle (cum m. t. O) et unguis caput ante tamen radis. Si autem recesserit a capite cutis oliue foliis coctis tritis cum melle cataplasmabis.

Ox 4r (tit.) Ad eas que in capite sunt scabies. Accipe rutam et stipt(er)eam teres cum melle et illinies capud ante tamen rades. Si autem recesserit a capite cutis oliue cortice et foliis (et corticibus *s.s.*) coctis tritis cum melle cataplasmabis.

P1 144vb Item aliut ad eaque in capite scauias sunt. ruta et stiptiria teris cum mel et inunguis caput | (145ra) antea tamen radis si autem recesserit a capitis cutis oliue folia admiscis sucum et inunguis (in- *s. s.*). et permittis ut siccet . . .

(145ra) XVII. (*spatium uacuum pro tit.*) Ad psydracia et ad ea que in capite scauias sunt. Ruta et stiptiria teris cum mel et inunguis capud antea tamen radis. Si autem recesserit a capite cutis oliue folia cocta trite cum mel catapl().

P2 9v Item ad eas que in capite sunt scabies (*corr. ex* -eas) rutam et stiptercam teres cum melle et illinies caput. Antea tamen rades. Si autem cutis a capite recesserit oliue foliis coctis cum melle tritis cataplasmabis.

P3 4r Item aliud ad eos quibus in capite scabies ueteres (ueteres *s. s.*) sunt. rutam et stiptercam t(er)is cum melle et inunguis caput. antea tamen radis. si autem cutis recesserit a capite cortice oliue et foliis coctis et (et *s. s.*) tritis cum melle cataplasmas.

(*Lib. pass.*) **s** p. 309 Item alia ad ea que in caput scabia sunt ruta et stiptiria teris cum mel et inlinebis et de folia oliuarum cum mel cataplab'

(*Ter.*) Par. lat. 11219, 49ra Item alia ad ea que in capite scabeas sunt. rute stipteria. teris cum melle et inunges caput anteponis rades. Si autem necesse est a capite cutis oliuae folia cocta trita cum melle cataplasmabis.

4.10.2. Book 1.18–19

(**A** 4vb; **B** 145r; **C** 8r; **D** 4vb; ***ed.*** 3r; **G1** 5r; **G2** 15r; **Ge** 148v; **L1** 13v; **L2** 7ra; **M** 289a; **Ma** 6v; **Mu** 2vb; **O** 5b; **Ox** 4r; **P1** 145ra; **P2** 9v; **P3** 4r; Greek text I, 461,11 Puschmann)

1.18.t. Ad ulcera in capite spissa et rubra modica[61] assimilantia titinulas ex quibus tabes quaedam defluit

1. Ante rades caput, et aqua +– frigida –+ et nitro delauabis, et sic postea sulfure uiuo cum humana urina trito uteris.
+– *another recipe* –+[62]
2. Item aliud. Melanteria cum aceto +– acro –+ inunges.

[61] *modice* M. This is surely *modica ulcera*=ἑλκύδρια rather than *modice assimilantia* all for παραπλήσια.
[62] Although he is reporting Greek ms. Mf at this point, Puschmann fails to say that this recipe is not in it.

(I, 461, 11–21) **t.** Πρὸς (ἄλλο πρὸς Mf) τὰ ἐν τῇ κεφαλῇ ἑλκύδρια πυκνὰ καὶ ἐρυθρὰ παραπλήσια θηλαῖς, ἀφ' ὧν ἰχῶρες ἀποτήκονται (ἀποτίκτονται Mf M L 2203)

1. Προξυρήσας τὴν κεφαλὴν καὶ ὕδατι καὶ νίτρῳ προαποσμήξας θεῖον ἄπυρον (θ. ἀπ. *abbr.* Mf) μετ' οὔρου ἀνθρωπείου (μετὰ οὔρου παιδὸς ἀφθόρου Mf) λείων χρῶ.[63]
+– Ἄλλο πρὸς τὰ ἐν τῇ κεφαλῇ. Λιθαργύρου δραχ. ιβ′ ψιμμιθίου δραχ. ιβ′ θείου ἀπύρου οὐγγ. η′. κηρωτῇ μυρσίνῃ ἀναλάμβανε καὶ χρῶ.–+
2. Ἄλλο· Μελαντηρίαν μετ' ὄξους +– (δριμέως Mf) –+ κατάχριε.

1.19.t. De acorae[64] signis

1. Acora passio est in ipsa[65] cute capitis facta, parua foramina habens ex quibus fluit humor similis quod icor[66] Graeci uocant, unde et ipsa passio acora appellatur,[67] quod nos tabem dicimus.
2. Est autem quod defluit aut[68] colericum aut flegmaticum interdum etiam et melancolicum.[69] Cognosci[70] ergo oportet passionis ipsius proprietatem, et ex hoc maxime curatio est adhibenda.
3. Colericus igitur abundans humor subtilior apparet[71] et subcolerico[72] colore.
4. Si autem non fuerit subtilis sed pinguis et glutinosus, flegmaticus humor salsus[73] augmentatus facit acoras.
5. Si autem nihil horum fuerit, sed appareant loca ex quibus fluit humor duriora magis +– et scirodia –+[74] et supereminentia cuti et constricta,[75] ut nihil ex his defluat aut uix[76] modicum, scias melancolicum esse humorem qui facit acoras.

(I, 463, 1–18) **t.** Περὶ ἀχώρων

1. Καὶ ὁ ἄχωρ πάθος ἐστὶ περὶ τὴν ἐπιφάνειαν τῆς κεφαλῆς γινόμενον, μικρὰς διατρήσεις ἔχον, ἐξ ὧν ἔξεισιν ὑγρὸν ἰχῶρι παραπλήσιον· διὰ τοῦτο καὶ ἄχωρ τὸ πάθος καλεῖται. **2**. ἔστι δὲ τὸ παραρρέον ὁτὲ μὲν χολῶδες ἢ φλεγματῶδες, ὁτὲ δὲ καὶ μελαγχολικόν. διαγινώσκειν οὖν χρὴ τὸ κυρίως αἴτιον· οὐχ ἡ αὐτὴ γάρ ἐστιν ἐπὶ πάντων θεραπεία. **3**. χολώδους μὲν γὰρ ὄντος τοῦ πλεονάζοντος περιττώματος,

[63] Puschmann seems to say here (I, 461 n. 3) that he has followed Guinther's reconstruction of this sentence from the Latin mss. and Paul. Aeg. 3.3, as the Greek mss. are corrupt at this point. Note, however, that the sentence is perfectly legible in Mf, with the interesting variant in the specification of the source of the urine.
[64] Latin *acora, ae* (f) for Greek ἄχωρ, -ος (m).
[65] ipsæ A
[66] icor η] ycor (-g- P1, -ch- G1) γ G1L2 Ox ycora (-ch- D) *cett.*
[67] appellant η′, prompted probably by the surrounding actives, *uocant* and *dicimus*.
[68] ut M A
[69] aut$_2$ . . . melancolicum *om.* A
[70] Active in γ, P3 and φ.
[71] It is surprising not to be offered some form of *consistentia/consistere* for Greek τῇ συστάσει.
[72] cf. ὑπόχολον, the reading of Greek ms. Mf. *cum* for *sub* in M, G1 and P3 may illustrate the proximity of γ′ to M rather than to P1.
[73] cf. ἁλμυρόν in Greek ms. Mf.
[74] This should perhaps be restored in the Greek text.
[75] There may be a trace of the Greek comparative in *constrictio* P1, *constricti* M, but it may be that the comparative form was ignored.
[76] uix γ B: uix et *plerique om.* φ. Cf. Greek μόλις ὀλίγον.

λεπτόν ἐστι τῇ συστάσει καὶ ὕπωχρον (ὑπόχολον Mf) τῇ χροιᾷ. **4**. εἰ δὲ μὴ λεπτὸν τῇ συστάσει, ἀλλὰ παχὺ καὶ γλίσχρον, φλέγμα (φλεγματῶδες νόει καὶ ἁλμυρὸν Mf) τὸ πλεονάζον καὶ ποιοῦν τὸν ἄχωρα· **5**. εἰ δὲ μηδὲν τούτων εἴη, φαίνοιντο δὲ οἱ τόποι, ἐξ ὧν ἀπορρεῖ τὸ ὑγρὸν, σκληροὶ μᾶλλον καὶ ὑπερέχοντες τῆς ἐπιφανείας καὶ στεγνότεροι, ὡς μηδὲν ἐξ αὐτῶν ἀπορρεῖν ἢ μόλις ὀλίγον, γίνωσκε μελαγχολικὸν εἶναι τὸ ποιοῦν αἴτιον τὸν ἄχωρα.

6. Ceterum autem et quae praecesserunt causae,[77] seu temperantia aegrotantis et aetas siue gustus.
7. Gustus igitur si amarus fuerit, colericus est humor; salsus[78] autem si fuerit,[79] flegmaticus est; *acetosus autem*[80] melancolicus.[81]
8. Sed et tactu cognoscere poteris +– qualis sit[82] humor–+. Calidior enim si tibi locus appareat, colericus inest[83] humor. Si autem frigidior, flegmaticus est. Minus autem frigidus, melancolicus inest humor. +– –+

6. λοιπὸν δὲ καὶ τὰ προηγησάμενα αἴτια, ἥ τε κρᾶσις τοῦ πάσχοντος καὶ ἡ ἡλικία καὶ ἡ γεῦσις. **7**. πικρότητος μὲν γὰρ αἰσθάνονται οἷς χολῶδές ἐστι τὸ αἴτιον· ἁλμυρᾶς δὲ ποιότητος, οἷς τὸ φλέγμα (φλεγματῶδες?[84]), ἰώδους δὲ, οἷς μελαγχολικός ἐστι χυμός. **8**. ἀπὸ τῆς ἁφῆς δὲ διαγινώσκειν ἐστί σοι δυνατόν· θερμοτέρα γάρ σοι φαίνεται ἐφ' ὧν ἐστι χολῶδες, ψυχροτέρα δὲ ἐφ' ὧν φλεγματῶδες, ἧττον δὲ ψυχρὰ ἐφ' ὧν μελαγχολῶδες. +–οὕτω μὲν διαγινώσκεις τοὺς τίκτοντας τὸν ἄχωρα χυμούς.–+

4.10.3. Book 1.85–88.2

(**A** 28rb; **B** 154v; **C** 20v; **D** 24vb; ***ed.*** 16v; **G1** 22r; **G2** 76r; **Ge** 170r; **L1** 59v; **L2** 22vb; **M** 315b; **Ma** 29r; **Mu** 11vb; **O** 18a; **Ox** 22v; **P1** 162rb; **P2** 26r; **P3** 19r; Greek text II, 3 Puschmann)

1.85.t. De oculorum passionibus[85]

1. Iam enim in aliis tribus libris a me script*um est*[86] de oculorum passionibus qualiter oporteat cognosci in eis consistentes passiones, et causas eorum et curationes et

[77] *uerba* considerande sunt (sunt considerande Ma) *add.* ε (*etiam* C) attendere oportet *add.* Ox Ge. γ and η have the same verbless sentence as the Greek. For the personal use of *considerandus*, cf. 1.124 *-anda qualitas et quantitas* (II, 105, 20 ἐπισκεπτέον).
[78] salsedo η
[79] si fuerit P1 Ma *om. cett.*
[80] These two words are omitted by γ and η, who after *flegmaticus est* have just *aut melancolicus*. The earlier presence of *acetosus* may account for *salsedo* in η. All the descendants of ε (but not C) have *acetosus* (ἰώδης, LSJ, s.v. II.). On the medieval Latin terminology for the flavours, see Burnett, 'Flavours'.
[81] That M omits *salsus ... melancolicus* perhaps indicates that *est humor* originally stood after *melancolicus*, as in the Greek, which would make M's fault a *saut du même au même*.
[82] This subjunctive is even in γ.
[83] Does *inest* reflect a misunderstanding of ἐφ' ὧν ἐστι?
[84] We expect a derivative, rather than just the base φλέγμα. -τῶδες could easily have been lost by haplography before ἰώδους.
[85] For *similia*, cf. Paul. Aeg. 3.22.3, p. 172, and Adams, *Paul. Aeg.*, I, 409ff., 423ff.
[86] scriptis Ox P3 scripta sunt *cett.*

diuersitates colliriorum,[87] et modus[88] qualiter oporteat adhiberi et qualiter conficiantur +– demonstratus est –+.[89]
2. Vndc nunc[90] benc hoc[91] mihi uisum est ut breuiter constricteque debeam de his dicere, ut legentes hunc librum +– –+ non quaerant ex alio codice quae ad oculorum curationem sunt[92] utilia. +– –+
3. +– Oportet ergo prius singularum in oculis passionum signa cognosci et sic adhiberi curationem.–+
4. Incipiamus ergo [nunc[93]] iam dicere de his[94] quibus in oculis contingere +– solent –+ dolores.
5. Nihil enim sic dolorosum est nec +– in alia passione –+ sic urgetur artifex ut succurrat, quomodo in dolore nimio oculorum.

(II, 3, 1–11) **t.** Περὶ θεραπείας ὀφθαλμῶν

1. Ἤδη μὲν οὖν ἐν ἄλλοις τρισὶ βιβλίοις ἀναγέγραπταί μοι περὶ τῶν ἐν ὀφθαλμοῖς παθῶν καὶ πῶς διαγινώσκειν χρὴ τὰ ἐν αὐτοῖς συνιστάμενα πάθη καὶ τὰς αἰτίας τούτων καὶ τὰς θεραπείας καὶ περὶ διαφόρων κολλουρίων καὶ τοῦ τρόπου τῆς χρήσεως αὐτῶν καὶ τῆς σκευασίας. +––+ **2**. ἀλλ᾽ οὖν ὅμως καὶ ἐνταῦθα καλὸν ἔδοξέ μοι κεφαλαιωδῶς καὶ συντόμως εἰπεῖν περὶ τῶν αὐτῶν, ὥστε τὸν ἐντυγχάνοντα τῷδε τῷ βιβλίῳ +– θεραπευτικῷ ὄντι –+[95] μὴ ζητεῖν ἐξ ἑτέρων ἀναλέγεσθαι περὶ τῶν ἐν ὀφθαλμοῖς χρησίμων. +– ἀλλ᾽ εἰ δύναιτό τις ὥσπερ καὶ ἄλλων πολλῶν παθῶν οὕτω καὶ περὶ τούτου πῶς δεῖ καὶ τὰ ἐν τοῖς ὀφθαλμοῖς ἅπαντα διαγινώσκειν τε καὶ θεραπεύειν πάθη. –+[96] +– (**3**.) –+ **4**. ἀρξώμεθα οὖν ἤδη τοῦ λόγου ἀπὸ τῆς ἐν ὀφθαλμοῖς συμβαινούσης ὀδύνης· **5**. οὐδὲν γὰρ οὕτως ἀνιαρὸν καὶ +– –+ κατεπεῖγον τὴν τέχνην[97] εἰς θεραπείαν, ὡς ὀδύνη σφοδρὰ συμβαίνουσα τοῖς ὀφθαλμοῖς.

6. Quando ergo dolores nimii et intolerabiles occupauerint oculos, +– –+[98] non, sicut multi faciunt, narcoticis confectis praesumendum est uti colliriis;
7. multi etiam et ipsum opium praesumpserunt inquimatizare, unde nullo modo paragorizauerunt dolorem sed adhuc etiam magis laeserunt.

[87] The accusatives *causas*, *curationes* and *diuersitates* are not appropriately governed by *cognosci*, and hang rather in the air.
[88] Probably originally *modos*.
[89] Added in the Latin along with the change of *modos* to *modus*.
[90] cf. Greek ἀλλ᾽ οὖν! Latin *nunc* could be for Greek νῦν (for οὖν), but the Latin fails to convey 'nevertheless'.
[91] *hic* in ϕ matches Greek ἐνταῦθα, but probably by chance. Could *hoc* be impersonal 'it'?
[92] sint P2 Ge ϕ
[93] Greek ἤδη: *nunc* is absent in γ, and probably entered the tradition as a gloss.
[94] eis A. The Greek refers to the pain, the Latin (with the addition of *solent*) to the patients.
[95] θεραπεύοντα?
[96] According to Puschmann (II, 3 n. 2), the foregoing sentence appears only in some of the Greek mss. including Mf, and is correctly omitted by L, as it is not original but (in Iwan Müller's view) based on marginal notes, including εἰ δύναιτό τις. Puschmann prints it only in the note, and adds, 'Vielleicht bietet der lat. Text (oportet ergo … curationes) einen Fingerzeig für den ursprünglichen Wortlaut dieser Stelle?'
[97] Latin *artifex* here is preferable to τὴν τέχνην, which should probably be corrected to τὸν τεχνίτην; cf. 1.85.13 below.
[98] But the Greek phrase at this point looks very much like a gloss on ἀκαρτέρητοι.

8. Contemplari ergo oportet qualitatem causae, et unamquamque causam attendens curationis praeuideas[99] species. Non enim est una qualitas causae, sed multae et uariae sunt.
9. Fit enim[100] plenitudo materiae supercurrens, ut solum ex hoc uideas fieri dolorem et qualitates.[101] Saepius autem ex utrisque fit, ex qualitate scilicet[102] et ex quantitate.
10. Prouidendum[103] est autem unde prorumpat quod supercurrit, utrum ex toto corpore aut de solo capite fluat, aut per arterias aut uenas +– aut per utrasque ministretur –+ et qualis utique[104] superfluitas est.[105]
11. Aut enim ex sanguine nigro[106] aut coleribus aut flegmate aut melancolia est quod fluit aut <ex?> uentositate [est?] spiritus,[107] et si[108] unus ex ipsis est qui molestatur humor aut duo commixti.
12. Contingit enim et unum solum fluentem facere flegmonem et dolorem nimium, et duo simul permixti faciunt +– dolorem uel –+[109] tumorem, ex quibus etiam differentia est causae.[110]
13. Ad unumquemque[111] igitur[112] eorum quae necessaria sunt artificem adhibere expedit existimantem[113] cognitionem singularum passionum.

(II, 3, 11–5, 17) **6**. εἰ (ὅταν 2203 M Mf) οὖν ὀδύναι σφοδραὶ καὶ ἀκαρτέρητοι περιέχουσι τοὺς ὀφθαλμούς, +–ὡς μὴ δύνασθαι καρτερεῖν τὸν πάσχοντα–+, μὴ ὡς πολλοὶ τοῖς ναρκωτικοῖς +– εὐθὺς Mf –+ σκευαζομένοις θαρρήσῃς κολλουρίοις· **7**. πολλοὶ γὰρ καὶ αὐτὸ τολμήσαντες ἐγχέειν τὸ ὄπιον, πρὸς τῷ μηδὲν ὅλως παρηγορῆσαι τὴν ὀδύνην ἔτι (ἔτι δὲ L) καὶ μεγάλως (μᾶλλον Mf) ἔβλαψαν. **8**. ἐπισκέπτεσθαι οὖν δεῖ τὴν ποιοῦσαν +– τὴν ὀδύνην Mf –+ αἰτίαν καὶ πρὸς αὐτὴν ἀποβλέποντα οὕτω καὶ τὸ τῆς θεραπείας ὁρίζειν εἶδος· οὐ γάρ ἐστιν ἓν τὸ ποιοῦν

99 -at M P3′ A P2 DOx -ant Mu -ere *cett. om.* O
100 Fit enim] Etenim γ Fit etenim η. The start of this sentence is very uncertain. The *et* (in the well-attested *etenim*) may have arisen from the *Fit*, which is needed as the main verb. In A, *etenim* normally comes first in its clause (although in a couple of cases it appears to come second, after a noun or an adjective.)
101 Latin *qualitates*, as if for Greek ποιότητας. That this was not corrected in the light of the next phrase suggests that the translator was working in haste at this point.
102 scilicet *om.* γ Ox P3
103 Peruidendum A
104 Here, as elsewhere in the Latin Alexander and the Latin Oribasius, *utique*=Greek ἄρα; cf. Langslow, '*utique*'.
105 sit B
106 Probably, μᾶλλον somehow lies behind this (in medical terms, unwanted) epithet *nigro*, which evidently troubled a medieval redactor: the words *uel puro* are added above *nigro* in P3, and follow *nigro* in L2, B and ϕ. Excluding polygenesis, we can draw from this seemingly trifling matter the important inference for the stemma that ϕ was a source, rather than a user, of B.
107 For the plain ablative, cf. 1.37 'manifestum est uentositate tumentis spiritus fieri' (Gk I, 487, 21 φυσώδους ἐγκειμένου πνεύματος γίνεται). Only G1, P3 and Ox have *ex uentositat*e (but perhaps from γ′ via θ). The fact that we are here talking about causes makes the phonetically- and palaeographically-plausible nominative *uentositas (e)spiritus* (with prothetic *e*-) less likely as the starting-point. For this translation, cf. Orib., *Syn*. 8. 41.1 La *ex uentositate[m] spiritus*=πνευμάτων φυσωδῶν.
108 et si unus M. I take it that *si* is the original, automatic, and nonsensical translation of Greek πότερον, variously corrected in the tradition.
109 This may well originally have stood in the Greek.
110 In the Greek, the sentence does not end here. Might the absence from γ of *igitur* in the next line be a trace of an earlier Latin version closer to the Greek?
111 Did the translator mistake the Greek neuter for masculine? Only D and P2 have *unumquodque*.
112 igitur] *om.* γ ergo D Ox P3
113 Only γ has the participle, necessary for the sense; the rest have *existimare*.

αἴτιον,[114] ἀλλὰ πολλὰ καὶ ποικίλα. **9**. καὶ πλῆθος ὕλης ἐπιρρέον μόνον οἶδε ποιεῖν ὀδύνην καὶ ποιότης, πολλάκις δὲ καὶ τὸ συναμφότερον, καὶ ποιότης ἅμα καὶ ποσότης. **10**. θεωρεῖται δὲ καὶ πόθεν ὁρμᾶται τὸ ἐπιρρεῦσαν, ἆρά γε ἐξ ὅλου τοῦ σώματος ἢ ἐκ μόνης τῆς κεφαλῆς, καὶ πότερον διὰ τῶν ἀρτηριῶν ἐκχεόμενον ἢ ἀπὸ τῶν φλεβῶν +––+ καὶ οἷον ἄρα τὸ ἐπιρρέον ἐστίν· **11**. ἤτοι γὰρ αἷμα μᾶλλον ἢ χολὴ ἢ φλέγμα ἢ μελαγχολικὸς χυμός ἐστι τὸ ἐπιρρεῦσαν ἢ πνεῦμα φυσῶδες· καὶ πότερον εἷς ἐστιν ὁ λυπῶν χυμὸς ἢ δύο συμπεπλεγμένοι· **12**. ἐνδέχεται γὰρ καὶ ἕνα μόνον ἐπιρρεύσαντα ποιῆσαι φλεγμονὴν καὶ ὀδύνην σφοδρὰν καὶ δύο ἅμα καὶ σύνθετον ἐργάσασθαι +––+ τὸν ὄγκον. ἐπεὶ οὖν διάφορά ἐστι τὰ αἴτια, **13**. πρὸς ἕκαστον αὐτῶν ἀνάγκη τὸν τεχνίτην ἐφαρμόζεσθαι. ἡγείσθω δὲ ἡ διάγνωσις ὁδηγοῦσα εἰς τὴν ὀρθὴν θεραπείαν.

1.86.t. Signa quando sanguineus humor facit flegmonem

1. Si ergo sanguineus fuerit humor qui supercurrens flegmonem fecerit, erit tibi manifesta cognitio ex specie ipsius flegmonis.
2. Rubra enim sunt omnia et sanguineo colore, et ipsa facies rubra, et in tumore magno sunt posita, et uenae apparent [apertius et] plenae,[115] et grauitas sentitur, et pigritia in omnibus consuetis actionibus accidit.[116]
3. Et si in his neque mordicans lacrima uel[117] acris uideatur, adhuc magis sanguineum humorem esse existima qui fluit et facit flegmonem.[118]

(II, 5, 18–25) **t**. Περὶ διαγνώσεως τοῦ εἶναι τὸν ποιήσαντα τὴν φλεγμονὴν αἱματικὸν χυμόν

1. Εἰ μὲν οὖν αἱματικὸς εἴη χυμὸς ἐπιρρεύσας καὶ τὴν φλεγμονὴν ἐργασάμενος, ἔσται δῆλόν σοι ἐκ τοῦ εἴδους αὐτῆς τῆς φλεγμονῆς. **2**. ἐρυθρὰ γὰρ ἅπαντα καὶ αἱματώδη καὶ τὸ πρόσωπον ἐρυθρὸν καὶ ἐν ὄγκῳ μείζονι καὶ αἱ φλέβες εὐρύτεραι καὶ βάρους συναίσθησις καὶ ὄκνος περὶ τὰς συνήθεις ἐνεργείας. **3**. εἰ δὲ πρὸς τούτοις μηδὲ τὸ δάκρυον δακνῶδες καὶ δριμὺ φαίνοιτο, ἔτι καὶ μᾶλλον αἱματικὸν εἶναι νόμιζε τὸ ἐπιρρεῦσαν αἴτιον καὶ ποιῆσαν τὴν φλεγμονήν.

1.87.t. Curatio +–flegmonis de sanguine facti–+

1. Si enim sanguineus esse tibi manifestus fuerit flegmon, incidenda[119] est uena magis capitalis.[120]

[114] *Pace* Puschmann, Mf at this point jumps to II, 21, 11.
[115] uenas afferent plenas M: uenas apparent eius plenas P1: might *apertius* somehow reflect *eius*, which corresponds to nothing in the Greek and might have been originally an addition above *apparent*? K.-D. Fischer suggests *uene apparentes et plene* (?).
[116] There is no verb in the Greek for the whole of this section.
[117] Understandably, *uel* is normalized to *neque* in all but γ and, I suppose, γ′, whence Ox and P3 find it in θ. For the very common use of *uel=et* in Late Latin, see Hofmann and Szantyr, 502 (their examples begin with Marcell. med.).
[118] flegmonem facit AC
[119] incendenda A
[120] The word-order of the last phrase is not nice but is that of γ and γ′ (reflected in P3L2 DOx) and the Greek.

2. Si autem colericus acer humor cum sanguine appareat mixtus, et catharticum postquam flebotomaueris dabis et colliriis[121] uteris intrinsecus +– –+[122] qui digerere possint flegmonis, quorum etiam confectiones uobis tradere non omittam.
3. Extrinsecus autem[123] superponenda sunt adiutoria haec. Lac mulieris cum oui uitello et oleo roseo superpositum +– –+ mitigat et digerit satis igneos oculorum flegmones. Similiter quoque et uiolae herbae folia praestant.[124]
4. A*d* autem <eum>[125] cui cum nimio flegmone uel tumore ingenti +– dolor fuerit ortus –+ bene facit crocus cum micis panis et uitellis ouorum +– –+. Similiter autem et dactili faciunt – postquam[126] autem repressum fuerit reuma – cum meliloto crocus et glaucion et ouorum uitella cocta et oleum roseum +– permixta superponantur. –+
5. Ad dolores autem et plenas epiforas oculorum: rosis siccis. L iiii, croco L i +– opio L i. –+ Cum sapa[127] ubi melilotum fuerit coctum colliges +– et uteris. –+

(II, 5, 6–7, 16) **t**. Περὶ θεραπείας +– –+

1. Εἰ μὲν οὖν αἱματικόν σοι φανείη τὸ τὴν φλεγμονὴν ἐργασάμενον αἴτιον, τέμνειν χρὴ τὴν φλέβα τὴν ὠμιαῖαν. **2**. εἰ δὲ καὶ χολώδεις καὶ δριμεῖς χυμοὶ σὺν τῷ αἵματι φαίνοιντο, καὶ κάθαρσιν μετ' ὀλίγον τῆς φλεβοτομίας παραλάμβανε καὶ βοηθήμασι χρῶ, ἔνδοθεν +– μὲν τοῖς ἀδήκτοις καὶ πραϋτάτοις, –+ ἔξωθεν δὲ τοῖς συμπέττειν δυναμένοις τὰς φλεγμονὰς, ὧν καὶ τὰς σκευασίας ὑμῖν ἐκθησόμεθα. **3**. Περὶ τῶν ἔξωθεν ἐπιτιθεμένων βοηθημάτων. Γάλα γυναικὸς μετὰ κρόκων ᾠῶν καὶ ῥοδίνου διατιθέμενον +–θαυμαστῶς–+ πραΰνει καὶ συμπέττει τὰς πάνυ ζεούσας τῶν ὀφθαλμῶν φλεγμονὰς, ὁμοίως δὲ καὶ τοῦ ἴου τὰ φύλλα. **4**. πρὸς δὲ τὰς μεγίστας φλεγμονὰς καὶ ἐν ὄγκῳ μείζονι ποιεῖ καὶ ὁ κρόκος μετὰ ψιχῶν καὶ τῶν κρόκων τῶν ᾠῶν +–καὶ ῥοδίνου.–+ τὸ αὐτὸ δὲ ποιοῦσι καὶ οἱ φοίνικες[128] μετὰ τοῦ ἐπέχειν τόν ἐπιφερόμενον ῥευματισμὸν μετὰ τῶν μελιλώτων καὶ κρόκου καὶ γλαυκίων καὶ πυρρῶν[129] ᾠῶν ἑφθῶν [ἐκζεστῶν][130] καὶ ῥοδίνου.+– –+

[121] More specific than the Greek βοηθήματα.
[122] *Saut du même au même*, whether in the translation or in the translator's Greek text. θ″ added *uel extrinsecus* (cf. *interius uel exterius* Ge).
[123] igitur γ γ′
[124] For this intransitive use, cf. 1.131 'quemadmodum in oculis frequens praestat inunctio' (not in Greek). For *praestare* in transitive use, cf. e.g. 2.43=Gk II, 293, 2 παρέχει; 2.73 (nothing corresponding in Gk II, 401, 26).
[125] A*d scripsi*] At η P2, Greek πρός; *addidi sensus causa*. Cf. 1.15 *At autem* (A: Ad *ed.*)=I, 459, 9 πρὸς δέ. (It is also possible that *at* reflects an old abbreviation for *autem*, which was somehow repeated. I owe this suggestion to Cloudy Fischer. Cf. 2.164 *De leguminibus. At offerenda sunt* (A: De leg. off. autem sunt *ed.*)=II, 193, 14 τῶν δὲ ὀσπρίων προσφερέσθωσαν.) A common opening in the Latin version is *Ad eos autem*, but for *Ad autem* …, cf. 2.243 *Ad autem non nimiam* … (A)=II, 515, 14 πρὸς δὲ τὰς μὴ πάνυ … I cannot parallel *Ad autem eum* …; *Ad eos autem quibus* … would be idiomatic, but is not reflected in the tradition!
[126] A mistranslation of μετά + genitive as 'after'.
[127] Usually for Greek ἕψημα, e.g. at 1.66=Gk I, 549, 10; 1.70=Gk I, 555, 9; 1.114=Gk II, 87, 22; 1.127=Gk II, 115, 3; 1.128=Gk II, 121, 1; for γλυκύ at 1.127=Gk II, 113, 22. Cf. Orib. *Eup*. 4.15.4 ἀναλάμβανε μελιλώτων ἀφεψήματι ἤ γλυκεῖ (Aa *cum sapa*, La *aut sapa*). Cf. also Cass. Fel. 29.14 Fraisse 'melilotum … in passo coctum.'
[128] This phrase goes better after ῥευματισμὸν.
[129] This variation in the word for 'yolk' so soon after two occurrences of κρόκοι may be a hint that μετὰ … ῥοδίνου is an addition, albeit one old enough to be in the Latin translator's text.
[130] Obviously a gloss, which is drawn into the text. The obscure word that it glosses is 'corrected' to ἑπτά.

5. Πρὸς περιωδυνίας καὶ μεγίστας ἐπιφοράς.
Ῥόδων νεαρῶν...... δραχ. δʹ
κρόκου...... δραχ. αʹ
+– –+
ἀναλάμβανε μελιλώτων ἀφεψήματι +–ἐν γλυκεῖ ἀφεψηθέντων.[131]–+

1.88.t. De colliriis +–mitigatiuis in doloribus oculorum ex sanguineo humore factis–+

1. Cataplasmata enim[132] extrinsecus ad flegmonem *talia quae*[133] *diximus* sunt utenda.
2. Superinunctiones autem et inquimatismata +–sequenti sermone sunt ordinanda.–+

(II, 7, 17–19) **t**. Περὶ κολλουρίων +––+
1. Ἐπιπλάσμασι μὲν οὖν ἔξωθεν ἐπὶ φλεγμονηθέντων[134] κεχρῆσθαι, **2**. ἐπιχρίσμασι δὲ καὶ ἐγχυματισμοῖς τοῖσδε.

4.10.4. Book 2.36–7

(**A** 62ra; **B** 182v; **C** 39v; **D** 59ra; ***ed.*** 38r; **G1** 52r; **G2** 178r; **Ge** 63r; **L1** 136v; **L2** 50ra; **M** 359a; **Ma** 66v; **Mu** 27rb; **O** 39a; **Ox** 50r; **P1** 186ra; **P2** 54r; **P3** 43v; **u** 320; **v1** 59r; Greek text II, 279,18 Puschmann)

2.36.t. De cardiaca passione[135]

1. Cardiaca passio stomachi[136] causa est.
2. Contingit autem his quibus pessimi et uenenosi cum mordicatione stomachi ibidem colliguntur[137] humores et dominantur,[138] maxime his[139] qui nimis sensibilem[140] habent stomachum, ita ut interdum etiam aliqui mox derepente moriantur, non ferentes insustentabilem mordicationem uenenosis humoribus.[141]
3. Scire autem oportet quia et[142] lumbrici saepius superiora petentes ex inferioribus partibus ad stomachum necesse est ut faciant cardiacam passionem et cum angustia +–

[131] ἐν γλυκεῖ ἀφεψηθέντων looks very much like an addition (possibly from another version of the same recipe).
[132] igitur γ γʹ autem Mu Ox
[133] quae γ γʹ P3] qualia *cett.*
[134] M inserts δεῖ. As it stands, the infinitive κεχρῆσθαι would have to be taken as imperatival: for a parallel, cf. I, 335, 7, but in the overwhelming majority of its more than 200 occurrences in the Greek Alexander κεχρῆσθαι is dependent and not absolute.
[135] For *similia*, cf. Adams, *Paul. Aeg.*, I, 511–13 (add Oribasius, *Syn.* 9.10), and, on worms, Adams, *Paul. Aeg.*, II, 145–50, and Krieger-Königsberg.
[136] Here *stomachus*=στόμαχος, but in 2.36.2, 4; 37.14 *stomachus* translates τὸ στόμα τῆς γαστρός.
[137] generantur φ
[138] *dominantur* corresponds to συρρεύσωσιν, but must reflect something like κυριεύσωσιν (kappa and sigma differing by only a single stroke).
[139] his *om.* A
[140] debilem γ P3 φ. Cf. 1.113 *sensibilitas*=II, 79, 9 αἰσθητικόν.
[141] We are clearly here reading the work of a superior translator! Might he have ventured the bare instrumental ablative after *mordicatio*? Or should we reckon with loss of *e(x)* before *uenenosis*?
[142] et *om.* A

–+ sincopos[143] ingerant, ita ut aliqui statim[144] a lumbricorum mordicatione pereant.[145]
4. Propterquod[146] oportet non omnino[147] existimare a pessimis +– et uenenosis –+ humoribus fieri subitaneas sincopas stomachi, in[148] qua re etiam lumbricorum signa sunt requirenda. +– –+[149]

(II, 279, 19–281, 5) **t**. Περὶ καρδιακῆς διαθέσεως

1. Καὶ ἡ καρδιακὴ διάθεσις τοῦ στομάχου πάθος ἐστί. **2**. συμβαίνει δὲ τοῦτο, εἰ μοχθηροὶ καὶ δακνώδεις καὶ ἰώδεις ἀθροισθῶσιν ἢ συρρεύσωσιν ἐν τῷ στόματι τῆς γαστρὸς χυμοί. ἐὰν οὖν εὑρεθῶσί τινες ἔχοντες τῆς γαστρὸς αἰσθητικὸν τὸ στόμα, παραυτίκα ἀπόλλυνται μὴ δυνηθέντες ὑπενεγκεῖν τὴν ἄμετρον δῆξιν τῶν χυμῶν. **3**. πολλάκις δὲ καὶ ἕλμινθες ἐκ τῶν κάτω μερῶν ἀναδραμόντες ἐπὶ τὸ στόμα τῆς γαστρὸς ἐργάζονται καρδιακὰς διαθέσεις καὶ λειποθυμίας +– –+ ἀμέτρους καὶ συγκοπάς, ὥστε τινὰς (II, 281) παραυτίκα ὑφ' ἑλμίνθων δακνομένους ἀπόλλυσθαι. **4**. διὰ τοῦτο οὖν χρὴ μὴ πάντοτε νομίζειν ὑπὸ μοχθηρῶν +– –+ χυμῶν γίνεσθαι αἰφνιδίους συγκοπὰς τοῦ στόματος τῆς γαστρὸς, ἀλλὰ καὶ τὰ τῶν ἑλμίνθων σημεῖα ζητεῖν· +– οὕτω γὰρ καὶ τὰ θηρία ταῦτα θανάτους αἰφνιδίους ἐργάζονται καὶ συγκοπὰς οὐδὲν ἧττον τῶν ὀλεθρίων χυμῶν.–+

2.37.t. [Curatio cardiace][150]

1. Nam[151] qui habent in stomacho mordicationem de malignis humoribus et propterea sincopos patiuntur, inprimis oportet eis cibos offerri qui et refrigerandi habeant aliquid,[152] et confortare possint locum qui solutus est.
2. Infrigdant igitur bene et corroborant[153] malogranati grana assumpta, siue sucus eorum acceptus, sed et mela[154] non satis dulcia sed mediocriter stiptica, et pira et persica[155]

[143] sincopos A O u P2 Ge (*cf.* sint copius P1 sine opus v1). Cf. *sincopas* in the next sentence.
[144] *statim* may be a hallmark of this translator. In A it occurs only twice in Book 1 and nine times (including this passage) in Book 2, compared with countless occurrences of *mox*.
[145] The Latin Alexander seems otherwise not to use *perire*, and the word is probably used here in the interests of *variatio sermonis*, after 2.36.2 *moriantur*. Contrast 1.113, where *mori* is used three times in quick succession, although the Greek has three different expressions (II, 79, 7; 12; 18).
[146] Unanimously attested here, although elsewhere often with the variant *propterea*. In Book 1, A attests *propterquod* twenty-four times, *propterea* eight times and *propter hoc* three times.
[147] A favourite word in the Latin Alexander, though here inferior to Greek πάντοτε.
[148] *in qua re* is unparalleled in Books 1 and 2 in A, although *de qua re* and *pro qua re* are quite common.
[149] The Greek sentence here omitted repeats what has gone before, and may be a later gloss.
[150] This title is in G1, B, D and ϕ only, in G1 at this point, in ϕ, before *Inprimis oportet*, in B and D, later still, before *Infrigdant igitur*. Like G1, P3 has a title at this point, a much longer one: *Curatio cardiacorum qui habent ... patiuntur*.
[151] I incline to read this particle, although it can be reconstructed only for β, as this translator seems to begin every sentence with a particle. (It is also in Ox, with a red dot above the N.)
[152] With *habeant aliquid* cf. the reading of Greek ms. M ἔχει τι, although Latin *et* ... *et* nicely translates Greek μετὰ ... ἔτι καὶ.
[153] cf. 2.37.1 *confortare* and note the *variatio* also between *assumptus* and *acceptus* a few words later, perhaps another feature of this translator's style.
[154] Ms A favours *mela* over *mala* by 3:1 in Book 1, but *mala* over *mela* by 16:11 in Book 2 (although in the latter many instances of *mala* are in the sections from Philumenus and Philagrius).
[155] persice η: another example of a divergent *a*-stem noun in η.

et[156] duracina[157] et uuae quae austerum aliquid et stipticum habent, et panis in aqua frigida aut in calida aqua,[158] si[159] is qui patitur sit temperantia satis calida, et in eius stomacho contineantur humores mordicantes et acres nimis.
3. His[160] ergo ab initio h*unc*[161] oportet uti qui cardialgiam[162] patitur.

(II, 281, 5–15) **1**. τοῖς οὖν ἔχουσι μοχθηροὺς καὶ δακνώδεις ἐν τῷ στόματι τῆς γαστρὸς χυμοὺς καὶ διὰ τοῦτο συγκοπῆναι κινδυνεύουσιν ἁρμόζει πρῶτον αὐτοῖς ἁπάντων ἐκεῖνα τῶν ἐδεσμάτων προσφέρειν, ὅσα μετὰ τοῦ ψύχειν ἔτι, καὶ ῥωννύειν δύναται τὸ μόριον ἐκλυόμενον. **2**. ἐμψύχουσι τοίνυν καλῶς καὶ ῥωννύουσιν οἵ τε τῆς ῥοιᾶς κόκκοι ἐσθιόμενοι καὶ ὁ χυλὸς αὐτῶν καὶ μῆλα δὲ τὰ μὴ πάνυ γλυκέα, ἀλλὰ μετρίως στύφοντα καὶ οἱ ἄπιοι καὶ περσικὰ καὶ ῥοδάκινα καὶ ἡ αὐστηρὸν καὶ στῦφον ἔχουσα σταφυλὴ καὶ ἄρτος εἰς ὕδωρ ψυχρὸν καὶ εὔκρατον, εἴπερ οἱ πάσχοντες ἦσαν τῇ κράσει θερμοὶ πάνυ καὶ οἱ περιεχόμενοι χυμοὶ δακνώδεις καὶ δριμεῖς ἄγαν. **3**. τούτοις μὲν οὖν κατ' ἀρχὰς δεῖ κεχρῆσθαι πρὸς τὴν καρδιαλγίαν.

4. Ceterum autem oportet eis[163] addere paulatim cibos qui tarde digeruntur +– –+, quale est [+–de piscibus–+] bulba[164] et pectines et astaci et isicia *et*[165] pectines et ciricia[166] et uentres anserini et pedes porcini et quaecumque non facile corrumpuntur sed repugnando uincere possunt malos qui continentur[167] humores.
5. Oportet autem his, cum requieuerit +– aut lenimentum acceperit –+[168] passio, suadere semper ut citius cibos accipiant.
6. Nullum enim est aliud maius iuuamen[169] quam cibi qui tarde digeruntur et difficile corrumpuntur accepti.[170]

[156] et M: *om. cett.*
[157] duracine η
[158] Note the repetition of *in aqua* and the chiasmus, further features of this translator's style(?).
[159] I run on at this point, partly because the Greek does also, and partly because of the absence of a particle in the Latin (cf. note 151 above).
[160] Huic η P2 (and therefore δ?), prompted by singular *qui patitur*.
[161] h*unc* Fischer: hoc β η *om. cett.*
[162] v1 along with δ has *cardialgiam* (which in view of the Greek καρδιαλγίαν is probably right), although γ, u and O have *cardiacam*: while this is an easy error, given that *cardiaca passio* is the subject of the chapter, and could have occurred several times independently, its distribution suggests that it was in β, and may be another hint that O knew a descendant of γ (cf. 4.8.3 above); v1 found *cardialgiam* either in a source higher than β or in a descendant of δ. (Cf. 2.37.8 below.)
[163] ei AMu G1P2L2B Ge
[164] bulba *plerique*] uulua M (ἥ τε βοῦλβα καλουμένη): is *uulua* (edible sow's womb) intended? Two parallel passages, in which the Greek has the diminutive βούλβιον, are unilluminating: II, 247, 27 οἷον στέρνιον καὶ βούλβιον καὶ δαμαλῶν πόδες=2.19 (A) 'qualia bubula sunt et sternion et de iunice pedes'; II, 495, 7 καὶ τῶν κρεῶν βούλβιον καὶ στέρνιον καὶ πόδες μάλιστα τῶν βοῶν=2.200 (A) 'et carnes steriles et pedes porcinos et maxime bouinos'.
[165] ad P1 adde M de *cett.*
[166] ciciria A
[167] Greek κρατοῦσαν would lead us to expect *dominantur/dominentur*, and *continentur* may reflect a misreading of a script in which *t* resembles *m*.
[168] Notice again the fullness of the translation. If this phrase was originally a gloss, it was incorporated very early.
[169] adiumentum A D
[170] Yet another double translation, but here the translator seems to have misunderstood βραδυσιτεῖν 'to eat late in the day' (LSJ) and the logic of ἀλλά, and consequently to have started a new sentence in the Latin.

7. His ergo hora tertia suadendum panem infusum in calida aqua ut assumant aut in aqua frigida infusum[171] aut mela aut citri[172] deforis[173] mundaturam.
8. Diaeta enim haec expedit eis[174] qui cardialgiam[175] patiuntur.

(II, 281, 15–25) **4**. λοιπὸν δὲ δεῖ προστιθέναι κατὰ μέρος αὐτοῖς, ὅσα δυσμετάβλητά εἰσι +– καὶ δύνανται πρὸς τὰ δακνώδη ἀντέχειν καὶ δριμέα τῶν λυπούντων χυμῶν,–+ οἷόν ἐστιν +– –+ ἥ τε βοῦλβα καλουμένη καὶ τὸ στέρνιον καὶ ἀστακοὶ καὶ ἰσικοὶ καὶ κτένια καὶ κηρύκια καὶ κοιλίαι χηνῶν καὶ πόδες συῶν καὶ ἁπλῶς, ὅσα δύνανται μὴ διαφθείρεσθαι ταχέως, ἀλλὰ καὶ μάχεσθαι καὶ νικᾶν τὴν κρατοῦσαν κακοχυμίαν. **5**. δεῖ δὲ τούτοις καὶ μετὰ τὸ παύσασθαι τῆς ἐπιχεούσης διαθέσεως ἀεὶ ταχύτερον συμβουλεύειν ἐσθίειν· **6**. οὐδὲν γὰρ αὐτοῖς οὕτω συμβάλλεται, ὡς τὸ μὴ βραδυσιτεῖν, **7**. ἀλλὰ περὶ ὥραν τρίτην ἢ τετάρτην ἄρτον εἰς εὔκρατον λαμβάνειν ἢ εἰς ὕδωρ ψυχρὸν ἢ μῆλον ἢ κίτρον ἐκτὸς τοῦ λέπους αὐτοῦ. **8**. ταῦτα μὲν ἁρμόζει τοῖς τὴν καρδιαλγίαν ὑπομείνασι.

9. Adiutorium autem magnum[176] est glicia,[177] cuius confectio recipit haec:[178] Aceti sext. unum semis, feniculi +–radicis corticis–+ ÷ vi,[179] aloe +–epatite–+ ÷ iii, melle attico lib. iS.
10. Conficies[180] ut mos est, et dabis ex eo coclearia duo aut tria. Malaxat autem[181] et confortat uentrem.
11. Hoc enim medicamen +–ad haec–+[182] optimum est, et non solum cardialgias[183] sanat sed et inchoantem epilempsiam et ypocondriacas passiones +– uel quibus stomachus flegmate repletus frigidus est,–+ sed et alia plurima de quibus nunc non est tempus[184] ad commemorandum.[185]

[171] Note again the chiastic repetition (cf. 2.37.2 above).
[172] citri β: citrie η P2′ citrium *plerique*: another *a*-stem in η.
[173] Mørland, *Oribasius*, 167 implies that in Oribasius *deforis* is only an adverb (as in Alexander at e.g. 2.143 *impositus deforis*, 2.238 *deforis desparso*). Here it seems at first sight to be a preposition + accusative=*extra* in the sense of *praeter*, *sine* (Hofmann and Szantyr, 230–1); cf. 2.200 (A) 'melones praeter semina'=II, 495, 8–9 καὶ τῶν πεπόνων ἡ σὰρξ ἐκτὸς τοῦ σπέρματος. If we take *deforis mundaturam* as 'without its rind', we have the problem of the case of *citrium* (or *citria* f.?), clearly genitive in β and η. This problem obviously prompted the rest of the tradition to substitute the accusative *citrium*, change *mundaturam* to the participle *mundatum* 'peeled' and take *deforis* as the adverb. An alternative, to save the reading of α, is to take *deforis* almost as adjectival, 'of a citron the outside skin'.
[174] eis δ] his β γ γ′
[175] cardialgiam] cardiacam γ O P3 Ma C cardia u. Again (cf. 2.37.3 above), v1 alone of the descendants of β has the correct reading.
[176] Did the translator's original have μέγα, perfectly idiomatic in Greek (attested in Pseudo-Democritus, Oribasius, Rufus)?
[177] Here and at 2.37.12 below, the tradition points fairly clearly to a *glicia*/*-ea* for Greek γλυκύ. The transfer to the 1st declension is striking.
[178] In this recipe, the Latin gives more detail than the Greek.
[179] radicis corticis] -um -ibus A OMu P2. Fennel-root is called for already at Cato, *Agr.* 127.1, but it is harder to parallel the use of the skin of the root (*cortex*). The Latin and the Greek disagree on the amount. The Latin tradition is unanimous.
[180] conficis β
[181] autem *om.* β: was it lost because abbreviated to *at* immediately after *-at* of *malaxat*? Or was it originally not there, as in the particle-less Greek?
[182] *ad haec* is not in the Greek. The Latin tradition is divided between *hec* and *hoc*, both branches being split, and some mss. having just an abbreviation (*h* with a dot, or a stroke through the tail).
[183] cardiacam M DOx P3 Ma: this time P1 and u (u has *cardian et alias*) reflect the correct reading as well as v1. Again, then, if DOx P3 Ma took *cardiacam* from γ′, we see the proximity of γ′ to M.
[184] tempus non est A
[185] This construction may be another tell-tale of this translator.

12. Scio autem quia et anacardion[186] +–antidotum–+[187] ad tales passiones bene facit et pigra data[188] iuuat sed nullum sic sicut glic*i*a adiuuat.[189]
13. Sufficiant haec de cardiacis dicta quae fiunt[190] de acredine + — + humorum cum mordicatione.
14. Ceterum uero de his dicendum quae proueniunt in stomacho simptomata aut ex qualitate[191] [accidentium][192] aut ex aegritudinibus diuersis augmentantibus[193] humoribus.

(II, 281, 25–283, 9) **9**. τῶν δὲ βοηθημάτων ἐστὶν αὐτοῖς ἐπιτήδειον τὸ γλυκὺ λεγόμενον φάρμακον, οὗπερ ἡ σκευασία ἔχει οὕτως· ὄξους ξεστ. α′ s″ μαράθρου οὐγ. α′ ἀλόης ουγγ. γ′ μέλιτος Ἀττικοῦ λιτρ. α′ s″. **10**. ἡ δόσις κοχλ. β′ ἢ γ′. μαλάττει καὶ τονοῖ τὴν γαστέρα. **11**. τοῦτο τὸ βοήθημα κάλλιστόν ἐστιν· οὐ μόνον γὰρ ἰᾶται καρδιαλγίαν, ἀλλὰ καὶ ἀρχομένας ἐπιληψίας καὶ ὑποχονδριακὰς διαθέσεις +– –+ καὶ ἄλλα πλεῖστα, ὧν οὐκ ἔστι καιρὸς μνημονεύειν νῦν. **12**. οἶδα δὲ, ὅτι καὶ ἡ δι' ἀνακαρδίων πρὸς τὰ τοιαῦτα ποιεῖ καὶ ἡ πικρὰ, ἀλλ' οὐδὲν οὕτως ὡς τὸ βοήθημα τοῦτο. **13**. τοσαῦτα περὶ τῆς καρδιακῆς διαθέσεως εἰρήσθω τῆς γινομένης ἐπὶ δήξει τῶν δακνόντων +– καὶ μοχθηρῶν –+ χυμῶν. **14**. λοιπὸν δὲ καὶ περὶ τῶν ἄλλων εἴπωμεν τῶν συμβαινόντων ἐν τῷ στόματι τῆς γαστρὸς συμπτωμάτων ἢ διὰ ποιότητα ἢ διὰ ποσότητα πλεοναζόντων χυμῶν.

4.10.5. Book 2.158

(**A** 98ra; **B** 175v; **C** 59v; **D** 92vb; ***ed***. 61v; **G1** 83v; **G2** 281r; **Ge** 100r; **L1** 213v; **L2** 78rb; **M** 401b; **Ma** 107r; **Mu** *om.*; **O** 59b; **Ox** 81v; **P1** 212va; **P2** 85v; **P3** 74v; Greek text II, 187 Puschmann)

2.158.t. Ad emoptoicos

1. Non scio si est alia peior passio ista,[194] id est qui sanguinem expuunt, non ob[195] hoc solum quia ipsa per se euacuando occidere potest hominem, sed quia pessima et diuturna +– cum terribili mentis turbatione[196] –+ passio generatur.

[186] anacardion β] anacardium *plerique*, anacardia η and, surely independently, P1 (*onicardia*). Again, η goes in for a 1st declension form.

[187] antidotus P1 v1: there is no ἀντίδοτος in the Greek. Can we trust P1's *-us*? Probably not! Equally, v1's *dianacardion antidotus* looks freakishly learned and should probably be ignored.

[188] data β P2 Ox] datum *cett.* Neither is satisfactory. We may have lost *antidotum* after *pigra*.

[189] Another instance of *variatio sermonis* (*adiuuat* ~ *iuuat*) in this translator?

[190] fiunt β γ γ′ Ox P3′ Ma] fit *cett.* There is no trace of *qui* in the tradition, so that we must either understand *passionibus* with *cardiacis*, or take *que* as the all-purpose relative. It was presumably the form of the relative that prompted several copyists to correct *cardiacis* to *cardiaca* and *fiunt* to *fit*.

[191] qualitate u θ″] -ibus *cett.* Cf. the singular in the Greek.

[192] This may have entered the Latin tradition as a gloss on *simptomata*. The Latin suddenly falls apart and departs dramatically from the Greek. On the other hand, the Greek appears to lack the article before ποιότητα, ποσότητα and πλεοναζόντων. The appearance of Latin *aegritudines* out of the blue makes one suspect that the translator's Greek text had νοσότητα. What does *diuersis* translate? Might there have been dittography of the first part of Greek πλεοναζόντων?

[193] augmentantibus β] -atis *cett.* It is easier to suppose that the perfect replaced the present than vice versa, especially as the Greek text has the present participle, πλεοναζόντων.

[194] ista] ab ista (abstam P1) γ P3

[195] ob] enim γ. In A, in all of Books 1 and 2, *ob* occurs only here and at 2.199 *ad fin.*, where it is difficult to see what it is translating of Gk II, 493, 22.

[196] turbatione] perturbatione A Ox Ge. Cf. Fischer ('Lib. Byz.', 290) on the phrase *cum terribili mentis alienatione* in parallel passages of Theodorus and the *Liber Byzantii*. What on earth is this phrase doing here?

2. Quam plurime[197] ergo festinare oportet inprimis[198] mox cognoscere passionem unde contingit[199] causa aut in quo loco querela facta est.
3. +–Quibus agnitis–+ sic curatio competens est adhibenda et differri[200] non oportet, quia omnium aegritudinum[201] est pessima +– –+.[202]
4. Ante omnia scire oportet quia tribus causis sputum uel uomitum sanguinis cognoscendum[203] est fieri, id est per rixin et diabrosin et anastomosin quae Graeci uocant.
+– **5**. Rixin dicunt[204] cum uena crepuerit.
+– **6**. Diabrosin dicunt quando uena,[205] amisso nutrimento,[206] caro desuper ipsam extenuatur,[207] et uena nudata subtiliorque[208] effecta, eius tunica a se ipsa comesta, multum desudat sanguinem, et sic effusus intrinsecus per os[209] redditur.
+– **7**. Anastomosin autem dicunt cum ora uenarum, uirtute amissa, apertiora effecta et laxiora sanguinem refundunt intrinsecus, et sic aut uomitur aut per uentrem deducitur in secessus.–+
8. Cognosces autem unamquamque passionem generatam his signis.

(II, 187, 2–12) **t**. Περὶ αἵματος ἀναγωγῆς

1. Οὐκ οἶδα πάθος εἰ οὕτως ἄλλο χαλεπόν ἐστιν ὡς ἡ τοῦ αἵματος πτύσις· οὐ γὰρ αὐτὸ καθ' αὑτὸ τὴν κένωσιν ἄμετρον ἐπιφέρον ἀναιρεῖν πέφυκεν, ἀλλὰ κακίστων καὶ χρονίων αἴτιον +– –+ γίνεται νοσημάτων **2**. ὡς ἐπὶ τὸ πολύ· σπουδάζειν οὖν δεῖ διὰ ταῦτα διαγινώσκειν τὸ πάθος τοῦτο πρότερον, πόθεν ἔσχε τὴν αἰτίαν καὶ ἐν ποίῳ τόπῳ συμβέβηκε, **3**. +– –+ καὶ οὕτω τὴν θεραπείαν ἐπιφέρειν καὶ μὴ ἀναβάλλεσθαι· ἐπὶ μὲν γὰρ πάντων τῶν νοσημάτων ἐστὶν ἡ ἀναβολὴ κακὸν πάνυ, +– πολὺ δὲ πλέον ἐπὶ τῆς τοῦ αἵματος ἐξαγωγῆς.–+ **4**. εἰδέναι τοίνυν χρὴ τοῦτο πρὸ πάντων, ὡς διὰ τρεῖς αἰτίας ἡ τοῦ αἵματος ἀνάπτυσις ἐγνώσθη γινομένη, διά τε ῥῆξιν ἀγγείων, δι' ἀνάβρωσιν καὶ δι' ἀναστόμωσιν.
+– **5**. –+
+– **6**. –+
+– **7**. –+
8. γνωρίσεις δὲ ἕκαστον τῶν πόνων[210] οὕτως.

[197] Note the divergent sentence-breaks in the Greek and Latin versions. For *quam plurime* 'in general' (= ὡς ἐπὶ τὸ πολύ), cf. e.g. 2.2=II, 147, 24.
[198] For *inprimis* 'first of all' in late medical Latin, see Mørland, *Oribasius*, 162–3 (including an example of *mox inprimis*). Here presumably for Greek πρότερον (or τοῦτο πρότερον, if this is an adverbial phrase).
[199] contigerit B (Ma?) ϕ — but *facta est*, a few words on, is indicative in all mss.
[200] dilatare γ P3
[201] aegr. *om.* A
[202] At best an obscure compression of 'of all diseases this is the worst to delay in'. A lost *dilatatio* (cf. ἀναβολή) would explain the variant *dilatare* (for *differri*) in γ, γ′ and P3.
[203] Does the gerundive reflect a misreading of Greek ἐγνώσθη (e.g. as an infinitive in –σθαι, an imperative in –θι, or a jussive subjunctive in –θῃ), or a sort of preservation of the notion of obligation in *oportet*?
[204] dicent γ (also in 6 and 7, immediately below).
[205] The nominative is best left (cf. 5 *cum uena*, 7 *cum ora uenarum*), notwithstanding the anacoluthon.
[206] Apparently a correctly used ablative absolute. Cf. immediately below *eius tunica a se ipsa comesta*, and *uirtute amissa*.
[207] extenuat γ fit extenuata η κ (!)
[208] et subtilior P3 (!)
[209] ore γ ora G1 P3′. *ora* (pl.) in the sense 'small holes in the vein' would not be absurd.
[210] πόνος seems odd here. It is otherwise attested in Alex. Trall. twice in the plural (II, 81, 7; 481, 8) and nine times in the singular (e.g. II, 75, 1; 579, 25), always meaning 'pain' (cf. ἄπονος 'without pain' II, 377, 14; 573, 23), never 'disease, affliction' (*passio*), as apparently here.

4.10.6. Book 2.235–6

(**A** 116va; **B** 194v; **C** 69r; **D** 110rb; **G1** 99v; **G2** 332v; **Ge** 119r; ***ed.*** 74r; **L1** 254r; **L2** 92va; **M** 424b; **Ma** 128v; **Mu** 48vb; **O** 69^{bis}a; **Ox** 97; **P1** 224vb; **P2** 99r; **P3** 90v; **v1** 75va; *Pod.*: **po** 60v; Greek text II, 501,7 Puschmann)

2.235.t. De podagra[211]

1. Podagrae passion*em*[212] sciri oportet ante omnia quia ex multis et ex diuersis causis[213] habet consistentiam, unde existimo quia propter uarietatem natiuitatis eius neque cognoscitur omnino neque curari potest[214] perfectius.
2. Relinquitur[215] enim eius[216] aliquid in ipsis locis, et ideo[217] nullo modo[218] ab artificibus[219] medicinae sanari potest +– quia eius ignoratur natiuitas.–+[220]
3. Ego autem existimo ut quicumque eius bene potuerit natiuitatem[221] cognoscere uel diuersitates aut ipsas species quaecumque fiunt et qualiter contingunt, bene et cito[222] possit[223] curari et facilius a medicis +– ab ipsis infirmitatibus liberari.–+[224]
4. Dicamus igitur primo cognitiones ipsarum et sic postea curationes ipsas exponemus.[225]

[211] For *similia*, cf. Paul. Aeg. 3.78 and Adams, *Paul. Aeg.*, I, 657ff., 666ff.

[212] -es *trad.* We really do not want the plural, which may easily have arisen from *-em* before *s-*, especially as the disease is referred back to with singular *eius*, *cognoscitur*, *potest*. The form with *-ica-* (*podagricam*?), which must have been in β and *Pod.*, deserves serious consideration. The type *-i(a)ca passio* is paralleled e.g. at 2.36 *cardiaca passio*, and is common in Cassius Felix (see Langslow, *Medical Latin*, Index, s.v. 'passio + –ica'). On the other hand, *podagrae passionem* nicely reflects the Greek τὸ τῆς ποδάγρας πάθος.

[213] β appears to have had *diuersarum causarum*; P3, Ox and φ have *causis*, but all could have it from γ′, and δ may have lost *causis* (*causarum*?). Are there parallels for the abstract use of the adjective (*multa et diuersa*)? The genitive *diuersarum causarum* is worth considering as a literal translation of διαφόρων αἰτιῶν without attention to its construction, although M and v1 repeat *ex* before *diuersarum*.

[214] Probably here and certainly in the next sentence, where Greek has the aorist stem of δύναμαι (both times the 'medical' gnomic aorist), some or all of the descendants of β have stem *pot(u)er-* for *potest*.

[215] The start of a terrible misunderstanding (the translator seeing, or understanding, ὑπόλειψιν for ὑπόληψιν?). The Latin just about makes sense, but bears no relation to the Greek. What went wrong?

[216] enim eius *Fischer*] eius A enim *cett.* If this is our superior translator, we want a particle, and *eius* nicely refers back to the disease.

[217] The translator's way back from desperation onto terra firma.

[218] Correctly for Greek μηδὲ ὅλως 'not at all'.

[219] Elsewhere (e.g. 1.85.13) the Greek has τεχνίτης; here the Latin has the practitioners, the Greek, the art (cf. 1.85.5).

[220] ignoratur natiuitas M v1 P3′] ignorantis natiuitatis P1 (making genitive forms to agree with *eius*?) ignorantur natiuitates *cett.* This is a rather otiose repetition of the second part of 2.235.1. It looks as if β had *ignoratur natiuitas*, and my instinct is to prefer the singular. Is the plural otherwise attested?

[221] Not in the Greek and presumably picked up from the sentence before. Again, I prefer the singular with β.

[222] et cito] citto P1 credo M v1 *om. Pod.* Three possibilities: (a) *credo* is right, and was inserted to give the sentence structure when *existimo ut* eighteen words earlier was in danger of being forgotten; then P1 and the rest agree in error against M and v1, and either P1 is contaminated or I must redraw the stemma!; (b) *cito* is right, *bene et cito* being another double translation of the superior translator; M and v1 would then agree in error against P1, unless we regard *credo* as an easy error for the no-longer-familiar adverbial form *cito*; (c) both are secondary, and *Pod.* preserves the original reading (*bene posse curare*). The fact that *Pod.* tends to summarize and abbreviate the Latin Alexander is a slight argument in favour of *cito* in *Pod.*'s exemplar, as a second adverb parallel to *bene* would have been much more easily omitted than *credo*.

[223] If *possit* is for Greek ἄν, this may be another sign of a superior translator, as elsewhere we might have expected the mechanical use of *utique* (cf. Langslow, '*utique*'). On the Greek use of future + ἄν, see Schwyzer and Debrunner, II, 351–2 with literature.

[224] *ab ... liberari* is not in the Greek. It is a common conclusion in the Latin version, occurring at least seventeen times in Book 1 alone. It illustrates the repetitiousness, *variatio sermonis* and fullness of expression characteristic of the superior translator.

[225] Note the chiastic word-order, another feature of the superior translator.

5. Credo[226] enim quia si ea quae scripta tradimus diligentius attend*antur*[227] [naturam uniuscuiusque[228]] [uoluerit operari],[229] multos poterit liberare,[230] et non solum eos quibus mox ab initio curationem adhibet[231] uerum etiam diuturnas iam existentes podagras[232] iuuare poterit.[233]

(II, 501, 8–19) **t**. Περὶ ποδάγρας

1. Τὸ τῆς ποδάγρας πάθος εἰδέναι χρὴ πρό γε πάντων ὡς ἐκ πολλῶν καὶ διαφόρων αἰτιῶν ἔχει τὴν σύστασιν, ὅθεν, οἶμαι, διὰ τὸ ποικίλον τῆς γενέσεως οὔτε διαγνωσθῆναι καλῶς οὔτε θεραπείας τελείας ἠδυνήθη ἐπιτυχεῖν. **2**. ὑπόληψιν δὲ ἐκ τούτου τὸ πάθος ἀνιαρὰν ἐκτήσατο, καὶ μηδὲ ὅλως ὑπὸ τέχνης ἰατρικῆς ἰαθῆναί ποτε δυνηθῆναι. +– –+ **3**. ἐγὼ δέ φημι, ὡς, εἴγε διαγνωσθεῖεν καλῶς αἵ τε διαφοραὶ καὶ τὰ εἴδη αὐτῆς, ὅσα τε καὶ οἷα τυγχάνει, εὐθεράπευτος ἂν ῥᾳδίως ὑπὸ τῶν ἰατρῶν γενήσεται +– –+. **4**. εἴπωμεν οὖν ἤδη τὰς διαγνώσεις αὐτῶν, εἶθ' οὕτω καὶ τὰς θεραπείας. **5**. ἐλπιζέτω (ἐλπίζω?) γὰρ ὅτι τοῖς γεγραμμένοις ἐάν τις ἀκριβῶς προσέχοι, ὠφελήσει πολλοὺς οὐ μόνον τοὺς ἀρχὴν ἔχοντας εἰς τὸ πάθος, ἀλλὰ καὶ τοὺς ἤδη κεχρονικότας ἐν αὐτῷ.

2.236.t.[234]

1. Multa igitur sunt uitia[235] in his qui insanabiles possident podagras.[236]
2. Etenim sanguis calidus supercurrens[237] in articulorum cauitates, extenduntur, et nerui[238] quos sindismos uocant dolores facere in pedibus solent[239] nimios.

[226] Sg. 1 indicative for sg 3 imperative ἐλπιζέτω — or did the translator's text have ἐλπίζω? This is the only occurrence of sg. 1 *credo* in Books 1 and 2. ἐλπίζω recurs at II, 109, 24, but is not translated. The Greek sg. 3 imperative is otherwise correctly understood and rendered with a sg. 3 jussive subjunctive, gerundive + *esse* or a jussive future. At II, 551, 28, the only other place where τις is the subject of the sg. 3 imperative, τις precedes. It would probably be better to read ἐλπίζω in the Greek text!

[227] attend*antur scripsi ut* Pod.] -endo α. The gerund/participle is an easy corruption of the pl. 3 passive. Perhaps the common phrase *naturam uniuscuiusque* was added to provide a clear object for *attendendo*. For *attendo*=προσέχω, cf. 1.137=II, 127, 20; 2.5.2=II, 149, 17; for προσέχω of attending to a prescription, cf. II, 309, 13 (unfortunately not translated at 2.47).

[228] For this phrase, cf. 1.35 *fin.*=I, 487, 11ff.; 1.131, twice (from Galen, not Alexander); compare also 1.144 '(curabis) si prius ad causam attendas et naturam ipsius passionis'.

[229] In general I remain very uncertain about this sentence. The text printed here dispenses with the elements not in the Greek text, but the translator's text may have had more (or the translator may have added to what he found). The bracketed words (*naturam uniuscuiusque*, *uoluerit*, *operari*) are all used elsewhere by the translator. cf. the remarks on this passage in 4.8.2 above.

[230] At first sight, the Greek would have been accurately and adequately translated with *liberabit*. But in the text here printed *poterit* must be impersonal (cf. however note 229).

[231] The subject of *adhibet* must be the doctor (cf. *habet* in P1, which could be impersonal, 'there is'). The Greek phrase τοὺς ἀρχὴν ἔχοντας εἰς τὸ πάθος denotes the patients, but seems very odd.

[232] The disease in Latin (and plural), the patients in Greek and *Pod.* However, the failure of *Pod.* to supply the right correction of *uitia* in 2.236.1 makes it clear that the maker did not have access to a sensible Greek text.

[233] Again, not in the Greek: cf. notes 221, 224. Note the chiasmus and the *variatio sermonis* (*poterit liberare ... iuuare poterit*).

[234] New chapter and title, *De causis podagrae*, only in φ.

[235] This looks suspiciously like Greek αἴτια! The Latin is barely intelligible.

[236] Again, the Latin appears to have the plural where the Greek has singular (the singular forms in M *insanauilem ... podagra* carry very little, if any, weight). Presumably, *insanabilis* is for a form of Greek ἀνιατός, and *possident* for κτῶνται (the first syllable of τίκτοντα perhaps being read as the enclitic and not translated).

[237] I take this as nominative absolute, and understand *cauitates* with *extenduntur*.

[238] neruis κ

[239] The subject of *solent* must surely be *nerui*. The Greek would be best rendered with *solet*, which is in Ox, Ge and P3 *ex corr.*, and could go back to γ'.

3. Similiter autem et colericus humor saepius supercurrens super neruos aut inter ipsos residens,[240] et +– maxime –+ in his quos sindismos diximus uocari +– qui et ossibus uicini sunt –+, ardorem simul et tensionem[241] locis qui dolent infert et magnos dolores.

(II, 501, 19–24) **1**. πολλὰ μὲν οὖν εἰσιν αἴτια τὰ τὴν ἀνιαρὰν τίκτοντα ποδάγραν· **2**. καὶ γὰρ αἷμα συρρεῦσαν ἐν τῇ τῶν ἄρθρων κοιλότητι θερμὸν καὶ διατεῖνον αὐτά τε καὶ τοὺς συνδέσμους ὀδύνην ἐργάζεσθαι πέφυκε σφοδράν. **3**. ὁμοίως καὶ χολὴ πολλάκις ἐπιρρυεῖσα μεταξὺ τῶν νεύρων καὶ +– –+ συνδέσμων +– –+ καὶ τῷ φλέγειν ἅμα καὶ διατείνειν ἐπιφέρειν οἶδε μεγάλας ὀδύνας.

4. Sed et flegma eodem modo[242] laedens dolores fortissimos facit simul et frigdorem,[243] et angustata loca extendit.[244]
5. Facit etiam sic et melancolicus humor: et non solum infrigdat et opprimit sed et grauitate sua facta sentitur <non> mediocris[245] commotio.
6. Non enim solum oportet[246] ut supercurrente[247] materia reumatismi +– –+ solent[248] fieri sed et per simplicem solam qualitatem +– efficitur, id est per distemperantias ipsarum[249] quae fiunt –+ ex calido, frigido, sicco et humido +– et duplicata distemperantia, id est aut calido et sicco, aut calido et humido, aut frigido et humido, aut certe frigido et sicco –+,[250] ex quibus distemperationibus[251] fiunt saepius reumatismi.
7. Oportet ergo diligenter, ut dictum est, omnia contemplari[252] quales sunt causarum singularum qualitates uel quantitates,[253] et sic singularum causarum[254] expedientem apponere curationem.

[240] Another nice chiasmus, *supercurrens … residens*.
[241] tensionem] intensionem η P2′ B Ma(?)
[242] This suggests that the translator read Greek τρόπ- instead of τόπ-.
[243] There is no support in the manuscripts for the tempting change to instrumental ablative *frigdore*, so I presume that the translator read Greek ἅμα τε τῇ ψύξει with what precedes.
[244] angustata γ] coangustata *Pod.* angusta *cett.* Alternatively, perhaps: et angusta*t* loca *et* tendit, allowing a main verb for each Greek infinitive. Greek διατείνω (to judge from ms. A at least) is sometimes *extendo* (with 2.236.2 above, cf. e.g. 2.195=II, 491, 1) and sometimes just *tendo* (with 2.236.3 *tensio* above, cf. e.g. 1.94=II, 31, 5. 7); at 2.185, it is first *extenditur* and then *tenditur* in the space of five lines (II, 477, 3. 7).
[245] mediocris] mediocris effecta M v1 *Pod.* mediocriter effecta P1 mediocriter *cett. om.* Ox Ge. In the Latin Alexander, *mediocris*, *-iter* is the standard equivalent of μέτριος, -ίως and occurs (as adjective and adverb) nearly 100 times. The occurrence of *non mediocris*=οὐ μέτριος at 2.30=II, 265, 11 and 3.58=I, 361, 7 makes it unlikely that the omission of the negative here was an error of the translator, but it could have failed in his Greek manuscript. I remain uncertain whether to regard *effecta* (β *Pod.*) as original.
[246] Presumably, somehow for Greek δεῖ, whether from δέ or διά.
[247] supercurrente] supra- η
[248] Apparently, *oportet ut* + indicative (corrected to *soleant* by D and Ge).
[249] Understand *qualitatum*, I suppose.
[250] The tradition makes a real hash of this list of qualities and combinations. I give the version of v1, changing only nominative (*calidus*, etc. — evidently present in β) to ablative (*sicco*, etc.) in the second part (after *duplicata distemperantia*, which I take to be instrumental ablative, parallel to *per distemperantias ipsarum*).
[251] distemperationibus] -antiis O P2 B Ma D Ge Ox. The commoner word must have been restored more than once (probably by O, θ′ and Ox). *distemperatio* must be right (being in γ and η), but is really very rare. *ThLL* cites only Ps. Garg. Mart p. 211, 20 (in a recipe which is also in Oribas., *Syn.* 3.66, p. 919). Its use here might be another instance of this translator's taste for *variatio sermonis*.
[252] The tradition is unanimous on *contemplo(r)*. Of five other occurrences of Greek ὑποπτεύειν in the *Therapeutica*, four are translated, one with *existimare* (1.76=I, 593, 13), two with *suspicari* (1.140=II, 143, 20; 2.7.2=II, 151, 5), and one with a combination, *existimanda suspicio* (2.214=II, 357, 30). In the Greek here, note the repetition of ἀκριβῶς — is this to be defended on the grounds that it is used in two different senses?
[253] A formula not in the Greek; presumably, *qualitas* was prompted by the first part of Greek ποιητική?
[254] A final chiasmus (*causarum singularum … singularum causarum*) followed by a formulaic ending with hyperbaton (*expedientem apponere curationem*).

(II, 501, 24–503, 7) **4**. ἔτι δὲ φλέγμα χωρῆσαν εἰς τοὺς εἰρημένους τόπους ὀδύνης ἰσχυροτέρας αἴτιον γίνεται ἅμα τε τῇ ψύξει καὶ τῷ στενοχωρεῖν καὶ διατείνειν αὐτούς. **5**. οὕτω δὲ καὶ ὁ μελαγχολικὸς χυμὸς οὐ μόνον τῷ ψύχειν καὶ θλίβειν, ἀλλὰ καὶ τῷ βάρους ἐπιτελεῖν αἴσθησιν, οὐ μετρίους ἐργάζεται τοὺς παροξυσμούς. **6**. οὐ μόνον δὲ διὰ ἐπίρροιαν ὕλης οἱ ῥευματισμοὶ +– τοῖς ἄρθροις –+ ἐπιγίνεσθαι πεφύκασιν, ἀλλὰ καὶ διὰ ψιλὴν ποιότητα μόνην +– –+ καὶ θερμὴν καὶ ψυχράν (ψῦξιν M)· ἔτι δὲ ξηρότης τε καὶ ὑγρότης αἴτια γίνονται πολλάκις ῥευματισμῶν. +– –+ **7**. δεῖ οὖν ἀκριβῶς, ὡς ἔφαμεν, ὑποπτεύειν, ἥτις ἀκριβῶς ἐστιν ἡ ποιητικὴ τοῦ πάθους αἰτία, καὶ τὴν ἁρμόττουσαν ἐπιφέρειν βοήθειαν.

4.10.7. Book 2.271

(**A** 129ra; **B** 200r; **C** 75v; **Ch** 128r; **D** 122rb; ***ed.*** 82v; **G1** 110v; **G2** 367v; **Ge** 128v; **L1** 281r; **L2** 102ra; **M** 442a; **Ma** 143v; **Mu** 54va; **O** 74a; **Ox** 107v; **P1** 233rb; **P2** 109v; **P3** 101v; Greek text II, 573, 24 Puschmann)

2.271.t. De localibus adiutoriis mitigatiuis et anodinis[255]

1. Haec ergo per os[256] sunt danda[257] quae mitigare possunt[258] dolores.
2. Qui autem propter stomachi imbecillitatem[259] non possunt continere ut accipiant,[260] sed mox ut[261] biberint in uomitum concitantur, seu pro[262] timore aliquo siue per[263] suspicionem aliquam medicaminum[264] +– – et hi in accessione dolores ferre non possunt – –+[265] aliqua[266] debemus[267] uobis exponere, quae in ratione et experimento utilissima nobis +– contra dolores –+ esse uidentur, +– cerotaria anodina, quae mox sine dolore faciant ordinamus –+.[268]
3. Cerotum, quod dum in statu accessionis fuerit superpositum, mox sine dolore locus efficitur.

[255] et anodinis γ Ch DGeOx *om.* A (η?: *titulum om.* O Mu C Ma L2) G1 θ″ φ
[256] os] ore γ
[257] The gerundive is rather stronger than the statement οἶδε in the Greek.
[258] possunt] -int γ. The subjunctive in γ is striking; usually, δ has the subjunctive and γ, the indicative!
[259] imbecillitatem] debilitatem P3 L2
[260] ut accipiant] quod accipiunt A: a good correction by A, but *ut* must have been in α, the phrase meaning 'cannot control themselves so that they can eat'. Note *se continere* in P3 L2.
[261] For *mox ut* 'as soon as', see Hofmann and Szantyr, 637, citing late authors from Florus on (and noting *ut mox* in Cael. Aur.).
[262] pro] per γ. The two prepositions fall together in part in Late Latin and Romance; see Hofmann and Szantyr, 270.
[263] per] pro A Ch G1P3 Ox
[264] Here *medicamina* is perhaps to be understood as a collective,=φαρμακεία. Cf. *medicamen*=θεραπεία in Ps. Sor., *Isag.* and the pseudo-Herophilean letter to King Antiochus (Fischer and von Staden, 95).
[265] This addition may refer back to 2.266 'Quoniam multi a magnitudine passionis urgentur, quoniam(?) non possunt nimios ferre dolores, a nobis anodina requirunt medicamina' (= II, 561, 13–15).
[266] I run on, as there is no trace of a sentence-particle, although the structure of the 'sentence' is loose, to put it mildly. Latin *aliqua* could be a faint reflection of Greek ἄλλης.
[267] Rather different from Greek ἐσπούδασα, unless the latter has developed nuances of obligation in the later language.
[268] The words *cerotaria . . . faciant* resemble an additional sub-heading in the Latin. Note that even P1 reflects a subjunctive (*faciat*).

4. Recipit autem haec:[269] croco[270] opio ana ÷ iiii,[271] panis L i, cera L i, oleo sext.
5. Crocum[272] et opium infundes in uino; panem uero[273] in aqua infundes et exprimens manibus admiscebis ubi crocus et opium trita sunt, et iterum teres[274] donec omnia misceantur, sic postea ceram +– –+[275] solutam supermittens teres[276] et uteris.

(II, 573, 24–575, 8) **t**. Περὶ τοπικῶν βοηθημάτων παρηγορεῖν δυναμένων

1. Ταῦτα μὲν οὖν παρηγορεῖν οἶδε διδόμενα διὰ στόματος. **2**. πρὸς δὲ τοὺς μὴ ἀντέχοντας, εἴτε διὰ τὸ τὸν στόμαχον πεπονθέναι καὶ μὴ δύνασθαι κρατεῖν τι τῶν προσφερομένων, ἀλλ' εὐθὺς εἰς ἔμετον ὁρμᾶν, εἴτε διὰ φόβον καὶ ὑποψίαν τινὰ φαρμακείας ἄλλης, ἐσπούδασα μὲν ἐκθέσθαι ὑμῖν, ἅ καὶ τῷ λογῷ καὶ τῇ πείρᾳ χρήσιμα ἡμῖν ἀπεδείχθη ὄντα, ἔχουσι δὲ οὕτω· **3**. Κηρωτὴ ἐν τῇ ἀκμῇ τῶν παροξυσμῶν ἐπιτιθεμένη, ἀνωδύνους ποιοῦσα. **4**. Κρόκου, ὀποῦ μήκωνος, ἀνὰ οὐγγ. δ′, ἄρτου, κηροῦ, ἀνὰ λιτρ. α′, ἐλαίου ξεστ. α′. **5**. τὸν κρόκον καὶ τὸν ὀπὸν ἀπόβρεχε ἐν οἴνῳ, τὸν δὲ ἄρτον ὕδατι. καὶ ἐκπιέσας ἐπιμελῶς μίσγε τῷ ὀπῷ καὶ τῷ κρόκῳ προλελειωμένοις. εἶτα τὸν κηρὸν +–μετὰ τοῦ ἐλαίου –+τήξας μίσγε τοῖς λοιποῖς.

6. Item aliud cerotum simile quod in statu passionis adhibeatur.[277] Cera ÷ iiii, litargiro ÷ ii, psimithio ÷ ii, strigni suco L i, oleo rosaceo L i. Supermittes[278] sucum donec totum[279] colligatur, et sic uteris.
7. Item aliud cerotum.[280] Et ipsum mitigatiuum[281] est: facit enim[282] ad omnem inflammationem[283] ignitam. Opium soluens[284] cum lacte muliebri, addes[285] olei rosei ÷ vi, cera ÷ vi, et sic miscebis[286] cerotum et uteris. +– –+

(II, 575, 9–17) **6**. Ἑτέρα κηρωτὴ ὁμοίως ἐν τῇ ἀκμῇ ἐπιτίθεσθαι δυναμένη. Κηροῦ οὐγ. α′ (δ′ M), λιθαργύρου, ψιμμιθίου, ἀνὰ οὐγγ. β′, ῥοδίνου, στρύχνου χυλοῦ, ἀνὰ

[269] *Recipit autem haec* must be for Greek ἔχουσι δὲ οὕτω, which Puschmann prints at the end of the preceding section.
[270] For the moment, I am writing ingredients in the form suggested by the tradition, alternately (apparently) ablative, genitive, accusative, even nominative. This is an issue which I deliberately postpone for now.
[271] This is a great deal of saffron, unless some other ingredient is intended. A very similar recipe in Oribasius (*Eup*. 4.116.14) also prescribes four ounces, although in Paul of Aegina (3.78.8) only one ounce is called for.
[272] Crocum enim η (A OMu Ch C) κ′ (Ox Ge) — presumably, the particle was added twice, independently?
[273] uero γ G1P3
[274] terens η D — perhaps rightly.
[275] We seem to have forgotten the oil, unless it is taken for granted that it is used to melt the wax. (On the ratio of wax to oil to be used for different types of application, see Orib., *Eup*. 4.118.)
[276] terens A
[277] adhibeatur] -etur γ *ed.*
[278] -ens η
[279] Did the translator see πᾶν in his Greek version? (Cf. 2.271.10 *omnes carnes* and note ad loc.). Greek ἀναλωθῇ would account both for ἂν λυθῇ printed by Puschmann and for the variant ἂν λειωθῇ that he reports, neither of which is satisfactory.
[280] cerotum ad podagram A Ch C
[281] ipse mitigatiuus γ: perhaps we should reckon with *cerotus* (masculine) in the early tradition of Alexander, as in the Latin Oribasius (Mørland, *Oribasius*, 64).
[282] enim *om.* γ
[283] cf. the chapters on coughing, where φλεγμονή is not translated but borrowed (e.g. 2.7, including in the phrase 2.7.3 *ignitus flegmo*=ζέουσα φλεγμονή). Is there a difference of sense, e.g. internal (*flegmo*) vs external (*inflammatio*)?
[284] soluens η P2 θ″ D Ge (*om.* Ox)] solues *cett.* Compare Greek λείου, which (*pace* Puschmann) cannot mean 'dissolve'.
[285] addes *om.* γ
[286] miscebis] misces (-is γ) γ P3 — *misces* could be a 3rd-conj. future; cf. Väänänen, *Lat. vulg.*, 145.

λιτρ. α′. ἀναλάμβανε τῷ χυλῷ, ἕως ἂν λυθῇ. **7**. Ἄλλη κηρωτὴ καὶ αὐτὴ παρηγορικὴ καὶ ποιοῦσα πρὸς πᾶσαν φλεγμονὴν ζέουσαν. Ὀπίου δραχ. δ′ ἐν ἄλλῳ η′ κηρωτῆς ῥοδίνου λιτρ. α′. λείου γυναικείῳ γάλακτι τὸ ὄπιον καὶ οὕτω μίσγε τὴν κηρωτὴν ἐν τῇ θυΐᾳ καὶ χρῶ +– ὡς πάνυ καλλίστη.–+

8. Item aliud cerotum ad podagram[287] mirabile experimentatum +– –+. Mittens[288] in caccabo oleum commune sext. ii, coques lignis de uitibus, id est de sarmentis, donec bulliat +– –+.
9. Et +– ubi iam desierit[289] bullire,–+ torpedinem[290] [piscem] maritimum uiuum[291] pensantem[292] L i mittes in ipso oleo et coques donec iterum[293] bullitionem faciat[294] secundam aut tertiam.
10. Et post hoc supermittes asphalaci[295] (animalis quem aliqui *madamus*[296] uocant) sanguinem ÷ iiii, et simul coques cum torpedine donec discoquatur et soluantur[297] omnes carnes[298] eius.
11. Et sublatum ab igne cum refrigerauerit colabis[299] et mittes in alio[300] uase,[301] et cum opus fuerit accipies ex[302] ipso oleo quantum sufficiat ad[303] utendum, et miscebis ceram et resolues in trulla et facies[304] cerotum mollissimum et linteo inductum superpones.
12. Coques autem oleum sicut dictum est[305] in hospitio pede plano[306] mense Martio quinta feria.[307] Sic enim facta coctio multum ualere[308] potest.

[287] ad podagram γ η (not C) G1
[288] Mittens η P2 P3] mittes *cett.* Only experience will show whether this is right, but I have already the impression that the pattern present participle + finite main verb may be right for the first two instructions.
[289] desierit] desinet M -it P1
[290] torpedinem φ] turpid- *plerique* turpitudinem de D Ox Ge B (!) torpedinis .i. φ. On the use of the stingray in medicine, see Gossen.
[291] uiuum γ] *om. cett.* Cf. Greek ζώσης.
[292] pensans A (A repeats the pattern present participle + future indicative).
[293] Strictly otiose in the Latin, given *secundam aut tertiam*. Could *iterum* have anything to do with Greek τὸ μέτρον? τὸ μέτρον is itself strange: might it have been added as a noun phrase to agree with δεύτερον ἢ τρίτον, when the latter were no longer understood as adverbs?
[294] Again, the tradition is unusually unanimous over *donec* + subjunctive.
[295] asphalaci] asfalacus (-icus P1) γ (Greek genitive singular).
[296] *madamus scripsi* (μαδαμούδαν Paul. Aegin. 7.17.77)] adamus γ manda(m)um η marida(n)um *cett.*
[297] dissoluantur A
[298] omnes *om.* γ (cf. Greek). It is tempting simply to regard *omnes* as an addition of δ, but this passage bears comparison with 2.271.6, where again a word for 'whole, all' in the Latin (*totum colligatur*) stands opposite not πᾶν but ἄν in the Greek (ἄν λυθῇ). So, too, here: *soluantur omnes carnes*:: ἄν ἀναλυθῶσιν αἱ σάρκες.
[299] colabis *trad. et* P3′] colas γ P3
[300] Reflecting Greek ὑέλινον?
[301] uaso M uasculo P1
[302] ex γ η] de *cett.*
[303] ad *om.* A (by haplography after *sufficiat*).
[304] et facies] faciens A G1 P2
[305] sicut dictum est γ] *om. cett.* Cf. Greek ὡς προγέγραπται.
[306] plano] plane (plene A) η P2 D φ. The *ThLL*, s.v. *hospitium*, 3043, 69, cites this passage as the only instance of *hospitium* denoting a 'hypogeum'. If this interpretation is correct, plainly, it must depend on the whole phrase *hospitio pede plano*, and not just the single word *hospitio*. The Greek must indeed refer to an underground room, but the Latin would naturally mean 'a room at ground level' (with an inversion of the phrase *plano pede* attested already in Varro and Vitruvius).
[307] die Iouis γ: the Latin, in either version, must mean 'Thursday' (on this use of *feria*, cf. *ThLL*, s.v., 505, 18ff.); both Puschmann and Thorndike, *History*, I, 582 take Greek πέμπτη to mean 'the 5th of the month' (i.e. the recipe may be made on only one day each year!).
[308] ualere] iuuare ε Ch(!). While *multum iuuare* is a frequent collocation in the Latin Alexander, *ualere* occurs apparently only here. The Greek and Latin are again some way apart.

(II, 575, 18–29) **8**. Κηρωτὴ θαυμαστὴ καὶ διὰ πείρας, +– ᾗ καὶ ἄλλοι πολλοὶ προσεμαρτύρησαν. –+ Βαλὼν εἰς κάκαβον ἐλαίου κοινοῦ ξε. β′ ἕψε ξύλοις ἀμπελίνοις, ἕως οὗ βράσῃ +– σφοδρῶς –+, **9**. καὶ +– –+ ἐπίβαλε τουρπαίνης θαλασσίας ζώσης λιτρ. α′ καὶ ἕψε, ἕως οὗ τὸ μέτρον τοῦ προειρημένου ἐλαίου βράσῃ δεύτερον ἢ τρίτον. **10**. εἶτα ἐπίβαλε ἀσφάλακος (τοῦ ζῴου ὅ τινες παλαμίδα καλοῦσι) τοῦ αἵματος οὐγγ. δ′ καὶ συνέψει τῇ τουρπαίνῃ, ἕως ἂν ἀναλυθῶσιν αἱ σάρκες αὐτῆς. **11**. καὶ ἐπάρας μετὰ ταῦτα ψῦξον καὶ διήθησον καὶ ἀνατίθει εἰς ὑέλινον ἀγγεῖον. ἐπὶ δὲ τῆς χρήσεως λαβὼν ἐκ τοῦ ἐλαίου ὅσον ἐξαρκεῖ πρὸς τὴν χρῆσιν, μίσγε κηρὸν καὶ λύσας ποίει κηρωτὴν ἁπαλωτάτην καὶ εἰς ὀθόνιον ἐπιπλάσας ἐπίθες. **12**. ἕψε δὲ τὸ ἔλαιον, ὡς προγέγραπται, ἐν οἰκήματι κατωγαίῳ, μηνὶ μαρτίῳ πέμπτῃ μηδαμῶς ὑπερτιθέμενος τὴν ἡμέραν· οὕτω γὰρ ποιῶν ἐπιτεύξῃ.

13. Sufficiat haec de anodinis et paragoricis cataplasmatibus[309] dixisse.

(II, 575, 29–30) **13**. τοσαῦτα περὶ τῶν ἀνωδύνων καὶ παρηγορικῶν ἐπιπλασμάτων μοι λέλεκται.

+–EXPLICIT LIBER SECVNDVS: INCIPIVNT CAPITVLA LIBRI TERTII.–+

[309] Note the contrast between Latin *cataplasma* and Greek ἐπίπλασμα (as at 1.88.1, above).

CHAPTER 5. AN EDITION OF THE LATIN ALEXANDER ON COUGHING

5.1. Principles and Conventions Used in the Edition

This chapter contains a provisional text of the first eleven chapters of the second book of the Latin Alexander, that is, most of the section on coughing, with full critical apparatus, English translation, the corresponding portions of Puschmann's Greek text (II, 147, 1–155, 28), and some notes on the text and language.

The presentation of this material is intended to serve two main purposes. In the context of the present work, it offers on the one hand in the very full critical apparatus (and in the accompanying notes) an extended illustration of the tradition of the text and the relations existing between the manuscripts argued for in Chapter 4, and on the other hand an opportunity to make some observations and raise a larger number of questions regarding the Latinity of the Latin Alexander, some of which are drawn together in 5.3 below. In the broader context of ongoing work on the Latin text, this chapter offers a sample of the form and content currently envisaged for the full edition.

In the text, I use, by and large, standard classical orthography for Latin words,[1] partly for the sake of clarity, partly because there is little to be gained — even if it were a feasible undertaking — from attempting to reconstruct the spelling of the original (see 5.2 below on the spelling of the manuscripts and the Appendix). In the case of Greek words in Latin letters, I have let myself be guided more by the forms in the manuscripts, thus making concessions to changes in the pronunciation and/or conventions in the spelling of e.g. *collyrium*, *dyspnoea*, *epiphora*: I write *collirium*, *dispnia*, *epifora*, and similarly *colera* (*colericus*, etc.), *emoptoicus* (αἱμοπτυϊκός), *icor*, *melancolia* (*melancolicus*, etc.) *scirodia*, and the unanimously-attested *inquimatizare* (ἐγχυματίζειν 'inject, treat by injections'), *pigra* (πικρά, an antidote), and *strigni* (στρύχνου[2]). In the text, I also make use of the following conventions:

[ ] enclose secondary material already in the archetype.
< > enclose original material already lost in the archetype.
italics signal material already corrupted in the archetype.
+– –+ in the Latin/Greek text enclose material absent from the corresponding portion of the Greek/Latin version.

In the apparatus, in general, unless they have a bearing on the reconstruction of the text or of a form attributable to the archetype, I ignore trivial orthographical variants (such as *-ti-* vs *-ci-*) and non-standard forms reflecting phonetic developments in Imperial and later Latin (e.g. alternation between *e* and *i*, *b* and *u*, *h* and zero), where these do not affect the grammatical or lexical form to be reconstructed (e.g. an isolated *conpedente* in P1 for *competenti*; again, on orthography, see 5.2 below). In the presentation of information in the apparatus, I have tried also to adhere consistently to the following conventions:

[1] This applies especially to the use of *ae*, *-ti-/-ci-*, *f* and *h*. I admit one or two departures from classical norms (e.g. *sulfur*, see 5.2 below). For now, I write *unges*, *ungere*, etc. and *urgetur*, etc., although γ at least seems to have spelled these verbs with *gu*.

[2] See André, *Plantes*, 251.

1. Variations affecting groups of words (e.g. points of word-order) are set out before those concerning individual constituent words.
2. Variants are cited in order of increasing distance from the chosen reading.
3. Illegible or partly illegible forms are reported only when they can contribute something, e.g. in virtue of their length by suggesting one reading rather than another.
4. '(?)' beside a reported form indicates that the reading is doubtful.
5. Manuscripts are cited in chronological order by family (γ before η before ε) and within each (sub-)family (e.g. D Ox Ge), although within ε, where things remain relatively uncertain, I tend to move from left to right across the stemma (θ′, θ″, κ); contaminated manuscripts are cited with the relevant family in each instance.
6. With reference to a single manuscript, **X′** = **X** *ante correctionem.*
7. *word-form*$_n$ (e.g. et$_2$) = the nth occurrence of the word-form (e.g. the second occurrence of *et*) in the section of text addressed by the apparatus at that point.

Finally, the notes are primarily philological and linguistic in nature. They contain very little on medical-historical aspects of the Latin Alexander, except in so far as these bear on the text and its interpretation. While in some senses regrettable, this is I think right and proper given the primary requirement of establishing a usable text (and of seeking linguistic criteria for identifying its date and place of origin), and especially because a new medical-historical commentary on Alexander must be based anyway on the Greek text, and on a new edition thereof (taking full account of the Latin version).

My first purpose in the notes is, then, to discuss significant manuscript variants, to justify the text that I have printed here, but also to consider alternative possibilities. This often depends to some extent at least on the usage of the Latin Alexander, which in the absence of an edition of the text is far from easy to determine. The information presented here in the notes (and elsewhere in the present study) is based for Books 1 and 2 of the Latin version on my own annotated electronic transcription of Angers 457, for Book 3 on a photocopy of the 1504 printing, and, for the Greek text, on Puschmann's edition (the Hakkert reprint and the text contained in the *TLG*) together with, for the relevant portions of the work (Section 2.1 above), a (rather faint) photocopy of the relevant folios of Venice, Marc. gr. 295 (Puschmann's Mf).

The second point of the notes is more strictly linguistic, having regard to the questions of the Latinity and the translation-techniques of the maker(s) of the Latin Alexander. At this early stage in the reconstruction of the text, observations offered under these headings are inevitably rather isolated and piecemeal. In that they are based on incomplete or imperfect evidence, they are often tentative and provisional, and they frequently raise implicitly or explicitly further questions which can be answered only in the course of further work on the edition. It seemed nevertheless preferable to include rather than to suppress these questions, in order both to make clear my proposed agenda and to invite help and comment from interested readers.

5.2. The Spelling of the Manuscripts

With the notable exception of the descendants of β, and P1 in particular, the spellings — including the erroneous spellings — of the manuscripts of the Latin Alexander are literary in nature and hence unpromising as evidence for contemporary pronunciation. In some cases, it seems plausible to reconstruct for the archetype α certain (non-classical) morphological and orthographical forms, but on the whole the tradition contains sufficient variation, even in the representation of a given word in a given manuscript, to render hopeless the notion of systematically reconstructing the orthography and morphology used by the maker of the archetype, let alone that of the original translation. I illustrate these general observations, both positive and negative, in a series of examples set out in Table 5.1 below.

Table 5.1: Some examples of orthographical variants in the manuscripts of the Latin Alexander

(Shading of a cell indicates that the word or form to the left with the spelling feature in bold is attested in the manuscript above; the sign '~' in a shaded cell means that the manuscript above attests both the 'abnormal' and the 'normal' spelling of the word or form to the left.)

ASPIRATED CONSONANTS

	P1	M	A	O	Mu	C	G1	P2	L2	B	P3	Ma	D	Ox	Ge	G2	*ed.*	L1
stoma**c**us																■ ~	■ ~	■
ca**th**aplasma						■			■						■		■	■
melan**c**olia	■	■		■				■				■				■	■	■
ca**t**articum	■	■		■	■	■	■	■			■	■ t-th	■ t-th	■	■	■	■	■
a**ch**ora	■ ~						■		■				■			■	■ ~	■ ~
i**c**or	y-	y-	■	■	■	■	y-	■ y-	■ y-	■ y-	■ y-	■ y-	y-	■ y-	■ y-	■ y-	■ y-	■ y-
torax	■ ~	■ ~		■	■ ~	■ ~	■ ~	■ ~			■			■ ~	■			
ni**ch**il		■	■ ~	■	■	■	■	■		■	■	■	■	■	■	■		■
mi**ch**i		?	■	■	?	?	■		■		?	■		?	■	■		■

i* AND *y

	P1	M	A	O	Mu	C	G1	P2	L2	B	P3	Ma	D	Ox	Ge	G2	*ed.*	L1
yc(h)or	■	■					■	■	■	■	■	■	■	■	■	■	■	■
sc**y**rod-	■		■				■	■	■			■	■	■ cy-	■ cy-			

NON-ETYMOLOGICAL /h/

	P1	M	A	O	Mu	C	G1	P2	L2	B	P3	Ma	D	Ox	Ge	G2	*ed.*	L1
habundans		■		■	■	■	■	■	■	■	■	■	■	■	■	■	■	■
his (= nom. sg. *is*)	■	■		■	■	■		■	■				■					
pro**h**icere				■	■			■	■	■	■	■	■		■			
ad_ibere	■							■ ~										

TWO PRONOMINAL FORMS

	P1	M	A	O	Mu	C	G1	P2	L2	B	P3	Ma	D	Ox	Ge	G2	*ed.*	L1
h**ii**s (= dat.-abl. pl. *his*)								■	■ ~	■ ~			■ ~	■ ~		■	■	■
his (= nom. sg. *is*)	■	■		■	■	■		■	■				■					

f* vs *ph

	P1	M	A	O	Mu	C	G1	P2	L2	B	P3	Ma	D	Ox	Ge	G2	*ed.*	L1
sulfur	■ -for	■ ~		■		■				■	■		■					

-gm- ~ -um-

	P1	M	A	O	Mu	C	G1	P2	L2	B	P3	Ma	D	Ox	Ge	G2	ed.	L1
fle**u**m-	■ ~	■ ~										■ ~				■		■ ~

SINGLE AND GEMINATE CONSONANTS

	P1	M	A	O	Mu	C	G1	P2	L2	B	P3	Ma	D	Ox	Ge	G2	*ed.*	L1
su**cc**us									■	■	■	■	■	■	■		■	■
o**pp**ium	■			■	■													
glu**tt**inosus		■ ~	■															
into**ll**erabilis					■	■											■	■
su**c**urrat								■	■									

WORD-FINAL *-d ~ -t*

	P1	M	A	O	Mu	C	G1	P2	L2	B	P3	Ma	D	Ox	Ge	G2	*ed.*	L1
se**t**											■							
uelu**d**																■		
aliu**t**	■																	
capu**d**	■												■	■ ~	■			

(continued)

Table 5.1: Continued

***-ci-* ~ *-ti-*: SOME EXAMPLES**

	P1	M	A	O	Mu	C	G1	P2	L2	B	P3	Ma	D	Ox	Ge	G2	*ed.*	L1
acciden**c**ia									■						■			
assimilan**c**ia									■	■		■				■		
distemperan**c**ia									■~	■				■~	■~			
nascen**c**ia									■	■				■	■			
sen**c**iunt									■	■		■						
fa**t**iunt						■~	■~	■					■					
suffi**t**iat						■	■	■										
pro(h)i**t**iunt						■	■						■					
ter**c**ia	■		■	■	■	■	■	■	■	■	■	■	■	■	■	■		
ac**c**io	■~			■	■~		■~				■~	■	■~	■	■~			
superun**c**cio												■			■			
cogni**c**io												■~		■~	■~			
cura**c**io	■~			■~								■~						
ini**c**ium	■~								■~	■		■		■				■
ui**c**ia				■					■	■		■		■		■		■
pa**c**iuntur	■				■~				■~	■~		■~	■~	■~				■~

A (SEMI-)PHONETIC ABBREVIATION

	P1	M	A	O	Mu	C	G1	P2	L2	B	P3	Ma	D	Ox	Ge	G2	*ed.*	L1
p(**er**)uus						■	■		■									■
p(**er**)agoriza-				■		■		■	■	■		■		■	■			

If we may ascribe to the archetype forms unanimously attested in the manuscripts, and in particular in the oldest manuscripts (P1, M, A and O), we may reconstruct with confidence, on the one hand, the following 'correct' spellings:

stomachus and *cataplasma* rather than *stomacus* and *cathaplasma*
flegm- (in *flegma*, *flegmaticus*, *flegmon*, etc.) rather than *fleum-*
sucus rather than *succus*
sed, *uelut*, *aliud* and *caput* rather than *set*, *uelud*, *aliut* and *capud*
-ntia rather than *-ncia* (at least in *accidentia*, *assimilantia*, *distemperantia* and *nascentia*)
sentiunt, *faciunt*, *sufficiat* and *proiciunt* rather than *senciunt*, *fatiunt*, *suffitiat* and *proitiunt*
and dative-ablative plural *his* rather than *hiis*.

On the other hand, we should be obliged also to write *melancolia*, *melancolicus*,[3] *catarticum*; nominative singular *his* (assuming correction in ms. A) for *is* 'he'; very probably *habundans* (discounting P1 and again supposing correction in A) for *abundans*; and *tercia* (standard in all the early witnesses, with the sole exception of ms. M) for *tertia*. And we should be uncertain whether to write *achora* or *acora*, *ichor* or *icor* or *ychor* or *ycor*, *thorax* or *torax*, *nichil* or *nihil*, *michi* or *mihi*, *sulphur* or *sulfur*, and *-ci-* or *-ti-* in a host of words containing etymological *-i-*, including the very common *patior*, *patiens*.

The examples of attested *-ci-* and *-ti-* forms reveal particularly clearly the extent to which spellings are tied to words rather than to sounds or sequences of sounds, and even then are subject to variation in the output of a single copyist (witness the variant forms of *actio*, *curatio*, *initium*, *thorax* in our oldest ms., P1). Given the special status of P1 (on which, more below), the long interval of time between the making of the Latin Alexander and the copying of M (the second-oldest witness), and the fact that we must still regard

[3] The patterns of spelling differ slightly even for such closely-related words as *melancolia* and *melancolicus* (to the extent that the later tendency to abbreviate the latter allows a pattern to emerge).

the question of the place of manufacture as open (in both geographical and sociolinguistic terms), for now at least I resist even those unanimously-attested non-classical spellings which are immediately clear and unambiguous (such as *habundans* and *tercia*), although I do report good manuscript evidence for non-standard spellings in the apparatus.

As already noted, the really interesting (i.e. non-standard!) orthography in the tradition of the Latin Alexander is more or less confined to descendants of β, and of these P1 has the lion's share. It is really only on this side of the tradition that one encounters in significant numbers the familiar written reflections of the sound-changes under way in Vulgar Latin/Proto-Romance, such as confusion of (a) (above all) *i* and *e*; (b) *u* and *o*; (c) the letters representing voiced and voiceless consonants; (d) single and geminate consonants.[4] Failing indication to the contrary, the examples in Table 5.2 below are all from ms. P1.

Table 5.2: Non-standard spellings in Par. lat. 9332 (and one or two other mss.)

(a) *i* for orig. long *e* (or unaccented short *e*):
humoris (nom. acc. pl.), *oportit*, *pectenis* (pl.; cf. *pectinis* v1), *qualitatis* ... *simplicis* (pl.), *refrigirandi*, *tussientis* ... *respirantis* (pl.), *ueninosis*; *aparit* (for *apparet*), *diffirentia*
e for orig. short *i* (or unaccented long *i*):
acedentia, *coleriis* (for *colliriis*), *contenentur*, *debelem*, *defferentia*, *deficele*, *humorebus*, *manefesta*, *mereto*, *netro*, *pegritia*, *pera* (also M u v1), *subcolorecus* (for *subcolericus*), *uetello*; *degerere* (for *digerere*), *insequente*, *requerantur* (for *requirantur*)

(b) *u* for orig. long *o* (or unaccented short *o*):
cognuscenda, *cibus* (for *cibos*), *multus* (for *multos*); *humur*
o for orig. short *u* (or unaccented long *u*):
confitemor, *eorom* (for *eorum*), *polmone*; *notrimento*

(c) voiced for voiceless:
agora (for *acora*), *agris*, *agro* (for *acris*, *acro*), *ygor* (i.e. *ichor*), *dracia* (for *trachea*), *sdrigno* (for *stricn-*), *grassitudinem* (for *crass-*)
voiceless for voiced:
clicia (for *glic-* = γλυκ-), *collicantur* (for *colligatur*), *expetientia* (for *exped-*), *meticatiuus* (for *mitiga-*)

(d) single for geminate:
acedentia, *aparit*, *cacauo* (*caccabo*), *coleriis* (for *colliriis*), *deficele*, *inflamationem* (also B), *reditur*
geminate for single:
oppium (also OMu)

Then there are (more isolated) examples of the syncope of short unstressed vowels (e.g. the familiar *calda* (also in mss. u and v1), *frigda*,[5] but also the less familiar *Fluminus*, *Flagrius* for *Philumenus*, *Philagrius*), the omission of *h* (e.g. *abere*, *abens*, etc., *abitudo*, *adibere*), the assimilation of certain consonant-clusters (*ss* for *rs*: *pessica*; *t* for *ct*: *petenes* (for *pectines*), and conversely *ct* for *t*: *tectinula* (for *titinula*); *(u)m* for *gm*: *aumentare*).

[4] This side of the family also throws up the occasional morphological or lexical vulgarism, such as the replacement of *differre* by *dilatare* (in P1, M and P3 and therefore in γ and γ′) or the 2nd-declension form *tenuus* (for *tenuis*) in M; these are in addition to the small number of banal late or vulgar forms to be reconstructed for the archetype, such as *acora*, *-ae* (fem.) for Greek ἄχωρ, -ος (masc.), *acro* ablative singular masculine/neuter of *acer*, *rubrus* for *ruber*, etc.

[5] On the other hand, *frigd-* seems to be the standard form in derivatives, such as *infrigdare* (for which only P1 and A sometimes, and L1 and *ed.* consistently, attest the stem *infrigida-*).

Ms. M has surprisingly few of these spellings in common with P1, and is characterized instead by other phonetically-conditioned ('vulgar') spellings which are rare in P1, notably uncertainty in the writing of word-final *s* (in e.g. *per arteria<s>*, nominative plural *humore*, nominative singular *lacrimas*, genitive singular *menti*) and above all confusion of *b* and *u*: note e.g. (with *b* for *u*) *bomitum, delabas, iubantur, mitigatibus* (for *-tiuus*), *solbis*, and conversely (with *u* for *b*) e.g. *inueccillitate* (cf. *inuecellitatem* in P1), and, above all, forms of *adhibere* and adjectives in *-bilis* (*deuilem, insanauilem, insustentauilem, intolerauilis, terriuili*); more isolated examples in P1 include *requieberit* on the one hand, and *beuere et* (for *biberint*), *souetaneas* (for *subitaneas*) on the other.[6]

Characteristic of the spelling rather than the pronunciation — the forms are in direct defiance of the pronunciation — of the makers of M and especially P1 is the non-assimilation of preverbs: both attest words beginning *ads-* (also in ms. u), *adt-*, M alone has *obp-*, and P1 alone regularly *adp-*, *conm-*, *conp-* (also, isolated, in ms. D), *conr-*, *inr-*; related to this almost hypercorrect non-assimilation is the consistent spelling *menbrum* (for *membrum*) in P1 (but contrast the assimilatory spelling *suptilis* in M). Curiously again, the digraphs *ae* and *oe* are almost exclusive to our 'vulgarest' of all witnesses, P1, where we find, for example, correctly *aegrotantis*, *haec* (also in ms. u), and hypercorrectly *astaciae tisicia* (for *astaci* et *isicia*!), *aemigranius, superfluaetatis, trahaere, ue(h)aementer, coeterum, uenoenosi.*[7] P1 attests hypercorrect use also of *y* (for etymological *i*), this in common with other manuscripts, on both sides of the family (e.g. *cybus* for *cibos* in P1, for *cibus* in P2). Apart from these and the other examples illustrated in Table 5.1 above, non-standard spellings occurring more than once in even a single manuscript are striking by their rarity: I might mention *exsistima* in Mu, *flecmaticus* in P2, and *accuta, melencolicus, significacio* in Ma, but the tradition is strikingly flat in this regard.

5.3. The Latinity of the Latin Alexander: Some Provisional Remarks

The following brief remarks on the Latinity of the Latin Alexander are naturally based almost entirely on the chapters so far edited, and are consequently provisional in the extreme. If the phonology and morphology of the descendants of β (with the partial exception of v1) are vulgar (see 5.2 above), there are repeated signs of a higher level of Latinity in their syntax and morphosyntax, so that I still incline to the general view[8] that the maker(s) of the Latin Alexander had a good command of a fairly high and 'correct' register of Late Latin. Another observation that seems to be receiving repeated confirmation is that of striking, and often enough apparently unique, lexical and grammatical agreements between the Latin Alexander and the Latin Oribasius. A third working hypothesis that I think deserves airing is that we should reckon with distinguishing the efforts of more than one translator (hence my frequent, cautious use of 'maker(s)'). I deal briefly here with each of these points in turn.

[6] Other, idiosyncratic forms in descendants of β that probably reflect both contemporary pronunciation and lack of familiarity with the target form include, in P1: *coare* (for *quare*), *sint copius* (for *sincopos*); in M: *inquismatismas* (for *inquimatismata*). There is a possible reflex of the palatalization of *d* and *g* before a front vowel in the forms *fatizium, fastigium* (for *fastidium* in P1) and *inierat* (for *ingerat*) in v1.

[7] There are isolated and generally incorrect examples of *ae* in other mss., e.g. *ipsae* in A, *oportaet* in O and P2, and a correct *ordinandae* in P3.

[8] Expressed and illustrated in Langslow, 'Alex. Trall.'.

5.3.1. A Relatively High Level of Latinity?

The Latin of the hyparchetype δ is of a much higher order than that of β, and the question arises whether β vulgarized or δ normalized what each found in his exemplar descended from α. A priori, it seems to me, the former alternative — namely that a relatively correct archetype was vulgarized in or before the making of β — is made more likely by the presence in β of morphosyntactic features of standard, 'high' Latin, especially in the absence of their hypercorrect use in β. So, for example, a correctly-used subjunctive or a construction such as the ablative absolute, the *ab urbe condita* construction, or *necessarium est* + accusative and infinitive or + *ut* with subjunctive, is much more likely to be a relic of something old and correct than an (at all events, sporadic) attempt to improve the Latin of an archetype even more vulgar than β.

The presence of features which in the classical period would have counted as vulgar need not tend against the general view of an at least reasonably high command of Latin on the part of the translator(s). The few secure non-classical forms so far identified, such as dative singular *acro*, nominative singular *rubrus*, may safely be regarded as standard by the fifth or sixth century at the latest (cf. Väänänen, *Lat. vulg.*, §234).

Nor is this general view of a relatively high level of Latinity in the Latin Alexander necessarily undermined by the steadily accumulating evidence of linguistic proximity between the Latin Alexander and the Latin versions of Oribasius (see the next section). Indeed, in my view, to raise this as an argument in favour of a vulgarizing Latin Alexander would be to beg the question of the linguistic register of the Latin Oribasius, texts which have arguably been ill served by their respective traditions and editors.

5.3.2. Agreements Between the Latin Alexander and the Latin Oribasius

Lexical and grammatical agreements between the Latin Alexander and the Latin Oribasius continue to multiply. To those that I have already recorded,[9] may be added yet further instances, both medical and non-medical, including (in alphabetical order):

alius alter 'other' (pleonastic; see 2.5.3 and note 98 below)
gargalio 'uvula' (also in the Latin Hippocrates; see 2.10.2 and note 172 below)
manifestum est quia (see 2.1.4 and note 35 below)
spissus (or *pinguis*) *et glutinosus humor* (see 2.10.t–1 and notes 161, 169, below)
uentositas spiritus, for Greek πνεῦμα φυσῶδες (at e.g. 1.85.11, Section 4.10.3 above).[10]

[9] In Langslow, 'Alex. Trall.': *acidonicus/acetonicus* 'bitter'; *aspratilis* (of fish) 'living in rocky places'; *bullitionem facere* 'bubble, boil'; *operatiuus* 'effective, drastic'; *princeps (neruorum)* 'main nerve' (or 'starting-point (of the nerves)', 'brain'?); *sablonosus* 'sandy'; *uirga* 'penis'; the spelling *mirti*-for Greek μυρσι-. In Langslow, '*utique*': *capitalis uena* (Greek ὠμιαία φλέψ) the humero-cephalic vein; *secessus* 'excrement'; *cataracta* (eye-disease); *lippes* (pl.; Greek λῆμαι); *amputo* 'allay, relieve, remove' (a symptom, disease); *euento* (with the derivatives *euentatiuus* in Alex. Trall., *euentatio* in Oribas. Aa, *euentatorius* in Oribas. La), used in both texts in tandem with *digerere* in 'double translations' of Greek διαφορεῖν 'dissipate, disperse', διαφορητικός 'discutient', etc.; *gutta prima a saponariis* (Alex. Trall. = Greek πρωτόστακτος κονία), *gutta de saponariis*, *gutta id est le<xi>ua a saponarios* (Oribas. Aa), *lexiua de saponariis* (Oribas. La = Greek κονία στακτή); *in antelatis* 'in the foregoing (discussion)'; *tricoscino*, *-are* 'sieve with a very fine sieve'; *absque* 'without'; *mox ut* 'as soon as'; *sic postea* 'then, after that'.

[10] I omit other features common to these texts which are attested more widely in later Latin, such as the use of *postea* = *postquam* (2.11.5 and note 194 below) or the use of *pus* 'pus' as a masculine noun (2.8.1 and note 133 below).

The evidence, then, continues to mount linking these texts in terms of translation-technique and hence by implication in space and time. Significant are not only unusual shared translation-equivalents for Greek terms (such as the last example above, or the double translation *digerere et/uel euentare* for Greek διαφορεῖν, note 9 above) but also the 'indirect', non-medical items including those in note 9 above or the particle discussed in detail in Langslow, '*utique*'. In that article, I was concerned to emphasize the differences between the older and the younger Oribasius (texts which, thanks in large part to the manner in which they have been edited, are standardly lumped together and spoken of in the same breath as out-and-out vulgar) and the differences between both versions of Oribasius and the Latin Alexander. Especially as the particle *utique* is attested in more than a few other late Latin texts, it was not part of my purpose in that article to argue with reference to these medical translations for proximity in their respective points of origin in time and space. Here, however, I would underline the importance of *utique* in two complementary if opposite respects: on the one hand, the very frequency of its use and the manner of one or two of its uses in the two versions of Oribasius and the Latin Alexander are surely significant links between these three texts; on the other hand, the fact that the overall pattern of use of the particle varies markedly from text to text is a salutary reminder that a single glossary, or set of translation-equivalents, may yield very different results in the hands of different translators. One would never think to suggest that the two versions of Oribasius were the work of a single man, and their respective uses of *utique* now constitute one documented divergence between them, with possible implications for their respective overall levels of Latinity. Equally, the possibility of multiple authorship is seldom raised in connection with late medical translations/compilations, even though the notion is a priori far from absurd and may find support in consistent stylistic differences between different parts of the 'same' text.

5.3.3. More Than One Translator?

Even in the short space of those few chapters of the Latin Alexander that I have attempted to reconstruct so far, I have been repeatedly struck by stylistic divergences that might just reflect the work of different translators. At this stage, most of the features that I think one can legitimately point to as potential tell-tales of the work of more than one translator concern sentence-structure, word-order and a tendency to *variatio*, rather than lexical choice in the matter of translating technical vocabulary.[11] Reading in text-order the sample chapters presented in 4.10 above and 5.4 below, I was struck first in 2.36–7 (and to a lesser degree in 2.235–6) by an apparently greater concern for and control of a certain higher style in the Latin manifested especially in the following features:

(a) the consistent use of a connecting particle to link each sentence to the preceding;
(b) hyperbaton apparently not suggested by the Greek, e.g. at 2.37.4 'malos qui continentur humores' (= τὴν κρατοῦσαν κακοχυμίαν);

[11] On the rare use of *statim* and the very frequent use of *mox*, see 2.36.3 and note ad loc. in 4.10.4 above). Other possible tell-tales include the use of *ad* + gerund at 2.37.11 'tempus ad commemorandum', and the use at 2.235.3 of a form of *possum* for potential ἄν instead of the automatic, translationese use of *utique*.

(c) chiasmus, e.g. at 2.235.4 'dicamus ... cognitiones, ... curationes ... exponemus'; 2.235.5 'poterit liberare ... iuuare poterit'; 2.236.3 'supercurrens super neruos aut inter ipsos residens';
(d) chiastic repetition, e.g. at 2.37.2 'in aqua frigida aut in calida aqua'; 2.37.7 'infusum in calida aqua ... aut in aqua frigida infusum'; 2.236.7 'causarum singularum ... singularum causarum';
(e) *variatio*, e.g. at 2.36.2–3 '... moriantur ... pereant'; 2.37.1–2 '... confortare ... corroborant'; 2.37.2 '... assumpta ... acceptus'; 2.37.12 '... iuuat ... adiuuat';
(f) double translation, e.g. at 2.37.5 'cum requieuerit aut lenimentum acceperit'; 2.37.6 'cibi qui tarde digeruntur et difficile corrumpuntur'; 2.235.3 'bene et cito curari et facilius ... liberari'.

Stylistically elevated Latin is no guarantee of a flawless, or even superior, translation of the Greek (the chapters on gout, for example, fall down over Greek ὑπόληψιν as early as the second sentence, 2.235.2 'Relinquitur enim ...'), and further study may falsify, or at least fail to substantiate, the hypothesis that at least two different men were responsible for translating 2.36–7 on the *cardiaca passio*, 2.235–6 on gout, and the very start of Book 2, set out below, on coughing.

5.4. AN EDITION OF BOOK 2, CHAPTERS 1–11

A 53vb; **B** 167r; **C** 35r; **D** 51ra; **G1** 45r; **G2** 154r; **Ge** 44v; ***ed.*** 32v; **L1** 118v; **L2** 44ra; **M** 349b; **Ma** 57v; **Mu** 23va; **O** 34b; **Ox** 43r; **P1** 180vb; **P2** 47ra; **P3** 38r (Greek text, II, 147 Puschmann)

2.1.t. De tusse

2.1.1 Tussis quidem[12]<est>[13] accidentia et ipsa, quemadmodum[14] et dispnia,[15] et[16] differentias[17] et ipsa habet qualitatis[18] causarum, [sed] quoniam[19] initium habet modo a calida distemperantia,[20] est autem quando[21] a frigida aut humida aut etiam sicca.

De tusse] De tussi ***ed.*****L1** Capitulum primum ad tussim **P3** *om.* **P1 O P2L2**

Tussis ... accidentia] T *deinde magnum spatium* **Ox** | quidem] equidem **M** si quidem **P1 AO Ma** (quidem **P1′**) | <est> *scripsimus* | accidentia] acedentia **P1** plurima accidentia **Ma** | et ipsa (et ipsas **AD**) quemadmodum **P1M AMu DOxGe**] quemadmodum et ipsa **ϕ** quemadmodum ***cett.*** *rasuram ante* quemadmodum *habet* **P2** | et$_2$] *om.* **M P3′ϕ** | dispnia (dipsnia (dipsinia **Ox** dipsnya **Ma**) **AOMu L2MaOxGe** disnia **D *ed.***)] de spuma **P1** disponet **M** | et$_3$ **G1L2BP3 Ma Ox** (*cf.* disponet **M**)] habet et **C** *om.* ***cett.*** | differentias] -tia (defe- **P1**) **P1M** differre scias **Mu** | et ipsa habet **MP2**] et ipsas habet **AMu Ma** et ipsas habuit **P1** et ipsas **C** habet et ipsas **L2B** habet ipsas **G1** habet et **DOxGe ϕ** habet ex **P3** (ex *add.* **m2**) habent **O** | qualitatis **P1 O**(?)] -e **P3** *corr. ex* -es **m2** qualitas *uel* qualitatis(?) **O** (*fort. corr. ex* -es) -es ***cett.*** | causarum] *om.* ***ed.*** causa (?) (*an ex* causarum *corr. uel abrasum?*) **O** | [sed] *seclusimus*] *om.* **P3Ma** | initium habet] h. i. **D** | initium] initio **O** | habet] -ent(?) **O** habuit **P1** | modo] hoc modo **Ox** | a] ad **P1** de **D** et **OMu** ex **P3Ma** *om.* **OxB** | calida distemperantia] -am -iam **O** | est autem **P1M AO P3Ma**] *om.* ***cett.*** | *inter* autem *et* quando *uerba* quando a calida distemperantia est quoque **AMu** (*dittog. notauit* **A**) | quando **P1M AO P3Ma**] quandoque **G1CP2L2B** *om.* **DOx ϕ** | a **A G1CP2L2**] aut **P1M O** autem **B** ex **P3Ma** modo a **OxGe ϕ** modo de **D** | *inter* frigida *et* aut *uerba* distemperantia est et humida *habet* **C** *uerba* uel calida *habet* **O** | aut] uel **Ma** | etiam] *om.* **OxGe ϕ**

[12] **quidem** *quidem* is one of several particles (including also *quippe* and *utique*) used very frequently in the Latin Alexander. It often answers a particle in the Greek, notably in the frequent chapter opening *Quoniam quidem*, which translates ὅτι μέν at 2.51 = II, 321, 2, 2.57 = II, 379, 1, 2.74 = II, 407, 6, ἐπειδὴ δέ at 2.16 = II, 245, 24, 2.211 = II, 353, 7 (note also 1.122 *solet quidem contingere* = II, 99, 8 ἐπειδὴ δὲ συμβαίνει). Also common are phrases of the type 1.41 *primo quidem ... postea autem* = I, 493, 10–11 πρῶτον μὲν ... ὕστερον δέ (cf. 1.47 = I, 501, 5 and numerous examples in Book 2), or 1.57 *sic quidem* = I, 517, 5 οὕτως μέν. But *quidem* is often used for emphasis when there is no corresponding particle in the Greek, as e.g. at 1.23 *et quidem* = I, 469, 8 καὶ τότε, and as apparently here. With the use of *quidem* here at the start of a chapter with no obvious match in the Greek, cf. 1.17 *Psidracia quidem sunt parui tuberculi* = I, 459, 22 ψυδράκιά εἰσι μικραὶ ὑπεροχαί; 2.204 *Pessima quidem passio* = II, 335, 5 δεινόν τι πάθος (unless here *quidem* is a corruption of *quaedam* for τι).

[13] **<est>** We obviously need the copula in the Latin (cf. Greek ἐστι). Its presence and its position matching that of Greek ἐστι may be reflected in the extra syllable between *tussis* and *quidem* seen in the variant readings *equidem* and *si()quidem*. On the other hand, it follows *quidem* in the similar chapter opening 1.17 quoted in note 12, and I tentatively follow suit here.

[14] **quemadmodum** In comparisons expressed in Greek with ὥσπερ, καθάπερ, in the Latin Alexander *quemadmodum* is apparently commoner and more widely used than *ut*, which in comparative function survives mainly in the fixed phrases *ut supra*, *ut dictum est*, *ut est* 'such as, for example'; note, however, *ut* for παραπλησίως at 2.11.5 *ut pthisici solent* (see below). *sicut* is also common, not only in the fixed phrases *sicut dictum est*, *sicut scripsimus*, and especially it seems in the chapters from Philumenus and Philagrius. The distribution of *quemadmodum*, *ut* and *sicut* may repay further attention. *quomodo*, on the other hand, is rare in the Latin Alexander in comparative function. I have

2.1.t. Concerning coughing

2.1.1 Coughing also, like dyspnoea, is a mere symptom, and it, too, has causes of different qualities. For it takes its beginning sometimes from a hot imbalance, sometimes, too, from a cold or a wet or even a dry imbalance.

II, 147, 1–4 (Book 5, ch. 1) Puschmann

Περὶ βηχός
Ἡ βὴξ ἐστι σύμπτωμα καὶ αὕτη καθάπερ καὶ ἡ δύσπνοια. διαφόρους δὲ καὶ αὕτη ἔχει τὰς ποιούσας αἰτίας· ποτὲ μὲν γὰρ ἄρχεται ἀπὸ θερμῆς δυσκρασίας, ἔσθ' ὅτε δὲ καὶ ἀπὸ ψυχρᾶς ἢ ξηρᾶς ἢ ὑγρᾶς.

---

found only three examples in Book 1 (plus two instances of indefinite *quomodo uolueris* 'however you like', at 1.110 and 119), and one in Book 2. Interestingly, three of these four instances have a negative first element (as does *Vitae patr.* 5.5.13, quoted by Hofmann and Szantyr, 649): 1.69 'nulla sic quomodo ista herba' (I, 551, 26 οὐδὲν οὕτως ὡς), 1.85 'nihil sic dolorosum ... quomodo' (II, 3, 9–11), 2.139 'non enim aliud inuenies melius quod sic possit malaxare duritias quomodo istud' (not in Greek); the fourth instance is 1.20 'similiter quomodo qui habent' (I, 463, 20 παραπλησίως τοῖς + participle). The distribution of *quomodo* 'as' in Latin generally, and the fact that it alone is continued in Romance (Ital. *como*, Fr. *comme*, etc.), suggest that it was stylistically lower than *quemadmodum* (already in Cicero, in casual registers; cf. Landgraf, 137–8); on the various replacements of 'comparative' *ut*, see Svennung, *Palladius*, 509–11, Hofmann and Szantyr, 648–50. The favouring of *quemadmodum* by the maker(s) of the Latin Alexander may be a further hint of relatively high linguistic pretensions.

[15] **dispnia** The Greek word is used only here and at 2.35 *dispnoici* (II, 273, 7 δυσπνοϊκοί). Otherwise, the following Latin equivalents are used: 1.143 *difficultatem spiritus*, *difficulter respirant* (II, 229, 6, 8); 2.7.1, 2.9.1 *difficultas spirandi* (II, 151, 2, 25); 2.7.2 *uix respirantes* (II, 151, 4 δυσπνοούντων); 2.259 *suspiriosi* (II, 543, 12). Of these, *difficultas spiritus* and *difficultas spirandi* are well attested as equivalents of δύσπνοια in earlier Latin texts, while *suspiriosi* is somewhat of a surprise, being earlier used to render ἀσθματικοί (cf. Langslow, *Medical Latin*, Index, s.vv.).

[16] **et differentias** This *et* may be a late addition (perhaps in θ″, whence G1 and L2, although it is also in B and Ox), or it may be original and reflected in *dispon<u>et</u>* M.

[17] **differentias** It is tempting to correct to *differentes*, but the Latin Alexander does not appear to attest the adjective *differens*! For a parallel where the Latin tradition has unanimously *differentia* + genitive for Greek adjective διάφορος, cf. 1.85.12 'differentia est causae' = II, 5, 16 διάφορά ἐστι τὰ αἴτια. The singular, *differentiam*, is thinkable here also.

[18] **qualitatis** The Latin does not translate Puschmann's text. Did the translator's Greek text have ποίας for ποιούσας? Or was the translator anticipating the content of the next clause? The low quality of his work in this chapter makes the latter possibility unlikely. For a parallel mismatch between Greek and Latin versions, cf. I, 441, 5–6 τὸ <u>ποιοῦν</u> αἴτιον τὸ πάθος = 1.1 *<u>qualitas</u> causae passionis*: *qualitas*, for *qualis*, for (ὁ)ποῖον, also illustrates the tendency of the Latin translator to nominalize.

[19] **[sed] quoniam** Presumably ποτέ is translated by *modo*, so does *quoniam* translate γάρ (as at e.g. 2.241 = II, 511, 25 (where NB *Pod.* has *quoque* for *quoniam*))? But why *sed*? It is tempting to suppose that *sed quoniam* is for ἀλλ' ὅτι in the translator's text: cf. the variant reading in Greek ms. L ἄλλοτε for ποτέ (reported by Puschmann); although in the Greek Alexander ἄλλοτε (well attested in the δέ clause) is unparalleled in the μέν clause, it would be an easy error. If this is right, *modo* must have been added by our translator to partner *est autem quando*. I tentatively take *quoniam* for γάρ and *sed* either as accidentally transposed from before *differentias* (for δέ) or as anticipating *sed quoniam* in 2.1.3.

[20] **calida distemperantia** On the Hippocratism of Alexander, see Temkin, 'Hippokratismus'.

[21] **est autem quando** For *est autem quando*, cf. 2.5.4 = II, 149, 19–20 ἐστιν εἶτα Puschmann but ἐστι δέ ὅτε LM (see note ad loc.); 2.41 = II, 289, 20 ἔστι δὲ ὅτε; 2.129 'in splene enim est quando et acetum mittimus' (not in Greek; Mihăileanu p. 171, 1 prints a comma between *est* and *quando*!).

2.1.2 Non solum autem secundum qualitates puras aut[22] simplices, sed et secundum humores[23] superfluentes[24] similiter exist*it*,[25] +– –+ seu calida[26] siue frigida aut alia aliqua qualitate assumpta.[27]

autem] *om.* **Mu ф** | qualitates] -is **P1** | puras] -a **P1** | aut] et **A** iam **P1** | simplices] -is **P1** | et] etiam **DGe P3** *in marg.* **m2** *om.* **M O P3′MaOx** | humores superfluentes **P3Ma**] humorum superfluentium **P1M** h. superfluitates ***cett.*** | similiter] etiam **C** | *post* similiter *habet uerba* habundantes uel **Ox** | exist*it scripsimus*] existens **C** existentes ***cett.*** | seu] sed **P1** | calida *scripsimus*] -as ***plerique*** -us **P1M O** -os **P3Ma** | siue (sibi **P1**) **P1M**] seu **AO G1CP2B MaD** aut **OxP3 ф** | frigida *scripsimus*] -as ***plerique*** -us **P1M O** -os **P3Ma** | alia aliqua **P1M A**] aliqua alia **CP2′** ab alia aliqua **O** ab aliqua alia **ф** alias aliquas **G1L2B P3′Ma** secundum alias aliquas **P3** (secundum *add. in marg.* **m2**) aliquas alias **P2** alias **DOxGe** (*sed deinde uerba* et humidas et siccas *habet* **D**) | qualitate assumpta *(abl. absol.) scripsimus*] sit (fit **A′**) qualitas (qualitas existens **Mu′**) assumpta **AOMuC** qualitas assumpta (adsum ta **P1**) **P1M P2′** (*ante* qualitas *habet rasuram* (sit?) **P2**) (ab ...) qualitate assumptas **ф** qualitates assumptas (assupmtas **Ma**) ***cett.***

[22] **puras aut simplices** Cf. 2.1.3 *pura uel simplex*. In both places, A alone has *et*, and here P1's *pura iam* suggests a corruption of *puras aut* rather than of *puras et*.

[23] **humores** More usually, *humores* translates χυμοί, but for *humores* = ὕλη, cf. 1.6 = II, 447, 10 and 2.185 = II, 475, 26 quoted in note 24.

[24] **humores superfluentes** I print for now the text of θ″. The correction of the reading of γ to *humorum superfluentiam* (suggested to me by Michael Reeve) is both minimal and elegant, but *superfluentia* is unparalleled in the Latin Alexander (and registered neither by Georges nor by Souter). A second neat alternative (suggested to me by Cloudy Fischer) is *humorem superfluentem* (the ending of *humorum* being occasioned by that of *secundum*). I would like to canvass also the possibility of reading *humorum superfluentium* <*qualitates*>. The Latin tradition appears to reflect two attempts to restore an accusative after *secundum* (viz. *humorum superfluitates* in δ, and *humores superfluentes* in θ″). The very form of the apparently secondary *superfluitates* could support an original sequence *superfluentium qualitates*. With *humorum superfluentium* cf. 2.185 *plenitudo humorum fluentium* (II, 475, 26–7 πλῆθος ὕλης ἐπιρρεύσαντος). Note that *superfluitas* (from the lexicalized adjective *superfluus*) is used not infrequently by our translator(s), but always to translate περίττωμα, περιττώματα, περιττός (e.g. at 2.12 (II, 157, 11), 2.40 (II, 287, 16), 2.152 (II, 441, 20), 2.205 (II, 341, 4), and cf. 2.39 (II, 285, 13 περιττόν) and 2.56 (II, 333, 13) ἀπερίττου); verbal and participial forms of *superfluo*, on the other hand, (and of *supercurro*, e.g. 2.5.1 below, 1.124 = II, 105, 21) are used to render forms of ἐπιρρέω, including the verbal adjective ἐπίρρυτος (if the Greek text here is sound). One should perhaps note the formal similarity of ἐπίρρυτον (the Greek form we are here translating) and περιττόν, and the fact that the former occurs (according to the *TLG*) only twice in Alex. Trall., here and on the very next page (II, 149, 14 = 2.5.2); verbal and participial forms on the stem ἐπιρρε-, on the other hand, number close to a hundred (according to the *TLG*). The Greek text should perhaps be emended.

2.1.2 But it emerges not only from qualities pure and simple but also similarly from the superfluous humours, when either a hot or a cold or some other quality has been taken on (by the condition).

II, 147, 4–7 Puschmann

οὐ μόνον δὲ κατὰ ποιότητα ψιλὴν, ἀλλὰ καὶ καθ' ὕλην ἐπίρρυτον ὡσαύτως συνίσταται +– παντὸς τοῦ ἐπιρρέοντος χυμοῦ –+ ἢ θερμὴν ἢ ψυχρὰν ἢ ἄλλην τινὰ ποιότητα προσειληφότος.

[25] **exist*it*** A plural form, *existunt* (or *existent*?, closer in form to the attested participles) is also thinkable, as the subject in the next sentence is the plural *tussiculae* 'coughs'. Finite forms of *existere* are not common in the Latin Alexander, but one may compare e.g. 1.114 'et maxime ubi inflammationes rubrae existunt', where *ubi . . . existunt* renders the genitive absolute at II, 87, 19 (cf. 1.125 = II, 107, 28); on the very frequent use of the present participle *existens*, see note below on 2.3.1 *existente*.

[26] **calida . . . frigida** What lies behind the *-us* endings in γ (whence presumably *-os* in θ″)? An accusative plural, or a late Latin nominative plural ending agreeing with *humores*?

[27] **qualitate assumpta** I have tentatively written an ablative absolute (for the Greek genitive absolute), as elsewhere we have seen some evidence that the translator controls this construction (cf. e.g. 2.5.4 *urgente causa*; 2.158.3 *Quibus agnitis*; 2.158.6 *amisso nutrimento . . . tunica comesta*; 2.158.7 *uirtute amissa*). η replaced the absolute participle with a finite periphrastic construction (*sit assumpta*, with the subjunctive after *seu*); this is faintly reminiscent of *fit extenuata* in η and κ for *extenuatur* at 2.158.6 (for the text see Section 4.10.5), although I have argued (above, p. 118) that *fit extenuata* is more probably original. The rest of the tradition made the participle conjunct in the accusative plural agreeing with *superfluitates*.

2.1.3 Scire autem oportet et hoc quomodo differunt abinuicem tussiculae secundum causas singulas[28] sed quoniam[29] et secundum loca, et quaequam quidem earum ipsa loca patiuntur, alia etiam compatiuntur.[30]

2.1.4 Propter quod[31] non una est causa tussis sed uaria, de qua re oportet nos accedere[32] cum omni studio ad cognoscendam uniuscuiusque ueritatem.[33] Confitemur[34] enim et manifestum est quia[35] sine cognitione non possunt bene curari.

autem] *om.* **D φ** | oportet] -it **P1** | hoc] hic **φ** hec **Ma** | abinuicem] ad- **MaOx φ** | tussiculae] -ae **M** -is **P1** | singulas] sineolas **P1** | sed quoniam (*s. s.* **Ma**)] sed **φ** *om.* **G1P3Ma′OxGe** | et$_2$] *om.* **O** et ipsa **Ox** | et$_3$] *om.* **AMuC G1P2L2B** *s. s.* **Ge** | quaequam **Ma**] quiaquam **M** quaquam **P1O** quanquam **AMuC P2L2B** quando **Ge** et quando *s. s.* **Ox m2** quam **φ** que **G1P3DOx** | quidem] quidam **Mu** quod(?) **P1** | earum **A P2CL2B φ**] eorum **G1MaDGeOx** erunt (erī̃) **M** eř **O** autem **P1** *om.* **P3** | ipsa loca] *om.* **G1P3** | patiuntur] -antur **AMuC P2L2BDGe** | alia etiam **M AOMu P2L2BD**] alia quidem **C** et que **G1P3Ma** et que membra **φ** (membra *in marg.* ***ed.*** *s. s.* **G2**) *om.* **P1Ox** | compatiuntur] -antur **CP2BGe** *om.* **P1Ox** |

propter quod **P1M O D**] propterea **AC P2L2B** et propterea **Ox** quoniam **G1P3Ma φ** | *inter* propter quod *et* non *habet uerba* per partes agnoscenda sunt quia **D** | una est] est una **G1CP2L2BGe** | causa] cura **L** *om.* **Mu** | *post* tussis *add.* cuiusque **P3 m3** | sed] sed et **D** | uaria] uarie **P1** | re] res **L** | oportet nos] nos oportet **Ox φ** | nos] et nos **P1** *om.* **O** | accedere] *super* c *alteram habet (fort. iocose) litteram* p **P1** accingere **O** accendere **D** attendere **Ox φ** occurrere **M** | cum] vi **P1** *om.* **C** | omni studio] omnem studium **P1** | cum omni studio accedere **G1** | cognoscendam (cognuscenda **P1**)] agnoscendam **A G2L** agnoscendum **Ox** gnoscendum **P3′** (ad *praeponit supra* **m3**) ad noscendum **Ma** | *post* uniuscuiusque *habent* tussis **Ox φ** | ueritatem **P1M AO B**] uarietatem ***cett.*** | confitemur] -mor **P1** | et] *om.* **P1** | quia] qua **P1** | cognitione] -em **P1** | curari non possunt bene **Ox** | bene] *om.* **OMu** | curari] curare **P1**

[28] **singulas** The reading of P1 *sineolas* presumably reflects an uncial model. The translation of κατὰ τὴν αἰτίαν μόνην as *secundum causas singulas* may seem rather free: we would perhaps expect rather *solus* for μόνος, as in a similar context at 2.236.6 (for the text, Latin and Greek, see 4.10.6 above). The meaning of the original is, however, well conveyed here ('according to each individual cause on its own'), and *singuli* (always plural) is common in the Latin Alexander in perfectly classical uses, so that I do not think we have to suppose the (Romance) use of *singulus* = *solus* (cf. *REW* 7945 *singulus* *'allein'). The fondness of our translator(s) for the word is seen in its gratuitous use twice within a line, again with *causae*, at 2.236.7 (*causarum singularum … singularum causarum*; for the text see 4.10.6 above), where there is nothing corresponding in the Greek.

On *abinuicem*, etc. for Greek ἀλλήλους, etc., see Hofmann and Szantyr, 177–8.

[29] **sed quoniam** This apparently simple sentence is replete with difficulties. At first sight one would take *quoniam* = *quod* or *quia*, in place of accusative + infinitive, a use well known in Late Latin (cf. Hofmann and Szantyr, 628). Furthermore, here the *sed* puts one in mind of the Late Latin *non quoniam … sed quoniam* (see Hofmann and Szantyr, 588), and in view of the Greek (ὡς οὐ διαφέρουσιν) one might hazard that we have lost a negative in the Latin. However, in spite of my translation I am as yet unable to parallel this use of *quoniam* in the Latin Alexander, and I have every sympathy with the maker of θ for ditching *sed quoniam*! Might *quoniam* be for ὅτι of the next clause (transposed in the translator's Greek text, or anticipated by the translator)?

[30] **et quaequam … compatiuntur** Although the Greek is not difficult, the translator appears to have made a complete hash of the second part of this sentence, where the subject should remain 'coughs'. Of course, we can only guess at what his Greek text contained, and indeed at his Latin version, which evidently caused such confusion in the tradition. On any account, the original translation appears to have meant something like, 'and that some of the coughs the bodyparts themselves suffer, other bodyparts also suffer in sympathy'. Clearly, we must have *et* followed by two short words beginning with *q-* followed by *quidem*. Alternatives to the printed text include: (1) *et quaequae quidem* (*quisquis*), with *quaequae* as object of *patiuntur*; (2) *et quaeque quidem* (*quisque*), with *quaeque* as object of *patiuntur* (I owe this idea to Cloudy Fischer: for *quisque … alius*, see Hofmann and

2.1.3 It is further necessary to know that coughs differ one from another according to their individual causes but that they differ also according to their locations. In the case of some of them, the locations themselves are affected, while other locations also are affected secondarily.

2.1.4 Therefore there is not a single cause of coughing, but (there are) various (causes), and for this reason we must proceed with all diligence to find out the true reason for each single cough. We admit, and it is obvious, that they cannot be treated well without recognition (of the underlying cause).

II, 147, 7–13 Puschmann

εἰδέναι δὲ δεῖ καὶ τοῦτο, ὡς οὐ διαφέρουσιν ἀλλήλων αἱ βῆχες κατὰ τὴν αἰτίαν μόνην, ἀλλὰ καὶ κατὰ τοὺς τόπους, καὶ ὅτι αἱ μὲν αὐτῶν κατὰ πρωτοπάθειαν, αἱ δὲ κατὰ συμπάθειαν συνίστανται. (**2.1.4**). ἐπεὶ οὖν οὐ μίαν αἰτίαν ἡ βὴξ, ἀλλὰ ποικίλην κέκτηται, δεῖ καὶ ἡμᾶς ἐλθεῖν μετὰ πάσης σπουδῆς ἐπὶ τὴν διάγνωσιν καὶ τὴν διάκρισιν τῆς ποιούσης αἰτίας· ὡμολόγηται γὰρ παρὰ πᾶσι τοῦτο καὶ δῆλόν ἐστιν, ὡς ἄνευ διαγνώσεως οὐχ οἷόν τε θεραπεῦσαι καλῶς.

Szantyr, 429); (3) *et quia quae quidem*, with *quae* as object of *patiuntur* (this probably stood in γ at least: at 2.1.4 Pl again has *qua* for *quia*; on this development, cf. Svennung, *Palladius*, 502). A fourth possibility suggested by the manuscript forms is (4a) *et quia quamquidem*, with *quamquidem* an emphatic equivalent of *quidem* = Greek μέν attested in the Latin versions of Oribasius, Rufus, *De podagra*, and Hippocrates, *De septimanis* (cf. Hofmann and Szantyr, 486, Mørland, *Oribasius*, 160f., Souter, s.v.) and αἱ not translated, or (4b) *et quia quaedam*, with *quaedam* = αἱ μέν as at 1.124 = II, 105, 23, although both variants are hard if not impossible to construe.

With *etiam* in the δέ clause (*alia etiam* apparently for αἱ δέ), cf. *adhuc* (in *sed adhuc* apparently for ποτὲ δέ at 2.9.1 below and note ad loc.

[31] **Propter quod** Here, in view of the following *de qua re*, and notwithstanding ἐπεί, the natural way to take *propter quod* is as a coordinating (rather than subordinating) conjunction, 'for this reason'. (For *propter quod* = *propterea quod*, cf. Hofmann and Szantyr, 246 (citing Chiron, Avell., Cassiod., Greg. M., Oribas.), Mørland, *Oribasius*, 180 (citing both the older and the younger translation of Oribasius) and Svennung, *Palladius*, 396–7.) Alternatively *propter quod* is resumed by *de qua re*.

[32] **accedere** The variant *attendere* in Ox and ϕ must be a correction of *accendere* (in D). M's *occurrere* could reflect either an early gloss or the careless substitution of a synonym.

[33] **ueritatem** Both *uarietas* and *ueritas* occur only once each in Books 1 and 2 (in ms. A), *uarietas* at 2.235 *propter uarietatem* = II, 501, 9 διὰ τὸ ποικίλον, *ueritas* at 2.68 *agnita ueritate diaeta ad unamquamque distemperantiam est ordinanda*, which corresponds rather roughly to II, 399, 4–5 καὶ ταύτην ἀκριβῶς διεγνωκότα οὕτω ποιεῖσθαι τὴν δίαιταν πρὸς τὴν ὑπαγορευομένην ὑπὸ τῆς διαγνώσεως διάθεσιν. I favour *ueritatem* both because of its distribution (γ η B) and because of the collocation with *cognoscere/agnoscere* here and at 2.68. The variant *uarietatem* was probably prompted by *uaria* (immediately above), and must have been introduced more than once independently in the tradition.

[34] **confitemur** Rather loose and brief for Greek ὡμολόγηται παρὰ πᾶσι.

[35] **manifestum est quia** Mørland, *Oribasius*, 180 mentions *manifestum est quia* as a 'feste Verbindung' in the Latin Oribasius. In Book 1 of the Latin Alexander I have counted five examples of *manifestum est quia* (1.36, 45, 110, 125, 131), five of *manifestum est quod* (1.35, 109 twice, 114, 145), and five of *manifestum est* with accusative + infinitive (1.93, 126, 128, 139, 140) (plus one possible example of *manifestum est ut* at 1.131), which suggests a greater variety of construction than Mørland reports for Oribasius.

2.2.t. De tussis cognitione quae de calida distemperantia generatur

2.2.1 Quod si de calida distemperantia pura uel simplici[36] generata fuerit tussis, sentiunt[37] enim merito[38] calorem, quasi[39] per aliquas qualitates taliter tussientes, et respirantes desiderium habent frigidi aeris.[40]

2.2.2 Etiam iuuantur magis si aeris ad se trahant frigdorem[42] plus quam[43] si aquam +– frigidam –+ bibant. Et uultus eorum rubrus[44] apparet, et caput +– similiter –+.

tit. om. **MaL2** | De - cognitione] *om.* **P1** De tussi (tusse **B**) **OxP3B** Si tussis fiat **D** | quae - generatur *om.* **O** | quae] Que *in initio capituli* **P1** que fit **Ge** si **B** Quemque *et in initio capituli* **M** *om.* **D** | de] ex **DP2** *om.* **Mu P3′** *add.* **m2** | generatur] generata tussis sit **M** est **G1** fiat **B** *om.* **P1 DGe**

Quod si - distemperantia *om.* **P1** | Quod si] Quod etsi ***ed.*** Quod **C** | distemperantia pura] p. d. **Mu** | pura] sola **Ox φ** pura sine humore **D** | uel] ns **P1** | simplici] -e **P1 P3** | generata fuerit tussis] f. g. t. **A B** g. t. f. **M** | sentiunt (-iant **P1**) enim merito (-eto **P1**) γ η] sentiunt et merito **P2L2B** et merito sentiunt **φ** merito sentiunt et **Ge** merito sentiunt **G1P3Ma** et in inicio sentiunt **Ox** sentiunt [obesse **D′**] calorem merito **D** | calorem] -e **P1O** colorem **C** *ante* merito *habet* **D** | quasi per] quas per **M** quem super **P1** quia per **G1P3′Ma** (quia *expung.* **P3 m2**) | aliquas qualitates (-is **P1**)] qualitates aliquas **Ox φ** qualitates **P3Ma** | taliter] et aliter **C** aliter **P1** tales **P3Ma φ** | tussientes] -is **P1** | et] sed et **Ox** | respirantes] -is **P1** | habent] *om.* **P1M** | frigidi] frigida **M** | aeris] acres **M** | frigidi aeris habent **P3MaD φ**

Etiam **P1M AO P2L2B**] et ***cett.*** *om.* **D** | iuuantur (iubantur **M**)] iuuantur quia **D** | si] sibi **M** *om.* **P1** | aeris (-es **M**)] uberis (ub- *an* ali-?) **P1** frigidi aeris **C** | ad se] *om.* **P3Ge′** | ad se trahant] trahant ad se **Ox** ad se aeris attrahant **G1** | trahant] trahunt **Mu G2L1** attrahant (atr- **Ge**) **G1Ge** trahit **P1M** thraent **D** | frigdorem] frigorem ***ed.*** frigdores **O** per frigdores **M** qualitatem **C** | plus quam] quam **M G1P3MaDGe φ** | aquam frigidam] aqua frigida **P1O** | rubrus (-um **M**) apparet (-it **P1**) **P1M AMu**] -ri -ent **O G1CP2L2BGe** rubei **D** rubeus **P3MaOx φ** | *post* similiter *uerbum* et *habet* **Mu**

[36] **pura uel simplici** For this translation of ψιλός, see 2.1.2 above and note ad loc.

[37] **sentiunt** … **calorem, quasi** … **tussientes** I take *tussientes* as dependent on *quasi* rather than directly on *sentiunt*. In the Latin Alexander *sentio* is common with accusative + infinitive (cf. 1.35 'Si ergo grauitatem sentiat sibi in capite fieri'; 1.62, 1.69, 1.117, 1.128; 2.3.2 'habere se sentiunt'; 2.7.4, 2.8.2, 2.10.1, 2.192, 2.204, 2.247), but I find no instance of *sentio* + nominative participle. This Greek construction can be paralleled in Late Latin prose, especially from Tertullian on (Hofmann and Szantyr, 364), but is regarded as highly literary. For *quasi* + participle, cf. 1.29 'et quasi imbecillior effectus humor' (I, 477, 21 καὶ οἶον ἀσθενεστέρα γενομένη), 2.152 'quasi … commotus' (II, 441, 3), 2.219 'quasi eum clisterians' (II, 363, 22). There is a question-mark also over the Greek construction, as I cannot parallel αἰσθάνομαι + (reflexive) nominative participle in the Greek Alexander (and note in passing the remarkable reflexive construction at II, 417, 24 τὸ … ἑαυτοῦ ῥωμαλεωτέρου τοῦ κάμνοντος αἰσθάνεσθαι 'the feeling of the patient that he is stronger').

[38] **enim merito** In the Latin Alexander, *merito* stands regularly (in ms. A, once in Book 1 and five times in Book 2) for Greek εἰκότως (which here would be an improvement on ἴσως in the Greek text!): cf. 1.136 = II, 125, 15; 2.49 = II, 311, 15; 2.194 = II, 489, 24; 2.204 = II, 335, 7; 2.214 = II, 359, 3; 2.257 = II, 535, 17 (at II, 321, 4 and II, 441, 20 εἰκότως is not translated in the Latin).

As *enim* is in both γ and η, it must have been in the archetype. Tentatively, I take it as standing for Greek μέν. At this point I can compare only 2.204 'Merito enim ei accidunt dolores nimii … Difficilis autem est ad cognoscendum' II, 335, 6–10 καὶ τὸ μὲν ἐπιφέρειν τὰς ὀδύνας σφοδρὰς εἰκότως τῷ κώλῳ προσγίνεται … τὸ δὲ δυσδιαγνωστικὸν …; and Dioscorides 1.9, p. 9, 10 M. 'sed ut scias utrosque discernere, fu enim fragilior est …, oximirsini uero durior … est' (quoted by Svennung, *Palladius*, 482 n. 2 without comment, and referred to by Hofmann and Szantyr, 509 d rather oddly as '*enim* im Nachsatz').

2.2.t. Concerning the recognition of a cough which arises from a hot imbalance

2.2.1 But if coughing arises from a hot imbalance pure and simple, they naturally feel heat, as if they are coughing in a way determined by particular qualities, and as they breathe they have a desire for cold air.

2.2.2 They are also helped more if they draw in cold air than if they drink cold water. And their face appears red, and the head likewise.

II, 147, 14–19 Puschmann

Διάγνωσις τῆς διὰ θερμὴν δυσκρασίαν βηχός
Ψιλῆς τοίνυν οὔσης τῆς θερμῆς δυσκρασίας αἰσθάνονται μὲν ἴσως διά τινος ποιότητος τοιαύτης, οἷον δυσκρασίας θερμῆς, βήσσοντες,[41] καὶ ἀναπνεῖν ἐπιθυμοῦσι ψυχρὸν ἀέρα. (**2.2.2**). καὶ ὠφελοῦνται μᾶλλον ὑπὸ τῆς εἰσπνοῆς ἤπερ ὑπὸ τῆς τοῦ ὕδατος πόσεως, καὶ τὰ περὶ τὸ πρόσωπον ἐρυθρὰ +– μᾶλλον –+ ὁρᾶται καὶ τὴν κεφαλήν.

[39] **quasi** Presumably *quasi* is for Greek οἷον, as at 1.29 (quoted in the note on *sentiunt*). Here, however, οἷον + noun appears to have its usual meaning 'such as' (introducing an example of a type), while *quasi* + participle (if this construal is correct) must mean 'as if' (or conceivably 'because': Hofmann and Szantyr, 675 δ).

[40] **desiderium habent frigidi aeris** I cannot parallel *desiderium habeo* + genitive in the Latin Alexander. Compare the translation of the very similar Greek phrase at 2.7.3 'ut frigidum desiderent aerem intrinsecus ad se trahere'.

[41] **διά ... βήσσοντες** Note the reading of Greek ms. L reported by Puschmann: διά τινα ποιότητα τοιαύτην δυσκρασίαν βήσσοντες.

[42] **si ... frigdorem** Considerably more elaborate than ὑπὸ τῆς εἰσπνοῆς. At 2.29 'Istos tantum infrigdatio iuuat quantum contineatur frigida aspiratio' (= II, 263, 12–13 ἡ μὲν γὰρ διὰ πνεύμονα δίψα οὐ τοσοῦτον ὑπὸ τῶν ψυχόντων ὠφελεῖται, ὅσον ὑπὸ τῆς τοῦ περιέχοντος εἰσπνοῆς), there are serious discrepancies between Latin and Greek versions, but εἰσπνοή is evidently rendered with *aspiratio*.

ad se trahant For *ad se trahere* 'inhale', cf. only 1.42 'et iube ut ad se trahat spiritum' = I, 493, 20 κελεύων ἀνασπᾶν, and 2.7.3 (quoted above in note 40) = II, 151, 7–8 ὥστε ψυχρὸν ἐπιθυμεῖν ἀέρα ἀναπνεῖν.

aeris ... frigdorem Literally 'coldness of air' for 'cold air'. For genitive + deadjectival abstract in place of noun + adjective, cf. 1.111.t. *ex frigdoris causa* = II, 77, 8 διὰ ψυχρὰν αἰτίαν.

[43] **plus quam** The manuscripts which omit *plus* all derive directly or indirectly from θ except M, and, if the change is not polygenetic, could all reflect a common ancestor of M and γ′. The collocation *plus quam* is common, especially in Book 2, and its separation from *magis* here renders it only mildly pleonastic. I have found only one example of *plus magis* juxtaposed, regarded by Mørland, *Oribasius*, 175 as characteristic of both older and younger Oribasius translations: 2.15 'et appetunt cibum et potum plus magis quam competit' (apparently mistranslating II, 245, 16–17 καὶ ὀρέγεσθαι μᾶλλον σιτίων ἢ ποτῶν).

[44] **uultus ... rubrus** Here Greek μᾶλλον is apparently not translated.

Perhaps surprisingly (cf. André, *Anatomie*, 36), *uultus* (seven times in Books 1 and 2: 1.26, 1.76, 1.121, 1.143, 2.2, 2.3, 2.70) is almost as frequent as *facies* (eight times: 1.7, 1.26, 1.69, 1.86, 1.133 twice, 2.72, 2.117). In A *uultus* is always singular. If the substitution of the plural here occurred only once in the tradition, then it was in ε, O finding it in θ. The manuscripts frequently vary between *rubrus* and *rubeus*. γ and η tend to have the former, which I incline to prefer also because it is the well-attested later Latin form of *ruber*, while *rubeus* is a different, and much rarer word. Ms. A has the classical form *ruber* only at 2.121 *fin.* twice (perhaps significantly in a chapter not from Alexander). Cf. the comparative *rubrior* at 1.128 (II, 119, 26 ἐρυθρότερον).

Note the Greek phrase τὰ περὶ τὸ πρόσωπον (in contrast with simple τὴν κεφαλήν): is the Latin translator right to render simply 'face', or is there more to it? (Cf. 2.3.1 below.)

2.2.3 Quod si[45] haec fuerint passi[46] et sola distemperantia[47] fuerit, nihil spuunt manifestum quod uideatur.[48]

2.2.4 Si autem et quod[49] expuerint,[50] salsa in eis[51] apparet qualitas, aut fumoso colore aut subcolericum[52] est, et hoc ualde[53] modicum et tenue apparet.

haec] haec **P1** | fuerint passi **AMuP2**] fuerit passus **P1M O** passio ***cett.*** | et **P1M AOP2**] et ex **Mu** ex ***cett.*** | spuunt **P1M AOMu P2D**] ex(s)p- ***cett.*** expuerint **C** | uideatur] -etur **P3′** (*corr.* **m2**) **φ**

autem] aut **G1** | et] *om.* **P3MaOx φ** | quod] quid **A′** que **D** aliquid **MaOx φ** aliquit **P3** *om.* **C** | expuerint (-ent **P1** -xsp- **G1 P2L2D**)] expuunt (-xsp- **G2L1**) **MaOxGe B φ** | salsa] et salsa **Ox** salsas **M** | in eis **P1M AOMuC DMa**] in eo ***cett.*** | apparet (-it **P1**)] -uerit **D** -eant **M** | qualitas] qualitates **M** | aut] uel **D** | fumoso **P1M AOMuC P2BD**] -a ***cett.*** (*incl.* **P2′**) | colore aut] aut colore **P3′φ** | colore] *om.* **Ma** | aut] autem **DOxGeP2 P3** (autem *add.* **m2**) | subcolericum] -us **C** subcolorecus **P1** [*illeg.*]ericus **O** solum colericus **M** subcolerico **DGe φ** colericum **Ma** | est] *om.* **Ma** | ualde modicum et tenue] modicum ualde et tenue **A** ualde tenue et modicum **OxL1** (et modicum *super* apparet *scr.* **Ox**) | tenue] -em **P1MO** | apparet] -it **P1**

45 **Quod si** ... **distemperantia fuerit** The Latin suggests that there is material missing from the Greek, and that the translator had in front of him something like εἰ μὲν οὖν οὕτως εἴη <καὶ> μόνη ψιλὴ <εἴη> ποιότης. Alternatively, the Latin is overtranslating and *haec fuerint passi* is simply rendering Greek οὕτως (an idea I owe to Michael Reeve).

46 **fuerint passi** Presumably, *passio* is a correction based on *passi* on the assumption that the first *fueri(n)t* is otiose. It may also reflect a formulaic phrase, for the sequence *xyz fuerit passio* (with hyperbaton) is strikingly common in ms. A, which here has *fuerint passi*: cf. e.g. 1.57 'Quando autem arguta (augmentata *ed.*; ἀκμάζῃ) fuerit passio' (I, 517, 12); 1.70 'Si autem diuturna fuerit passio' (I, 553, 21–2); 1.77 'quibus ex sola plenitudine sanguinis melancholica fuerit passio' (I, 597, 2–3); 1.91 'Quod si diuturna facta fuerit passio' (not in Greek II, 29, 2–3); 2.80 'Quod si iam diuturna fuerit passio facta' (not from Alexander); 2.81 'si malitiosa fuerit passio' (not from Alexander); 2.116 'si iam timpanitis facta fuerit passio' (not from Alexander). The frequency of this pattern could explain the substitution of *passio* for the participle (as parallels for the latter I have found only 1.68 'Quod si stomachus fuerit passus' (I, 549, 22); 1.77 'cum unum membrum fuerit passum' (not in Greek)). Since in *spuunt* a few words later the tradition unanimously has the plural, I am not tempted by *fuerit passus* (in γ and O) as a singular form, but I wonder whether the ending might not reflect a late nominative plural form in /-ọs/.

47 **distemperantia** As if δυσκρασία alone stood in the translator's Greek text.

48 **uideatur** Note the subjunctive in γ.

49 **quod** Late Latin *quod* for indefinite pronoun *quid*.

50 **expuerint** The alternation at so short an interval between 2.2.3 *spuunt* and 2.2.4 *expuerint*, both for Greek ἀναπτύω, is on the face of it striking. In fact, at this date, the two forms represent mere phonetic variants, with and without prothetic vowel, of a single stem (*(e)spu-* or *(i)spu-*). It would be interesting to see whether the selected form correlates with the sound at the end of the preceding word (here: no prothesis after a resonant [*nihil spu-*] vs prothesis after a stop [*quod expu-*]; but contrast 2.5.1 *quod spui*tur).

51 **in eis** Presumably, αὐτοῖς in the Greek refers to the patients, but (although plural) has been taken by our translator to refer to what is spat: perhaps his text had ἐν αὐτοῖς (cf. Latin *in eis*). The unambiguous reference of *in eis* to the spittle prompted the relatively early change (in θ′) of *eis* to *eo*; conversely, D corrected the antecedent *quod* to plural *que*.

2.2.3 But if they have this condition and there is only an imbalance, they bring up nothing that can be seen.

2.2.4 But if they really do bring something up, its quality seems salty, it is either smoky in colour or slightly bilious, and it appears very little in quantity and thin.

II, 147, 19–22 Puschmann

εἰ μὲν οὖν οὕτως εἴη μόνη ψιλὴ ποιότης, οὐδὲν ἀναπτύουσιν ἄξιον λόγου ἢ οὐδ' ὅλως. (**2.2.4**). εἰ δὲ καὶ ἀναπτύουσιν, ἁλμυρὰν αὐτοῖς ἔχον ποιότητα τὸ πτυόμενον φαίνεται ἢ καπνῶδες τῇ χροιᾷ ἢ ὑπόχολον καὶ τοῦτο σφόδρα ὀλίγον καὶ λεπτόν·

[52] **subcolericum** For *subcolericus* of a colour, cf. 1.19 *-o colore*. Greek χολερικός seems not to be used as a colour-term, the Greek for 'yellowish' being the (originally possessive) compound ὑπόχολος, so that *subcolericus* is an essentially Latin formation, one which shows that Latin adjectives in *sub-* 'slightly, somewhat' are not mere calques on Greek forms in ὑπο-. The greater productivity of the Latin type is seen in Alexander also in *stipticus*: *substipticus* (2.103, 164) = Greek στυπτικός: ὑποστῦφον. Other *sub-* formations in the Latin Alexander include 1.17 *subalbidus*, *subrubrus*, 1.26 *subtumidus*, 1.72 *subnubilis*, 1.95 *subflauus*, 2.70 *subsimilis*. On the formation, see Svennung, *Wortstudien*, 125f., Langslow, *Medical Latin*, 336–8, with further references.

[53] **ualde** Apart from *ualde* (in A, ten times in Book 1, seventeen times in Book 2), the Latin Alexander employs a range of intensifiers, notably *nimis* (in A, twenty-seven times in Book 1, forty times in Book 2; see Mørland, *Oribasius*, 162; Hofmann and Szantyr, 163), but also *satis* and adverbial *multum* and *nimium*. Soundings suggest that our translator was not dependent on a list of fixed translation-equivalents, but used each intensifier freely and variably for a range of Greek forms: for instance, *ualde* translates πάνυ (e.g. 1.57 = I, 515, 19) and λίαν (e.g. 1.115 = II, 91, 6), as well as σφόδρα (here and e.g. 1.144 = II, 233, 21), while *nimis* renders πάνυ (e.g. 1.23 = I, 469, 3), σφόδρα (e.g. 1.60 = I, 531, 24), and ἄγαν (e.g. 1.23 = I, 469, 10), which in turn may be rendered also by *satis* (e.g. 1.29 = I, 477, 22).

2.2.5 Sic enim[54] erit cognoscenda calida distemperantia[55] a praedictis[56] signis.

2.2.6 Nihil igitur[57] minus et a praecedenti[58] qualitate calidi aeris, sicut etiam[59] quam plurime, et nimium si sit calidum balneum et diaeta calida, et ex furore magis quam ex sollicitudine praecedente, hoc contingere solet.

enim] *om.* **OxP3B** | erit] *om.* **MuC** | cognoscenda (-gnusc- **P1**)] agnoscenda **P3MaD** cognoscetur **C** cognoscentia **G1P2L2BGe** | *ante* calida *uerbum* qualitas *habet* **A** | calida (colerica **Mu**) distemperantia] -ide -tie **A G1P2L2B** distemperantia **P3′Ma** (*post* dist. *add. in marg.* calida **P3 m2**) | a] ex **D** | praedictis] -dis- **Mu′**

igitur] enim **L2** | *ad* igitur *gloss. habet* cognoscenda erit ***ed.*** | minus] inuenus **P1** *post* minus *addunt*: cognoscenda erit **G2L1** contingit tussis **P2MaDGe** contingit tussis et fit ex **B** | et] ex **DOxGe** et ex (ex *s. s.*) **P2** fit ex **G1L2** *om.* **OP3′Ma ϕ** quam *in marg.* **P3 m3** | a **P1M** | praecedenti **AMuCP2BD**] -nte ***cett.*** | *super/ad* praecedente *habent* .i. si praecedat **ϕ** | qualitate (-tem **P1**)] -tis **O** | calidi aeris (calidi *om.* **L2**)] -o -e **O** -um -em **P1M** calida ex his **C** | sicut] sic **P3** fit sic **Ox** | quam plurime] quam plurimum *add. in marg.* **P3 m2** | et (*add. in marg.* **P3 m3**)] contingit et **D** | si sit] sicut **P1** | calidum balneum] calidus balneus (ual- **M**) **P1M** balneum calidum **ϕ** | diaeta (diae- **P1**)] die **P3′** (*corr.* **m3**) | et ex] etiam ex **C** | quam ex sollicitudine praecedente] p. q. ex s. **Mu** | sollicitudine] soli- **P1** | praecedente (-em **P1**)] -ium **ϕ** | hoc **P1M Mu**] hec ***cett.*** | solet **M Mu P3**] -ent ***cett.*** *et* **P3′**

[54] **enim** With *praedictis signis*, this is in a sense a conclusion, and it is hard to see any regular force of *enim* here. I incline, however, to regard it as a slavish translation of γάρ rather than as an instance of 'end-of-recipe' *enim* (cf. Langslow, 'Particles'), although the latter use of *enim* is well attested in the Latin Alexander.

[55] **distemperantia** Note the absence of the cough (βῆχα) from the Latin. The fact that A inserts *qualitas* and θ′ changes *cognoscenda* to *cognoscentia* could be taken to imply that δ had the genitive *calide distemperantie*, and it is tempting to supply <*tussis*>.

[56] **praedictis** Latin *praedicta* vs Greek παρόντα! Adjectival and substantival use of *praedictus* is common enough in the Latin Alexander, but I cannot parallel its use with *signa* (cf. *supradicta signa* at 2.58, 2.133, 2.142). It bears noting that if the Latin had *praesentibus signis*, the *enim* introducing this sentence would be more natural, not to mention the logic of the passage and the connection with 2.2.6. The one comparable use of *praesens* in the Latin Alexander (and incidentally the one parallel for the use of Greek παρόντα in the present passage) is in a quotation from Hippocrates: 2.158 'Oportet ergo peruidere ut dixit Hippocrates et praesentia et futura et praeterita' (cf. II, 461, 4–5).

[57] **igitur** Greek δέ here is clearly adversative, given the contrast between παρόντα and προηγησαμένα. In Imperial and Late Latin *igitur* frequently renders δέ in both its adversative and its weaker connective functions (see Mørland, *Oribasius*, 158–9; Hofmann and Szantyr, 513). The usage of our translator(s) remains to be established, but cf. 2.4.2 below.

2.2.5 Thus will a hot imbalance have to be recognized from the aforementioned signs.

2.2.6 Furthermore, this regularly occurs also from a preceding quality of hot air, as is very often the case, and from too hot a bath and a hot diet, and from a preceding state of high emotion (*furore*) more than from anxiety (*sollicitudine*).

II, 147, 22–6 Puschmann

οὕτω γὰρ ἔστι τὴν διὰ θερμὴν δυσκρασίαν βῆχα ἀπὸ τῶν παρόντων σημείων διαγινώσκειν. (**2.2.6**). οὐδὲν δὲ ἧττον καὶ ἀπὸ τῶν προηγησαμένων ἐξ ἐγκαύσεως, ὡς ἐπὶ τὸ πολὺ, καὶ θερμῶν βαλανείων καὶ διαίτης θερμῆς καὶ ἐπιθυμιῶν μᾶλλον ἢ φροντίδος τοῦτο συνέβη γενέσθαι.

[58] **praecedenti** The epithet *praecedens* is idiomatic of antecedent causes in late medical Latin, (as is προηγησαμένος in Greek: see LSJ, s.v. προηγέομαι, 4.f., and cf. Alex. Trall. I, 463, 13; I, 489, 7; II, 191, 2 and often); note already Cels. pr. 70 'causa quae ante praecesserat', compare Oribas., *Syn.* 9.12.1 Aa p. 296 'sine aliqua praecedente causa' (ἄνευ τοῦ προηγήσασθαι), and see *ThLL*, s.v. 'praecedo', 401, 37ff. Of many similar instances in the Latin Alexander, cf. e.g. 1.40 'ex praecedentibus causis', 1.83 'ex tristitia et sollicitudine praecedente' (= I, 605, 23), 1.111 'praecedente frigido uento' (= II, 77, 9). Cf. *antecedens* in Cass. Fel. and Cael. Aur.

Note the (chiastic) repetition of *praecedens* after *sollicitudine*, at the end of the list of possible causes, and compare the (similarly chiastic) repetition of *apparet* in 2.2.4: neither προηγησαμένος nor φαίνεται is repeated in the Greek. Are the repetitions in the Latin accidental, or are they a deliberate point of style? Fraisse, lxviii, observes a similar feature in the prose of the fifth-century African medical writer Cassius Felix, and the phenomenon promises to repay further attention.

[59] **etiam** Does *etiam* reflect ἔτι in the translator's Greek text (for ἐπὶ in Puschmann's)?

2.3.t. De tusse quae[60] ex frigida distemperantia fit

2.3.1 Tussiunt[61] etiam plurimi[62] ex frigida distemperantia existente[63] in thorace pura uel simplici[64] qualitate. Hi ergo magis pallidi sunt in uultu et in capite,[65] et neque sitim habent neque[66] salsum[67] expuunt.

2.3.2 Et laeduntur ex frigidis et iuuantur ex calefactionibus,[68] et acidonicum[69] magis quam amaritudinem +– –+ habere se sentiunt.[70]

De - fit] *om.* **P1 MaL2** De frigida distemperantia thoracis **G1** | ex frigida distemperantia fit] fit ex f. d. **Ge** | tusse] tussi **Oxϕ** | quae] qui **M** si **B ϕ** | ex] de **OxC** | fit] oritur **B ϕ**

Tussiunt] Tussent **P1** Tussem **M** Tusse **O** Si autem tussis **P3Ma** | etiam] aetiam **P1** *om.* **P3Ma** | plurimi] -e **P1** -a **O** quam plurimi **OxCϕ** *om.* **P3Ma** | frigida distemperantia existente in thorace] f. e. in t. d. **G1** | frigida] -am **P1** | distemperantia] -iam **P1** diss- **M** | existente] -em **M** | thorace] -ae **P1** | pura] et pura **Ox** pura pura **L1** | uel] et **A** | qualitate] -em **P1** qualitate fit **P3MaOx** *om.* **A** | Hi ... uultu] hi magis uultu pallidi sunt **P3** hii uultu magis pallidi sunt **Ma** | Hi ergo magis] *om.* **O** | ergo] uero **P2** *om.* **P3Ma** | pallidi sunt] sunt pallidi **C** | in$_2$] *om.* **O P3Ma** | uultu] -o **P1** | in$_3$] *om.* **P3Maϕ** | et$_2$] *om.* **P3MaOxϕ** | neque sitim] sitim nullam **C** | sitim habent] h. s. **Ge** | sitim] -em **P1M** | habent] abent **P1** | neque$_2$] nec **MC** | salsum] -as **O** salsidinem **P1**

ex] et **M** | et iuuantur - et] et calefactionibus iuuantur et **Ox** | calefactionibus (calf- **M** calefat- **A**)] calefacientibus (-fat- **DC**) **DC** ***ed.*** | et acitonicum magis] quia magis citonicum **Mu** | acidonicum (acit- **A** acet- **OP2BCG1L2D** aced- **Ge** cit- **Mu**)] accidinoso **P1** acetosum (-am **Ma**) **P3MaOx ϕ** acidum **M**; *s. s. habent*: acetosum **B** .i. acetosum saporem **D** .i. saporem acetosum **MaGe** uel acedonicum **Ox** | magis quam] tam quam **P1** quam **OP3′** *ante* acetosum *add.* magis **P3 m3** magis citonicum quam **Mu** quidem et **M** | habere se sentiunt] habere (abere **P1**) sentiunt **P1M Mu** se sentiunt habere **P3MaOxG2** sentiunt habere **L1** sentiunt ***ed.***

[60] **quae** The headings of 2.4, 5, 6, 7, and 8 are with *si-* rather than relative clauses. B and ϕ seem to anticipate the shift by having *si* here.

[61] **Tussiunt** The readings of γ and O, and the correction by θ″ (why change *Tussiunt*?), suggest the existence of an old variant with a stem *tusse-*: a form of the noun? or was βήσσουσι taken as a future (*tussient*)?

[62] **plurimi** It is unlikely that *plurimi* is meant to be for Greek ὅσοι δέ. This clause-opening is common in Greek medical prose from the Hippocratic corpus on, recurs several times in the Greek Alexander, and is otherwise always correctly translated with a form of *Qui(cumque)* + *autem* (so e.g. I, 525, 21 = 1.58 *Qui autem*, II, 101, 6 = 1.123 *Quibuscumque autem*, II, 553, 16 ὅσοις δέ = 2.263 *Quibus autem*). An alternative — if on the face of it rather far-fetched — account would be to see *plurimi* (for *quam plurime*?) as misplaced from 2.3.2 for ὡς ἐπὶ τὸ πολύ, which is not there translated (and cf. 2.2.6 *quam plurime*).

[63] **existente** *existens* serves as the present participle of the verb to be in the Latin Alexander (cf. note 186 below); on *exsisto* = *sum*, cf. Hofmann and Szantyr, 395, and the *ThLL*, s.v., 1873, 31ff. (on the use of the participle in particular, 1875, 33ff.). Usually, but to judge at least from Puschmann's text by no means invariably, it stands opposite a form of Greek ὤν: so e.g. at 1.72 'in uesica ouis aut caprae urina adhuc plena existente' (I, 563, 22–3); 1.57 'caput ipsum calidum existens' (I, 517, 10 τὴν κεφαλὴν, ..., θερμὴν αὐτὴν οὖσαν); 1.76 'Horum enim existente plenitudine' (I, 593, 12 ὄντων); 1.113 'humor enim ... frigidior simul et spissior existens' (II, 79, 15 ὤν); 1.114 'Mediocribus autem flegmonibus existentibus' (II, 81, 18); 1.146 twice (II, 239, 27, 28). At 1.108 'ex flegmone intrinsecus et extrinsecus existente in meatu' it translates II, 71, 5 συστᾶσαν; cf. 2.1.2 *existit* = συνίσταται (above).

Here there is no participle in the Greek, although the Greek arguably needs it more than the Latin. Other instances where there is no corresponding word in Puschmann's text include 1.57 'Ego uero sic sanaui aliquem ualde freneticum existentem' (I, 515, 19–20); 1.83 'Fit enim haec passio ex tristitia et sollicitudine p(rae)cedente aut animi alia aliqua passione existente' (I, 605, 24); 1.114 'iuuenibus et calida temperantia existentibus' (II, 83, 18); 1.125 'In profundo autem existentibus (sc. parotidibus)' (II, 109, 14–15); 1.146 'igneo satis iam non existente flegmone' (II, 241, 3–4 ζεούσης πάνυ μηκέτι τῆς φλεγμονῆς). The last example shows particularly well the use of *existens* as a Latin form independent of the Greek.

2.3.t. Concerning coughing which occurs as a result of a cold imbalance

2.3.1 Again, very many people cough as a result of a cold imbalance located in the chest and of a pure and simple quality. These then are more pallid in the face and head, and neither are they thirsty nor do they bring up salty matter.

2.3.2 And they are harmed by cold substances and benefited by warming applications, and they feel that they have a sharp taste rather than bitterness.

II, 149, 1–6 Puschmann

Περὶ βηχὸς διὰ ψυχρὰν δυσκρασίαν γινομένης
Ὅσοι δὲ βήσσουσι διὰ ψυχρὰν δυσκρασίαν ἐν τῷ θώρακι διὰ (κατὰ τὴν L) ψυχρὰν ποιότητα, μᾶλλον ὠχρότεροί εἰσιν οὗτοι τὰ περὶ τὸ πρόσωπον καὶ τὴν κεφαλήν. καὶ οὔτε διψώδεις εἰσὶν οὔτε ἁλμυρὸν ἀναπτύουσι. (**2.3.2**). καὶ βλάπτονται μὲν ὑπὸ τῶν ψυχόντων, ὀνίνανται δὲ ὑπὸ τῶν θερμαινόντων, καὶ ὀξίδος μᾶλλον ἢ πικρίας, +– ὡς ἐπὶ τὸ πολὺ, –+ αἰσθάνονται.

64 **pura uel simplici** The repetition of διὰ ψυχράν in the Greek is much less satisfactory than the Latin epithet. Might the second ψυχράν be for ψιλήν?

65 **in uultu et in capite** For *uultus* = τὰ περὶ τὸ πρόσωπον, cf. 2.2.2 above.

66 **neque** ... **neque** I have yet to investigate the usage of our translator(s) with regard to *neque/nec*, *siue/seu* (cf. e.g. 2.5.2 below), *atque/ac*. Here manuscript support for the longer forms is obviously overwhelming. Even in sub-literary texts *neque* survives especially in responsion, as here (see Hofmann and Szantyr, 451–2).

67 **salsum** Were it not for the simple Greek form ἁλμυρόν, one would incline to prefer the reading of P1 *salsidinem* as the *lectio difficilior*, which cannot possibly be the invention of the maker of P1! Even with the Greek, however, *salsido* deserves further consideration because it illustrates the fairly common substitution of abstract noun for adjective (type *frigdor* for *frigidum*). With the reading of P1 here compare ms. A at 2.174 'salsedinem uel acredinem', where Puschmann's text has simply II, 207, 26 ἁλμυρόν!

68 **calefactionibus** An example of *concretum pro abstracto* with an 'instrumental' case-relation between concrete and abstract senses, i.e. 'things *by means of which* heating occurs' (Langslow, *Medical Latin*, 171–2). Good medical Latin (cf. *collutio*, *purgatio*), even if less true to the Greek than *calefacientibus*, and paralleled at 2.208 *calefactiones* = II, 345, 1 θερμαίνοντα; for this concrete sense, cf. Theod. Prisc. 2.29, 94 p. 194, 4, and the *ThLL*, s.v., citing only veterinary and medical authors, from Chiron to Oribasius (but omitting Alexander), apart from four examples from jurists and two from Christian ecclesiastical writers. The substantival participle appears to be used at 2.238 = II, 503, 28, but otherwise *calefaciens* is always adjectival (with *res*, *adiutorium*, *medicamen*, etc.).

69 **acidonicum** Note the very similar contrast at 2.70 (= II, 399, 26) 'neque amaritudinem in ore sentiunt sed magis acidonicum sentiunt', where ms. A attests the form I adopt here. The word is found in other late medical texts, including Rufus and Oribasius (see Mørland, *Oribasius*, 130, who derives it from *acidus*). I hesitate to segment this word: **acido*, *-onis* would fit nicely into a derivational type which seems to recur in late Latin medical texts, and which is clearly important in Proto-Romance — namely, the formation of new *n*-stems in *-o*, *-onis*. The Latin Alexander appears to attest *flegmo* 'an inflamed tumour, boil' (2.7; cf. Greek φλεγμονή) and possibly *fymo* 'a growth' (2.9.1 and note ad loc.; cf. Greek φῦμα, -ατος), Pelagonius and Oribasius, *acro*, plural *acrones* 'the extremities' (cf. Greek ἄκρα; ἄκρων) and Oribasius also *testo* 'testicle' (of animals; cf. André, *Anatomie*, 178) and Adams, *Sexual Vocabulary*, 67, who mentions also *coleo* = *coleus* 'testicle' and *posterio* = *posteriora*. Then there are two derivatives common to Alex. Trall. and Oribasius and certainly built on new *n*-stem nouns: *sablon-osus* 'sandy' (*sab(u)lo* 'sand'), *sapon-arius* 'soap-seller' (*sapo* 'soap', a Germanic loanword). Svennung, *Wortstudien*, 97 n. 1 takes *acidonicus* from *acidus*, by colloquial lengthening of the suffix (*-icus* → *-onicus*?). (At II, 309, 23 Greek ὀξίς is rendered by *acida ructatio* (2.48).)

70 **habere se sentiunt** One of the very few places where the descendants of φ disagree. I take it that L1 omits *se* before *sentiunt* by mistake; *ed.*'s omission of φ's *se* ... *habere* on the other hand could be deliberate.

2.3.3 Et praecessit[71] eos[72] magis frigdor quam calor, et balneo non in tempore competenti et potionibus et cibis usi sunt frigidis.

2.3.4 Sic enim ex frigida[73] distemperantia generata cognoscitur tussis.[74]

praecessit] precedit (*add.* .i. precessit) ***ed.*** precedet **M** | frigdor] frigor ***ed.*** | balneo] balneum **OP3** (al. ‘balneo’ **P3 m2** *in marg.*) ualneum **M** balneis **Ma** balneorum (*fortasse pro* balneo non) **Mu** | non] *om.* **Mu** | tempore competenti] c. t. **MaOx ϕ** competenti usu (usu *add.* **m2**) tempore (*expunct.* **m3**) **P3** | potionibus] -em **M** putionis **P1** | et_2] aut **P1** | cibis ... frigidis] -us ... -idus **P1** -is ... -idos **M** -o ... -ido **D** | usi sunt] usis **P1** ut sunt **M**

ex] *om.* **P3′** *add.* **m2** | frigida distemperantia] -is -iis **Ox** | generata cognoscitur tussis **A**] c. g. t. ***plerique*** c. t. g. **Ma** t. g. c. **OxGe** t. esse g. c. **ϕ**

71 **praecessit** The unusual use of the perfect here seems to be confirmed by *usi sunt* at the end of the sentence. There is a possible parallel for *praecessit* at 1.90 ‘Praecesserunt etiam et acres cibi’ = II, 25, 18 (προηγοῦνται), where the perfect may be triggered by the immediately preceding relative clause *ex his quae praecesserint* translating the Greek aorist participle.

Alternatively, given that for Greek χρῆσις we expect the noun *usus* (as at 1.79 = I, 597, 24–5, 1.81 = I, 603, 5, 1.91 twice = II, 25, 26 (with a past participle!) and 29, 2, 1.97 = II, 41, 14, al.), we might suppose that the corruption of *usus* to *usi sunt* prompted the correction of an original *precedit* (cf. *precedet* M) to *precessit*; *ed.*’s reading *precedit* probably has nothing to do with M’s reading but is rather a ‘correction’ of the *precessit* in his exemplar (hence the note *.i. precessit*, which most unusually is not shared with G2 and L1).

72 **eos** The pronoun evidently refers to the patients in the Latin, but in the Greek τούτοις can only refer to the morbid conditions. This is not an important discrepancy, as alternation, even confusion, between patient and disease is frequent in ancient medical texts. Cf. 2.2.4 *eis* and note.

73 **frigida** The Greek (with ἢ θερμὴν) is summing up 2.2 and 2.3 together, and contrasting (with μέν ... δέ) cold/hot with (2.4) dry/wet. The Latin, as it stands, concludes 2.3 only, and we may have lost *aut calida*.

74 **generata cognoscitur tussis** I follow A’s word-order, although most of the manuscripts have *cognoscitur generata tussis*, partly in order to keep the participle with its prepositional phrase, but mainly because hyperbaton is so much a feature of the style of the Latin Alexander. The Greek appears to lack γινόμεναι corresponding to Latin *generata*.

2.3.3 And they have experienced in advance cold rather than heat, and they have taken a bath at an unsuitable time and cold drinks and foods.

2.3.4 In this way a cough arising from a cold imbalance is recognized.

II, 149, 6–9 Puschmann

καὶ προηγεῖται μᾶλλον τούτοις ψῦξις ἢ ἔγκαυσις καὶ λουτρῶν ἀκαίρων καὶ πομάτων καὶ ἐδεσμάτων ψυχρῶν χρῆσις. (**2.3.4**). οὕτω μὲν αἱ διὰ ψυχρὰν αἰτίαν ἢ θερμὴν διαγινώσκονται βῆχες.

2.4.t. De tusse si ex sicca aut[75] humida distemperantia fuerit facta

2.4.1 Si autem ex siccitate aut humectatione[76] distemperantia[77] fuerit generata, operatiuis[78] similiter cognoscitur qualitatibus.

2.4.2 Differunt[79] igitur[80] quod magis operatiu*ae*[81] habent manifestas significationes,[82] material*es*[83] autem [si accesserit tussis][84] amitroter*as*,[85] et non oportet <t>alia[86] iterum dicere.

De - facta] *om.* **P1 MaL2** | De - humida] De sicca tusse ex humida **P3** (tusse ex *add.* **m2**) | De tusse] *om.* **B** | si] *om.* **G1Ox** | ex] de **M Ox** *om.* **G1** | sicca aut humida] calida **Mu** | sicca] siccitate **Ge** | aut] et **M A Ge** uel **OxBL1** an **D** | distemperantia fuerit facta] fuerit d. facta **O** | distemperantia] temperantia **A′** *om.* **G1 P2** | fuerit] fit **C** sit **Ge** fiat **B** *om.* **OxP3** | facta] *om.* **CB**

siccitate] -em **P1** | aut] et **P1** | humectatione (-em **P1**)] humec[tationib?]us **O** humiditate **G1Ox ϕ** humectatione cognoscitur **Mu′** | distemperantia fuerit generata (f. g. *om.* **M**)] g. f. d. **Ox** f. g. tussis **D** d. g. f. **ϕ** | operatiuis] -as **M** operatiuis .i. actiuis **ϕ** | *ad* similiter *habent in marg.* .i. similiter cognoscitur (cognoscitur tussis **G2L1**) ex passiuis qualitatibus sicut ex actiuis **ϕ** | cognoscitur] -gnusc- **P1** | qualitatibus] et qualitatibus **M**

Differunt (Defferent **P1**)] Differtur **A′** | igitur] autem in eo **C** | quod] quia **ϕ** qui **O** | magis operatiu*ae*] operatiue magis **ϕ** | *super* magis *habet uerba* quam humiditas et siccitas **P3 m4** | operatiu*ae* (-e **Ox**(?) **B**(?) **ϕ**] -am **M** -i **P1** -as ***cett.*** | habent manifestas] manifestas (magni- **L**) habent **C ϕ** | habent] abit **P1** | manifestas] -a **P1** -am **M** cal. et frig. *s. s.* **P3 m4** | significationes] -is **P1** -em **M** cognitiones **C P2** -es uel cognitiones **B** uel cognitiones *s. s.* **Ma** | *ante* material*es trad. 2. 5. t.* | material*es scripsimus*] -is ***cett.*** -iter **Ox** | si] sic **Mu′** | amitroter*as scripsimus (fort. cf.* a materia est **M**)] -a ***plerique*** (amet- **P1** amyt- **P2** amicr- **G2L1**) amitro terea **O** amicio tera ***ed.*** amitrota **Ge** a materia **M** *om.* **Mu** (*post* a. *habent* est **MD P3** *add.* **m3**) **G2** | et] *om.* **OMu** | oportet] -it **P1** | <t>alia iterum (<t>alia ***Fischer***)] alia iterum **P1MA O**(?: alia *illeg.*) iterum alia **MuCP2L2BOxGe P3** (iterum **m2** *add. in marg.*) iterum taliter **ϕ** iterum **G1** aliter **Ma** | dicere] *om.* **Ge′** dici **P3Ma ϕ** (*ad* dici *habent* .s. signa (signa .s. **G2**) quibus (e quibus **L1**) cognoscatur si materialis est **ϕ**)

[75] **sicca aut humida** The agreement of A and M in favour of *et* rather than *aut* is outweighed by the overwhelming support for *aut* in 2.4.1 and by Greek ἢ in both places.

[76] **humectatione** A favourite word of the Latin Alexander, selected despite the anisomorphism with *siccitate*, which perhaps prompted the late correction *humiditate* in G1 and Ox (and hence ϕ). *humectatio* occurs five times in each of Books 1 (21bis, 42, 63, 69) and 2 (42, 50bis, 152, 200), the underlying verb four times in Book 1 (29, 59, 80, 145) and twenty-four times in Book 2 (25, 29bis, 40bis, 41, 47, 49, al.), including several times in Philagrius but never in Philumenus; the adjective occurs only at 1.109, 2.72 and 2.82. Both noun and verb are used nearly always of the (Hippocratic) state of the body or the humours, the verb of bringing this state about by means of foods or medicaments. There are parallels for the medical use in Cael. Aur., *Chron.* 3.2.18 and Theod. Prisc., *Log.* 27 p. 124, 11 (Theodorus also attests the adjective); *humectatio* is a variant for *humidatio* at Oribas., *Eup.* 2.1 Aa p. 485. (Otherwise, for the abstract noun, Georges cites Cassiod., *Var.* 10.26.2, and Isid., *Orig.* 4.7.4, and Souter, *Iren.* 1.30.3 and 'saec. v on'). In Classical Latin *umectare* is attested on the one hand in Lucretius, Vergil (once in the *Georgics* and twice in the *Aeneid*) and a few later poets, on the other in the (technical) prose of Columella, the Elder Pliny (of eyes watering at *Nat. Hist.* 11.145) and Aulus Gellius. The adjective *umectus*, on the other hand, is found both early (in Cato and Varro) and late (in Apuleius, Gellius, Palladius, and Macrobius).

[77] **distemperantia** Again (cf. 2.2.5 and note), we are surprised by the absence of a reference to coughing (this time in the Greek, too), an absence which evidently prompted D's correction of *distemperantia* to *tussis*.

[78] **operatiuis** Apart from one example in an excerpt from Augustine (*Divers. quaest.* 63), *operatiuus* is apparently (*ThLL*, s.v.) found otherwise only in the Latin Oribasius (frequently: see Svennung, *Wortstudien*, 103; Mørland, *Oribasius*, 123–4) and the Latin Hippocrates (*De aere* 24 *fin.*). The word is used fifteen times in the Latin Alexander.

2.4.t. Concerning coughing if it arises as a result of a dry or a wet imbalance

2.4.1 If, however, it is as a result of dryness or wetness that an imbalance has been caused, it is recognized likewise from its active qualities.

2.4.2 They differ in that the active tend rather to have clear signs, while the material ones have more indistinct signs. And it is not necessary to say this again.

II, 149, 10–14 Puschmann

Περὶ βηχὸς διὰ ξηρὰν ἢ ὑγρὰν δυσκρασίαν γινομένης
Αἱ δὲ κατὰ ξηρότητα ἢ ὑγρότητα δυσκρασίαι ταῖς δραστικαῖς ὡσαύτως διαγινώσκονται ποιότησι. (**2.4.2**). διαφέρουσι δὲ τῷ (*correxi ex* τοῦ) μᾶλλον τὰς δραστικὰς ἔχειν ἐναργέστατα σημεῖα, τὰς δὲ ὑλικὰς ἀμυδρότερα, καὶ οὐ χρὴ ταὐτὰ πάλιν λέγειν.

[79] **Differunt** Presumably, the unexpressed subject are qualities of *distemperantia* rather than types of cough?

[80] **igitur** Note *igitur* again (cf. 2.2.6 above and note) for Greek δέ, which must be at least weakly contrastive (ὡσαύτως διαγινώσκονται vs διαφέρουσι).

[81] **operatiu*ae*** I have adopted the correction of B, Ox and ϕ.

[82] **significationes** All the Latin manuscripts which transmit the heading 2.5.t. *De tusse si ex humoribus fiat* have it at this point, between *significationes* and *materiales*. It must belong at the start of the next sentence.

[83] **materiale*s*** For *materialis* = ὑλικός, cf. 2.74 ‘Materiales autem aliae qualitates id est siccae et humidae distemperantiae’ = II, 409, 12 τὰς δὲ ὑλικὰς ποιότητας οἷον ξηρότητας καὶ ὑγρότητας.

[84] **[si accesserit tussis]** I take it that this addition, which I have bracketed although it was evidently already in the archetype, was prompted by the reading of 2.5.t. before *materiale*s.

[85] **amitroter*as*** There may conceivably be support for the feminine accusative plural in M’s *a materia est*. More probably, however, the transmitted forms (nearly all) in *-a* are in agreement with *tussis* in the Latin addition *si accesserit tussis* (see note 84). ἀμυδρός ‘faint’ is transliterated also at 1.59 ‘Pulsus etiam raros et breues et amidros habent’ (= I, 529, 11 καὶ τοὺς σφυγμοὺς ἀραιοὺς καὶ μικροὺς καὶ ἀμυδροὺς ἴσχουσιν) and 3.41 (I, 345, 25); cf. 3.45 (I, 347, 21) where ἀμυδρός is confused with ἄμετρος and translated *absque mensura*. That the word was less than familiar is seen clearly at 3.48 ‘pulsus . . . paruus autem et amidros in ethica febre’, where the Latin version adds the note: ‘Amidros autem pulsus dicitur defectus, qui solutam habet uirtutem et percussionem facit imbecillem’. (The marginal gloss at this point — of Jacques Despars(?) — reads ‘.i. imbecillis seu debilis. Gal. in lib. de differentiis febrium’.)

[86] **<t>alia** For *talis* = *hic*, cf. Hofmann and Szantyr, 205–6, and Svennung, *Wortstudien*, 129–30 (the latter mainly on *hic talis* = *is* in Oribasius, which I have not found in the Latin Alexander).

2.5.t. <De tusse si ex humoribus fiat>

2.5.1 Supercurrente[87] igitur materia efficitur tussis, et quod[88] spuit*ur* plenitudo, certa et manifesta apparet, quia ex reumatismo ex alio in alium transmittitur[89] locum, et[90] exinde nascentiam tussis habet.

2.5.2 Vnde et ex quibus transmittitur locis, haec utique omnia[91] contemplari oportet et attendere seu de capite fluit qui[92] mouet tussem, siue[93] ex altero membro, et qualis suscipit *locus*.[94]

<De - fiat> *transposui ex 2.4.2*] *om.* **P1 P3L2Ma Ox** | tusse] tussi **G1 ϕ** | si] qui **M** | humoribus] hu. **C** | fiat] sit **O**

Supercurrente] -em **P1** Succurrente **G1** | efficitur tussis] t. e. **Ox ϕ** | quod **P1M AOMu P3′**] eo quod **P2** ex eo quod ***cett.*** (*in* **P3** ex eo *add.* **m2**) | spuit*ur scripsimus*] spuit ***cett.*** ex(s)puit (-et **O**) **M O DP3** fluit **L** | *post* spuit *habet* ḟ **Mu** certa **D** | plenitudo] -tuto **B** *om.* **M** *illeg.* **O** | manifesta] magnifesta **L** | apparet] -it **P1** quia **M P2**(*ex corr.*)] quod **O** que ***cett.*** Quod si **D** | reumatismo] reumatissimo **Ox** | ex] et **P1P3′** | alio] alia **P1** | in alium transmittitur] transmutatur in alterum **P3** | in] ad **Ox** | alium] alio **M** alterum **DP3** altero **P1** | transmittitur (-miti- **Ge**)] transumitur **Ox** transmutatur **P3 ϕ** | locum - (**2.5.2**) transmittitur] *om.* **P1** | locum] loco **M** | et$_3$ **O P3MaDOx**] *om.* ***cett.*** | nascentiam tussis habet] tussis nascitur **P3Ma ϕ** | nascentiam] -ia **M**

Vnde - locis] *om.* **P3Ma** | Vnde et] *om.* **G1L2B D** *rasura* **P2** | et] *om.* **Ox** *et* **O**(?) | ex] de **M** *habet litteram* i *super litteram* x **Ox** | haec utique omnia] *om.* **ODOx** | haec (haec **P1**)] hec enim **Ge** | utique (utei- **P3′**) omnia (omnia et **Mu**) **P1P3′AMu**] utique ante omnia **P3** (ante *add.* **m2**) omnia utique (itaque **L2**) **M G1CP2L2B Ge ϕ** | contemplari] -are **P1** | oportet] -it **P1** | attendere] adt- **P1M** | *post* attendere *habet* ex quibus transmutatur locis **P3 m2** *add. in marg.* | fluit **P1M D**] -et(?) **O** -at ***cett.*** fuerit **Ox** | qui (que **P1**)] quod **G1CP2L2B MaDOx** humor qui **P3** (humor *add.* **m2**) **Ge ϕ** | mouet tussem (uomitussim **P1**)] t. m. **D** | siue] seu **Ox** | ex] de **Ox** | altero] alio **L2** | qualis **P1M AMu D**] quale **P2CL2BMaOxGe ϕ** (*post* quale *add.* membrum **ϕ**) qualis quod **O** quale quod **G1P3′** (*post* quale *add.* est **P3 m2**) | suscipit] -cepit **P1 Ox** -cipiat **Ge ϕ** | *locus* **DOx**] solum **M** solus ***cett.***

[87] **Supercurrente** See note on 2.1.2 *humores superfluentes*.

[88] **quod** (Cf. 2.4.2 *quod* 'in that'.) My impression is that causal *quod* is not very common in the Latin Alexander. The tradition has normalized it with, successively, *eo quod* (P2) and *ex eo quod*.

[89] **transmittitur** Presumably, P3 (followed by ϕ) misread *transmittitur* as **transmutitur* and corrected the latter to *transmutatur*. It is remarkable that none of them corrected *transmutatur* in the light of 2.5.2 *transmittitur* ten words later.

[90] **et** (before *exinde*) An easy omission, especially before *ex-*, *et* may have been lacking already in the archetype. Its distribution in the tradition could imply that it is a correction in θ (or even that it had survived in γ′).

[91] **haec utique omnia** It is striking that a classical particle such as *utique* should be common in the Latin Alexander and in both older and younger translations of Oribasius (Mørland, *Oribasius*, 161–2). Mørland states that in both Oribasius translations *utique* stands in the majority of cases for Greek ἄν. I have tried to show in detail elsewhere (Langslow, '*utique*') that the use of *utique* is more complicated than Mørland implies, that his summary statement applies better to Alexander than to either the older or the younger Oribasius, and that there are differences in its use between the two Oribasius translators and between them and the translator(s) of Alexander. Common to all three texts, however, are the use of *utique si* 'especially, even if' for Greek κἄν, and, remarkably, the erroneous use of *utique* to render κἄν, the first syllable of κἀνταῦθα, which is what we must have here.

On the assumption that *utique* here stands for Greek κἄν (by a false segmentation of κἀνταῦθα), I prefer the word-order of P1 AMu MaP3 (*haec utique omnia*); it is also more likely that *haec* and *omnia* were secondarily brought together than that they were secondarily separated.

omnia Did the translator's Greek text have πάντα? Or does *omnia* reflect παντ- rather than κἀντ- (in κἀνταῦθα)? In the latter case *utique* would be hard to explain.

2.5.t. Concerning coughing if it arises from humours

2.5.1 If, then, there is an overflow of material, coughing is brought about; and, because there is an abundance of spitting, it appears certain and manifest, because (?) as a result of a flux it is transmitted from one place to another, and from there the cough has its origin.

2.5.2 Whence and from which places it is transmitted, all of this in particular it is necessary to consider, and (it is necessary) to observe whether that (humour) which sets the coughing in motion flows from the head or from another body-part, and which part receives it.

II, 149, 14–19 Puschmann

αἱ δὲ κατ' ἐπίρρυτον ὕλην ἐπιγινόμεναι βῆχες αὐτῷ τῷ ἀναπτύεσθαι πλῆθος εὔδηλοι ἢ καὶ φανεραὶ τυγχάνουσιν, ὅτι κατὰ ῥευματισμὸν ἐξ ἑτέρων ἐπιπεμπόντων τὴν γένεσιν ἔχουσιν· (**2.5.2**). ὅθεν δὲ καὶ ἐξ ὁποίων ἐπιπέμπονται μορίων, κἀνταῦθα διορίζεσθαι δεῖ καὶ προσέχειν, εἴτε ἐκ τῆς κεφαλῆς ἐπιρρεῖ τὸ κινοῦν τὴν βῆχα εἴτε καὶ ἐξ ἑτέρων, καὶ ποῖα <μᾶλλον δέχεται μόρια M>·

[92] **qui** On the strength of the transmitted forms, especially the correction (perhaps by ε, if not polygenetic) of *qui* to *quod*, I think we must understand (from 2.5.t.?) rather than read *humor* (added in λ or in P3 and Ge independently).

[93] **seu** ... **siue** Here at least the tradition is virtually unanimous on the respective forms (as it happens, *seu* before consonant, *siue* before vowel).

[94] **suscipit *locus*** For the collocation, cf. 2.39 *qui suscipit locus* (II, 285, 13). Our translator must have had something like the text of Greek ms. M before him (perhaps without μᾶλλον). I have put *locus* in italics, because the evidence we have indicates that it must have been corrupted in the archetype; we have no reason to suppose that D and Ox had access to another, superior copy in which they would have found *locus*: I take it rather that κ conjectured *locus* on the basis of the context (cf. *locis* at the start of this sentence).

2.5.3 Etenim[95] pulmo suscipit primum,[96] est autem quando[97] et thorax et latera uel praecordia et alia altera[98] patiuntur membra.

2.5.4 Et hoc per partes[99] cognoscendum est, simul autem et curationes uniuscuiusque dicendae sunt, et omnino nihil praetermitti debet de tusse sed magis perquirere,[100] ut facile curatio urgente causa[101] adhibeatur.

Etenim] enim **Mu P3L2Ma** et quandoque **Ox** | pulmo] pulmon **M** pulmos **P1** | suscipit primum] p. s. **DOx** | suscipit (-cep- **P1**)] *pos. ante* pulmos **P1** *post* thorax **Ge ϕ** | primum] prima **AMu** | autem] ergo **B** | et$_1$] *om.* **G1P2L2** | uel] siue **P1** et **Mu G1L2B** | altera **P1M AMu P2 Ox**] etiam **D** *om.* ***cett.*** | patiuntur membra] m. p. **G1 ϕ** | patiuntur] pascuntur **C**

hoc] hec **DOx P3 ϕ** (per partes hec **Ox**) | partes] -is **P1** | cognoscendum est] est cognoscendum **C** | cognoscendum] -a (-gnusc- **P1**) **P1 O DOx P3′ ϕ** (*punct. sub.* a **P3 m2**) | est] sunt **O DOx ϕ** *om.* **P1 AMu P2** | simul] similiter **P2** (*corr. ex* simul) **G1L2 MaGe ϕ** | curationes] -is **P1** | dicendae sunt **M P2 P3Ox ϕ**] sunt dicende ***cett.*** | dicendae] -a **P1** | sunt] *om.* **Mu Ge′** | omnino] *om.* **G1L2** | nihil] *om.* **M** | praetermitti debet de tusse] p. de t. d. **A** d. de t. p. **Mu** d. p. de t. **Ox** praetermittendum (p. est **P3**) de tusse **P3 ϕ** | praetermitti (-e **P1**) debet (-it **P1**)] -endum est **P3Ma** -endum **ϕ** | de] *om.* **M** | tusse] -i **DOx** | perquirere (-quer- **P1**) **P1M O P3 ϕ**] perquiri ***cett.*** | facile] -is **G1L2B P3MaGe ϕ** | urgente] -em **P1** | adhibeatur] ex- **L2**

[95] **Etenim** This conjunction is used at least nine times in Book 1 and twenty-three times in Book 2, usually for καὶ γάρ in Puschmann's text (e.g. 1.55, 57, 63, 74), occasionally apparently for καί (e.g. 1.21, 27), almost invariably in clause-initial position, which supports the reconstruction here.

[96] **suscipit primum** The translator's Greek text must have had δέχεται πρῶτος (with or without πολλάκις); and see the next note.

[97] **est autem quando** Presumably, our translator's Greek text had ἐστὶν δὲ ὅτε, and since this is reported as well by Puschmann for Greek mss. L and M, ἐστὶν εἶτα must be a late innovation, albeit an attractive one (of Zipser's π); a simple *TLG* search finds seventy-three examples of εἶτα in the Greek Alexander, as a rule (as here) clause-initial and without a connecting particle. Ox prepares for *est autem quando* by beginning the sentence with *Et quandoque* 'sometimes (on the one hand)'! On *est quando* for ἔστιν ὅτε see Hofmann and Szantyr, 520, and now Adams, *Bilingualism*, 496, on its use by Anthimus.

[98] **alia altera** Cf. 1.69 'ab alio altero membro' (I, 551, 15 ἄλλου). The pleonastic *alius alter* is otherwise attested only in Solinus and both versions of the Latin Oribasius (Mørland, *Oribasius*, 138–9; Hofmann and Szantyr, 208).

[99] **per partes** The phrase *per partes* is well attested in the Latin Alexander as the equivalent of κατὰ μέρος 'severally, in turn; gradually, bit by bit'. Cf. 2.9.1, 2.11.7 below, and e.g. 1.140 = II, 141, 23 (of blood-letting); 1.148 = II, 243, 14 (of purging); this is further illustrated by the mistranslation at 2.163 'si per partes auferatur sanguis' = II, 191, 5 ἡ ἐκ τῶν κάτω μερῶν ἀφαίρεσις, where κάτω μερῶν must be right but has been misread as (or corrupted to) κατὰ μέρος and so translated. In the present passage, *partes* could be taken to refer to body-parts, but this is an accident of the context and I have not so translated it; at 2.101 (Philumenus) 'body-part by body-part' is *per partes membrorum*, with an additional word for body-part.

[100] **perquirere** All the attestations of the active form may have their source in β, partly by way of γ′, so that this is probably a case of a straightforward disagreement between β (*perquirere*) and δ (*perquiri*). I provisionally prefer the active as in a sense the *lectio difficilior* so soon after *praetermitti*, and for lack of a good parallel for the impersonal passive. For the active form in a similar context, cf. 2.57 'Iterum contemplari oportet et perquirere'; and, with a curious change of construction, 2.39 'Contemplandum est ergo omnis corporis habitudo et alia signa inquirere'. Note that, while *debet* can on the face of it be taken impersonally with both *praetermitti* and *perquirere*, the Latin Alexander seems not to use impersonal *debet*, so that we must take *nihil* as subject of *debet* and reckon with a slight anacoluthon before *perquirere*.

[101] **urgente causa** For the use of the ablative absolute, cf. 2.1.2 *qualitate assumpta* and note. For *causa* 'disease', cf. 2.36.1 'Cardiaca passio stomachi causa est' (II, 279, 18 πάθος).

2.5.3 For the lung receives it first, but sometimes the chest and the flanks and/or the *praecordia* and some other parts suffer.

2.5.4 And this must be diagnosed each type in turn, but at the same time, too, the treatments of each single condition must be stated, and absolutely nothing must be omitted on the subject of coughing, but it ought to be looked into all the more closely, so that treatment can easily be applied when the disease is acute.

II, 149, 19–23 Puschmann

καὶ γὰρ ὁ πνεύμων ἀδικεῖται πολλάκις· πρῶτος γάρ ἐστιν, εἶτα ὁ θώραξ ἢ πλευρὸν ἢ τὸ διάφραγμα ἢ ἄλλο τι μόριον· (**2.5.4**) εἴπωμεν οὖν καὶ τούτων τὰς κατὰ μέρος διαγνώσεις, ἅμα δὲ καὶ τὰς θεραπείας, ὡς πανταχόθεν ἀπαράλειπτον εἶναι τὸν περὶ τῆς βηχὸς λόγον καὶ μᾶλλον εὑρίσκειν ἅπαν εὐχερῶς τὸν εἰς θεραπείαν ἐπειγόμενον ἰατρόν.

2.6.t. De tusse si ex capite fluat humor

2.6.1 Si igitur de capite defluat[102] humor, necesse est ut per uuam in[103] tracheam[104] arteriam irritationem quandam moueat cum sonitu in faucibus existente.[105]

2.7.t. Signa si de capite in pulmonem fluat

2.7.1 Quod si[106] in pulmonem[107] fluat, difficultas subsequitur[108] spirandi, et febris acuta apparet,[109] interdum autem[110] et lingua aspera et mela rubra, et grauitas sentitur +– in pectore –+.

De - humor] *om.* **P1 MaL2** | De] *om.* **Ox** | tusse] -i **ϕ** *om.* **Ox** | si] *om.* **C** | ex] de **P3** | capite] -is **M** | fluat] defluat **M** fluant **P3** fiat **P2** *om.* **C** | humor] humores **P3** humor qui est in causa **Ox** *om.* **C**

defluat (diff- **O**) **M O Ma**] -et **P1** -it **G1CP2L2D** fluat **AMu Ox P3 ϕ** fluit **BGe** | ut **M OC P3Ma DGeOx**] *om.* ***cett.*** | per uuam] p(er)uam (*i.e.* paruam) **L2** | uuam] unam ***ed.*** gulam **Mu** *spatium* **P1** | in tracheam] in tracia (dracia **P1**) **P1M** intra **AMu** | arteriam] -ia **P1M A** | quandam] quedam **P1M** | sonitu] -o **P1** s[--]um **O** | in faucibus (falc- **Mu**) existente] e. i. f. **ϕ**

Signa - fluat] *om.* **P1 L2BMa** De eodem **Ox** | Signa] *om.* **C** *ed.* | pulmonem] -e **M P2P3D** | fluat] fluat humor **P3Ge ϕ** h. fluat **C**

Quod si] Quod si amplius **Ge ϕ** | pulmonem] -e **M G1P2L2 P3** pleumone **P1** | fluat] -it **P1M Mu** fluat de capite **B** fluat hu. **Ox** | subsequitur] sequitur **Ox L2** sola sequitur **O Ma** | spirandi **P1 AMuC P2**] -i *an* -o **M** (?) inspirandi ***cett.*** respirandi **Ox** in spirando ***ed.*** | febris] -es **M** | acuta] accuta **Ma** -e **M** | apparet] -it **P1** -ent **M** | autem] *om.* **P3Ma** | et] *om.* **P3Ma** | lingua aspera] -am -am **P1** | mela **P1A**] male **Mu** mala ***cett.*** (*punct. sub priore* a **P2**) *addunt uerba* .i. maxilla **ϕ** .i. maxille sunt **Ma** maxilla **B** .i. gena **Ox** | rubra **P1M AO DOx P3 m2** *in marg.*] rubre **Mu** rubea **G1CP2L2BGe ϕ** rub̆ (rubea (?)) **P3'** nigra (*.s. s.* uel rubea) **Ma**

[102] **defluat** Note the discrepancy between *ex capite fluat* in the heading and *de capite defluat* in the text. Given *fluat* in the title, I tentatively regard *defluat* as the *lectio difficilior*, the agreement of P2 and γ as decisive in favour of *deflu-*, and the simplex as a (polygenetic?) correction based on the title.

[103] **in** It is tempting to supply <*aut*> for Greek ἤ, but the Latin version is rather different from the Greek, and makes good medical sense as it stands.

[104] **in tracheam** Given that C and O each had an accessory model from which they could have recovered *in tracheam* (see 4.8.4), *intra* could have been in η, and need not imply a common ancestor for A and Mu lower than η.

[105] **cum sonitu in faucibus existente** The phrase *sonitus in faucibus existens* must translate γαργαρισμόν (transmitted by Greek ms. L) or a similar word, and refer to a sound made while breathing; *sonitus* is used of ringing in the ears at 1.117, 118. I hesitate to give *existens* more force than 'being, existing'; on the use of *existens*, see the note on 2.3.1 *existente* above.

[106] **Quod si** The addition of *amplius* (in Ge and ϕ) is typical of a late recension seeking to smooth the argument. The Latin is fuller and smoother than the Greek here. Is this because the Greek tradition has faithfully preserved the notes of a busy doctor (cf. Section 1.3)? Or were words lost in the branch of the tradition used by Puschmann?

[107] **pulmonem** I am uncertain whether to prefer accusative or ablative. The form *pleumone* in P1 resembles Greek πλεύμων 'lung', but late borrowing of the Greek word is apparently not otherwise attested (cf. André, *Anatomie*, 119–20). On the other hand, P1 offers the same form *pleumone* in the very next sentence for 2.7.2 *flegmonem* (see note ad loc.), which could not be right here.

2.6.t. Concerning coughing if humour flows from the head

2.6.1 But if humour should flow from the head, it is bound to cause a certain irritation over the uvula into the trachea, with a noise present in the throat.

2.7.t. Signs if it flows from the head into the lung

2.7.1 But if it flows into the lung, there ensues difficulty with breathing and an acute fever appears, and sometimes also the tongue (is) rough and the tonsils red, and a heaviness is felt in the chest.

II, 149, 24–151, 3 Puschmann

Διάγνωσις, ὅτι ἐκ τῆς κεφαλῆς ἐπιρρεῖ
Εἰ μὲν οὖν ἐκ τῆς κεφαλῆς εἴη τὸ ἐπιρρέον, ἀνάγκη κατὰ (περὶ M) τὴν σταφυλὴν ἢ τὴν τραχεῖαν ἀρτηρίαν ἐρεθισμόν τινα (καὶ γαργαρισμὸν *add.* L) γίνεσθαι. (**2.7.t.**). Φλεγμονῆς ἐν τῷ πνεύμονι σημείωσις
Δύσπνοιαι δὲ καὶ πυρετὸς ὀξὺς ἐπιφερόμενος (ἐπιφαινόμενος M), ἔσθ' ὅτε δὲ καὶ γλῶττα τραχεῖα καὶ μῆλα ἐρυθρὰ καὶ βάρους συναίσθησις +– –+

[108] **subsequitur** The variant *sola sequitur* presumably rests on the graphic similarity between 'b' and 'la', and arose independently in Ma and O (cf. conversely *subinfrigdat* for *solum infrigdat* in P1 at 2.236.5). In the Latin Alexander *subsequor* regularly translates παρακολουθέω (1.33 = I, 483, 18; 1.57 = I, 519, 3) or ἐπακολουθέω (1.119 = II, 97, 2; 1.122 = II, 99, 9 (v.l. παρ- in ms. M)).

[109] **apparet** Again, our translator's text must have been closer to Greek ms. M (with ἐπιφαινόμενος) than to Puschmann's.

[110] **interdum autem** ... **rubra** This looks like a word-for-word translation of the Greek nominal sentence, with *interdum* for ἔσθ' ὅτε (cf. 2.1.1 *est quando* and note ad loc.) and *autem* for δέ. The Latin version has three additional finite verbs (*subsequitur*, *apparet* and *sentitur*), but there is no trace of *est* at this point. *autem* does not properly introduce the clause with *sentitur* (and is probably for that reason omitted by θ″).

2.7.2 Et post[111] haec, si nihil dignum sputent[112] uix respirantes, flegmonem[113] necesse est de his omnibus signis suspicari nos in[114] pulmone esse factum.

2.7.3 Si autem et sitis sit nimia,[115] et frequenter[116] ad haec signa et calor sentiatur[117] multus[118] in thorace, *ita* ut[119] frigidum desiderent aerem intrinsecus ad se trahere,[120] et adhuc magis[121] existimari[122] oportet ignitum esse flegmonem[123] in pulmone.

Et post] postea **Ox** | haec] hoc **D** | si] *om.* **D** | nihil] quicquam **Mu** | dignum] eger(un)t **Mu** *om.* **ϕ** *super* dignum *habet* unde leuior fiat **P2** | nihil dignum] *om.* **P3′** nihil digne *add. in marg.* **m2**, dignum *corr. ex* digne **m3** | sputent] spuent **Ma** sputant **M** sputet (putet **Mu**) **AMuC G1P2L2** spuet **B** | uix] et uix **M** uix digne **P3′Ma ϕ** (*punct. sub* digne *habet* **P3**) | respirantes (-entes **P1** -ant ex **M**)] respirans **AMuC G1P2L2B** | flegmonem . . . factum] necesse est de his omnibus signis suspicari flegmonem in pulmone (-em **L2**) esse factum **G1L2** | flegmonem] pleumone **P1** pulmone **M** | necesse est *habet post* signis **Ma** | suspicari] -are (-ecare **P1**, -icaere(?) **Mu**) **P1M OMu Ox** | nos] *om.* **O G1 MaP3′ Ox** | suspicari nos] n. s. **P3** (nos *add.* **m3**) **ϕ** | esse factum] f. e. **Mu P3** (esse *add.* **m2**)

et] *om.* **CP3 ϕ** *post* autem *add.* ad hec signa **P3 m3** *in marg.* | sitis sit nimia] sitis nimia **P1 O P3′MaOx** (sit *add.* **P3 m2**) sit sitis nimia **ϕ** sitis nimia est **M** | et frequenter] frequenter **DMa′** frequenter et **O OxP3** | *post* frequenter *habent* respirent et **ϕ** etiam exspirent **D** expirent **MaGe** (*add. super* et calor) | ad haec signa] *om.* **P3′MaDGe** | haec] hoc **ϕ** | et_3 **P1M AMuC Ma D**] *om.* ***cett.*** | calor] calorem **M** | sentitur] -iatur **P1 A G1CP2B Ox** (**O** *illeg.*) | multus] magnum **M** | sentitur multus] m. s. **P3Ma ϕ** | *ita* ut **P3 m2** *in marg. ad* et] id est ut **AMuC G1P2B** intus et **M** intus **P1** ut **OGeϕ** et **P3′Ma DOx** | desiderent] -ant **Ma** -et **AMu G1P2L2B** | intrinsecus] extrinsecus **C** | trahere] trahaere **P1** thraere **D** | adhuc magis] *om.* **P3Ma** | et (sed **Mu**)] *om.* **M OCDOx** | existimari] -are **P1M O D** estimare **Ox** | ignitum] -etum **P1** | esse flegmonem] f. e. **P3Ma** | flegmonem] fleumonem **P1M** | pulmone] -em **P1M**

[111] **post** For *post* 'besides', Georges cites Calp., *ecl.* 10.22, Hofmann and Szantyr, 243 cite Gaius, *dig.* 30.65. Cf. 2.7.3 *ad haec* for πρὸς τούτοις.

[112] **sputent** Whether indicative or subjunctive, singular (as in δ) or plural (as in γ and γ′), we have here a form of *sputare* (rather than *spuere*), and the Latin has active for the Greek passive. (Cf. 2.7.4 *sputant*, 2.8.3 *sputetur*, 2.11.t. *sputato*.)

[113] **flegmonem** Apparently, a new *n*-stem in *-o*, *-onis*, attested also at Veg., *mulom.* 2.48.1. Cf. 2.3.2 *acidonicum* and note.

Are the errors in M and P1 related? Both have a word for 'lung', but each could have arisen very differently, P1's *pleumone* for *fleumonem* (but cf. 2.7.1 where P1 has *pleumone* for *pulmonem*), M's *pulmone* by anticipation of *pulmone* in the next line. Alternatively, they could reflect a word for 'lung' (*pulmonem* or *pleumonem*?) in γ. Note that both P1 and M (and therefore γ) have *fleumonem* for *flegmonem* at 2.7.3.

[114] **in** Once here, and twice in 2.7.3, we have Latin *in* for Greek περί + bodypart.

[115] **sitis sit nimia** Presumably, *sit* was omitted in γ and γ′. M supplied indicative *est* after *sitis nimia*; ϕ supplied *sit* before *sitis nimia*.

[116] **et frequenter** Latin *et frequenter* was surely prompted by the form in the translator's text corresponding to Puschmann's συνέχοιτο (cf. συνέχεται M): perhaps συνεχῶς τε?

[117] **sentiatur** Subjunctive (with P1, η and most of the tradition), as this is a further symptom in the Greek. ϕ (presumably following P3) and θ″ (conceivably following γ′: cf. M) by using the indicative effectively make it a result, which we do not want until the diagnosis, beginning *et adhuc*.

[118] **calor . . . multus** The Latin *calor multus* makes better sense than Greek αἴσθησις πολλὴ: we should perhaps correct πολλή to πολλῆς.

2.7.2 And besides these (signs), if they should spit nothing of note while breathing with difficulty, we are obliged from all these signs to suspect that inflammation has arisen in the lung.

2.7.3 But if there is also excessive thirst, and frequently in addition to these signs a great heat is felt in the chest, i.e. with the result that they long to breathe in cold air, even more is it right to conclude that there is a blazing inflammation in the lung.

II, 151, 3–9 Puschmann

καὶ πρὸς τούτοις, εἰ καὶ μηδὲν ἄξιον ἀναπτύεται δυσπνοούντων αὐτῶν, φλεγμονὴν ἐξ ἀνάγκης ἐκ πάντων τούτων ὑποπτεύειν ἡμᾶς περὶ τὸν πνεύμονα γεγενῆσθαι προσήκει. (**2.7.3**). εἰ δὲ καὶ δίψῃ σφοδρᾷ συνέχοιτο πρὸς τοῖς σημείοις τούτοις καὶ θέρμης αἴσθησις αὐτῷ γίνοιτο πολλὴ περὶ τὸν θώρακα, ὥστε ψυχρὸν ἐπιθυμεῖν ἀέρα ἀναπνεῖν, ἔτι καὶ μᾶλλον ὑπονοεῖν δεῖ ζέουσαν εἶναι τὴν φλεγμονὴν περὶ τὸν πνεύμονα.

[119] ***ita* ut** I adopt P3's correction *ita ut*, although *id est ut* is favoured by the tradition (arguably even by M and P1), as *ita ut* is so common for Greek ὥστε, while *id est ut* occurs otherwise only in an explanatory note ('that is to say, like ...') at 2.69 'id est ut aqua in qua caro recens lauatur', not in the Greek (II, 399, 17).

[120] **frigidum** ... **trahere** Very similar content and form is translated more briefly at 2.2.1. Here *intrinsecus ad se trahere* appears in addition for Greek ἀναπνεῖν as at 2.2.2 (see note ad loc.).

[121] **adhuc magis** Adverbial *adhuc magis* is common in the Latin Alexander (I have counted sixteen instances in Book 1 alone): cf. e.g. 1.57 'adhuc magis iuuandum est' (I, 517, 13 ἔτι μᾶλλον βοηθεῖν), 1.58 (I, 525, 23), and in diagnosis as here 1.76 'adhuc magis existimandum' (I, 593, 15). On *adhuc* = *etiam*, see Hofmann and Szantyr, 464–5.

[122] **existimari** I favour the passive infinitive after *oportet* (against γ, O and κ, which may reflect γ′), although my impression is based at this stage mainly on A, which has the impersonal passive at 1.39, 76, 143; 2.186, 192, and the active (after *expedit*) only at 1.85.

[123] **ignitum** ... **flegmonem** For *ignitus flegmo* = ζέουσα φλεγμονή, cf. 1.114 = II, 85, 26 (and in a mistranslation at 1.88 of II, 7, 23 ἐν τῇ φλεγμονῇ ζέοντος παυσαμένου 'when the heat has subsided'). The same Latin phrase translates πυρώδης φλεγμονή at e.g. 1.128 = II, 123, 18. For *ignitus* = πυρώδης cf. e.g. 1.58 = I, 525, 21 ἀήρ; 1.128 (*ignitior*) = II, 119, 27 ὄγκος; for *ignitus* = ζέων, e.g. 1.112 = II, 77, 27 δυσκρασίαι. (Svennung, *Wortstudien*, 88 notes the form *ignatus* (= πυρώδης) in the older Latin Oribasius.)

2.7.4 Si autem et colericum sputant nec nimis grauiter angust*a*[124] sentiunt se habere +– praecordiae loca –+, sed magis calida esse, erisipilas manifeste scito in pulmone consistere.[125]

2.8.t. Signa si tussientibus pus[126] in thoracem fluat et humor

2.8.1 Manifestum est enim quod[127] sit pus ex ipso colore solo et ex aliis signis[128] ex quibus didicimus[129] puris cognitionem: et ab odore[130] ex ustione fact*o*,[131] et ab hoc[132] quia soluitur missum[133] in aqua et non proicitur[134] quemadmodum[135] flegma et crudus humor.

et] *om.* ***ed.*** | colericum] colerum **P1** | sputant (putant **P1**) **P1M**] spuant **O** spuent **Ma** sputent **P3DOxGe** **ϕ** sputet ***cett.*** | nec] neque ***ed.*** et **O** **G1P3′MaDOx** | grauiter] *om.* **A** | angust*a* ***Fischer***] angustias **P3′MaDOx** -ia **P1** -iam ***cett.*** | sentiunt se] se sentiant **Mu** | sentiunt **P1M O**(?)**P3Ma**] -iant **AMu DOx** **ϕ** -iat **G1CP2L2B** | se] sed **P1** | habere (abere **P1**)] ualere ***ed.*** *om.* **Ox** | praecordiae (-ia **Mu**) loca **P1 AMuC**] in p. l. **M P2** in precordiorum locis **G1L2BGe ϕ** circa precordiorum loca **O P3Ma DOx** | sed] *om.* **O P3′Ma DOx ϕ** | calida **P1M AMuC P2B**] calidam **Ge** calidas ***cett.*** calore **P3 m2** *in marg.* | esse] *om.* **G1P3Ma ϕ** | erisipilas] -am **Ge P3** (*corr. ex* -as **m3**) eripilas **G1** | manifeste] -is **P1** | pulmone] -em **M**

Tit. om. **P1 L2Ma** | si tussientibus] t. si **P3** si ex t. ***ed.*** | tussientibus *eqs*] tuss. in thoracem pus fluat **G1** pus in toracem fluat tuss. **Ox** in t(h)orace tuss. fluat pus et humor **P2′ D** | pus] *om.* **M C P2** thus **L1** | thoracem (-e **MOP2P3D*ed.***)] pulmonem **Ge** | et humor **A Bϕ**] ex humore **O** humor **M MuC P2** humorum **G1** pus et humor **P2′D** *om.* **P3Ox**

est] *om.* **ϕ** | enim] autem **Ge** *om.* **P1Mu** | quod sit (fit **G1P2 L2** (*corr. ex* sit) si **P1 C B′Ge**)] quia sit **Ox ϕ** quod **M DOx** *om.* **O P3Ma** | pus] plus **P1′** | ex] et **P1M** fluat non ex **Ge m2** | ipso] -um **M** -us **P1** *om.* **Ge ϕ** | colore] -em **M** -es **P1** calore **O G1P2′ L1** | solo] -um **P1M** *om.* **Ox** | et ex] sed ex **Ge** ex **P1M** et **OP3′MaOx** | aliis signis] -a -a **P1M** | ex] *om.* **P1** | didicimus (dedicimus **P1**)] deducimus **M** didiscimus **BGe** | puris] poris **P1** | cognitionem] significationem et c. **Mu** c. habet **Ox** c. haberi **D** | et] nam **O** .s. (scilicet) **Ge** | ab] ob **M** ex ***ed.*** | odore] hoc dare **M** hoc **P1** odore et **Ox** *ad* odore *habent in marg.* .s. quando pus proicitur super carbones fetet **G2L1** | ex ustione fact*o* **O**] exustionem -am **CL2** exustione facta ***cett.*** | et] etiam (etiam et **L1**) **ϕ** | ab hoc] ob hoc **G1CBMaD** ob **L2** adhuc **P1M** | quia] quod **MaOx** | *uerba* soluitur missus in aqua *bis scripsit* **Mu′** | soluitur] soluit **D** | missum] -us **P1 AMuC** | aqua] -am **DOx** | quemadmodum] -amm- **M** | flegma] fleuma **P1 G2L1** | humor] humoris **P1**

[124] **grauiter angust*a*** In order to achieve a defensible text, I have adopted Cloudy Fischer's correction of *angustiam* in the archetype to *angusta* and left *praecordiae loca* without a preposition. The alternative would be *angustiam … in praecordiae loca*, with M and P2; I have yet to investigate systematically case-usage after prepositions, but my clear initial impression is that the translator would here have used *in* + ablative (cf. the examples quoted below). In any case the patients, and not the body-parts, must be the subject of *sentiunt se habere*. Cf., from the present treatment of coughing alone, 2.3.2 'habere se sentiunt'; 2.10.1 'sentiunt coangustata praecordia se habere'. Conversely, when the symptom is the subject, *sentio* appears in the passive: 2.7.1 'grauitas sentitur in pectore'; 2.7.3 'calor sentiatur multus in thorace'; 2.8.2 'grauedo sentitur fieri'.

Latin *grauiter* suggests either that the translator thought he was rendering βαρῶς (βάρους Puschmann), or that the original translation had the abstract nouns *grauitas et/uel angustia* (which should then have had a passive form of *sentio*, as above), and we have to reckon with a change of construction or serious corruption.

[125] **consistere** Like *existo*, *existens* (cf. 2.3.1 and note ad loc.), *consisto* and *consistens* are favourite words of the Latin Alexander. For *consisto* = συνίστασθαι, cf. e.g. 1.52 'Vnde ergo consistit (sc. frenetis)' = I, 509, 3 ὅθεν δὲ συνίσταται; 1.53 = I, 509, 18; 1.85 'in eis (sc. oculis) consistentes passiones' = II, 3, 3–4 τὰ ἐν αὐτοῖς συνιστάμενα πάθη.

[126] **pus** This heading looks like an invention of the Latin tradition: there is no break in the Greek text here. It is obviously based on recent headings, and attempts to combine *pus*, an accompaniment of inflammation and the main new topic, with *humor*, the subject since 2.5.t. The heading is unconvincing in that *pus* does not flow *in thoracem*! On the other hand, *pus* is absent only from M and C. It must have been in δ; without the evidence of P1 we cannot know whether it was in α.

2.7.4 But if they produce bilious sputum and do not feel that the area of the diaphragm is too heavily constricted, but rather that it is warm, then know full well that erysipelas is established in the lung.

2.8.t. Signs if in the midst of coughing pus flows into the chest, and humour

2.8.1 Now it is evident that it is pus both from the colour itself alone and from other signs from which we have learned the recognition of pus: both from the smell that is made when it is burnt and from the fact that it dissolves when put in water, and is not brought up like phlegm and raw humour.

II, 151, 9–15 Puschmann

εἰ δὲ χολῶδες ἀναπτύοιτο, μὴ πάνυ δὲ βάρους ἢ στενοχωρίας συναίσθησις γίνοιτο +– –+, ἀλλὰ μᾶλλον θέρμης, ἐρυσίπελας εἶναι σαφῶς ἐν τῷ πνεύμονι γίνωσκε. (**2.8.1**). δῆλον μέν ἐστι τὸ πῦον καὶ ἐξ αὐτῆς τῆς χροιᾶς μόνης καὶ ἐξ ἄλλων δὲ σημείων, ἐξ ὧν ἐμάθομεν πῦον διαγινώσκειν, καὶ ἀπὸ τῆς ὀσμῆς τῆς ἀπὸ τῆς καύσεως γινομένης καὶ τοῦ διαλύεσθαι βαλλόμενον ἐν ὕδατι καὶ μὴ ὑφιζάνειν (ἐφιζάνειν L M), ὥσπερ τὸ φλέγμα καὶ ὁ ὠμὸς χυμός.

[127] **manifestum est . . . quod sit** Cf. 2.1.4 'manifestum est quia', and note ad loc. The omission of *quod sit* by O and θ″ (did both find it in θ?) has the effect of bringing their text closer to the Greek.

[128] **ipso colore . . . signis** Note the (?seventh/eighth-century) Vulgar Latin of γ in the string of accusative forms for ablative in *ipsum colorem solum . . . alia signa* in M (cf. *ipsus colores solum . . . alia signa* P1).

I confess, I am puzzled by Puschmann's δέ in Greek καὶ ἐξ ἄλλων δὲ σημείων (unless it is a simple misprint for δή).

[129] **didicimus** Cf. 1.127 (II, 113, 10ff.); 2.186 (II, 481, 4ff.).

[130] **ab odore** Unusually, the explanatory note in G2 and L1 (and therefore surely in φ) is not in *ed.*, presumably an oversight.

[131] **ex ustione fact*o*** All the manuscripts except O write this as one word and with a feminine form of the participle. That we should read it as two (in *ab odore ex ustione facto*), with a prepositional phrase rather than an ablative absolute (and with *facto*, rather than *facta*, agreeing with *odore*, as in O), is suggested not only by Greek ἀπὸ τῆς καύσεως but also by the overwhelming preference in the participle (the nominalization in *-tio* occurs apparently only here) for the simplex *ust-* over the compound *exust-* (the latter is attested in A only three times, in quick succession, 1.80, 81, 82).

[132] **ab hoc** The tradition shows a neat division between *ab hoc* in δ and *adhuc* in γ. I favour the former because *hic* quite frequently translates the Greek definite article (here τοῦ), while *adhuc* regularly stands for Greek ἔτι, which here fails (but cf. 2.8.2 *adhuc*, which was perhaps anticipated here in γ). I cannot parallel *ab hoc quia*, but cf. the very similar *ex hoc quod* at 1.90 'Primo quidem ex hoc quod non plethoricum apparet totum corpus' = II, 25, 13 πρῶτον μὲν ἐκ τοῦ μὴ πληθωρικὸν φαίνεσθαι τὸ σῶμα ὅλον.

[133] **missum** Pending further collation, I treat *pus* as a neuter (cf. the probable accusative at 2.8.2 *supercurrens* (*pus*)), but I am impressed by the agreement of P1 and η here in treating it as masculine. Note that *pus* is among the neuters treated as masculine in the Latin Oribasius (Mørland, *Oribasius*, 66).

[134] **proicitur** Again, the translator's text seems to have had a variant in common with Greek manuscripts L and M, although even for ἐφιζάνειν 'form a deposit' the translation 'is brought up' is rather approximate.

[135] **quemadmodum** Cf. 2.1.1 and note ad loc.

2.8.2 Si ergo fuerit in[136] thorace, manifestum est ex multis aliis signis, adhuc etiam et ex grauedine quae sentitur fieri[137] in altera parte membri,[138] et supercurrens[139] ex subitaneis mutatis euersionibus[140] et sonos aurium cum obclusione saepius patiuntur.[141]

2.8.3 Haec enim sufficiat dixisse, si consistat[142] in thorace et ibidem contineatur. Quod si ad ea[143] quae dicta sunt praecedat pleuritis, nihil manifestum spuentes,[144] et hoc ipsum uiolenter sputetur,[145] manifeste[146] confi*t*endum[147] est quia pus est quod in thorace continetur.

fuerit] fuerit pus **Ox** | manifestum est (est *om.* **D**)] manifesta erunt **P1M** | ex] ex his et **G1L2DGe ϕ** his et **P2** *ex corr.* ex his et ex **O P3MaOx** | multis aliis] a. m. **G1** | etiam]etiam (*s.s.*) magis **Ox** | et ex **AOMu P3Ma**] et **M** ex ***cett.*** | grauedine] grauidinem **P1** grauedinem **M** | quae] *om.* **M** | fieri (fierit **P1**)] fiat **P3′** (fieri *add.* **m2** *in marg.; ante* fiat *add.* si **m3**) | *ad* in *habent in marg.* .s. quando eger (epar ***ed.***) iacet supra partem sanam sentit quasi pondus aggrauari super eam **ϕ** | altera parte (-am -em **P1**)] alia p. **ϕ** | et] *om.* **G1L2** | supercurrens] *habet litteras* te *super* -ens **P3 m3** (*hoc est* -ente?) *s. s.* pus **ϕ** | ex subitaneis **AMuC G1P2B**] subitaneis **Ox** subitaneas (-bet- **P1**) **P1M O D** subitas **P3 ϕ** subitat **Ma** | mutatis euersionibus] e. m. **Mu** | mutatis] -as **M P3Ma** mutatur **P1** mutat **O DG2L1** immutat ***ed.*** *om.* **G1L2** *ad* (im)mutat *habent* .i. inducit **ϕ** | euersionibus **AMuC G1P2BOx**] -es (-is **P1**) ***cett.*** *ad* e. *habent in marg.* .i. nauseas uel subuersiones stomachi **ϕ** | sonos **AMu DOx** (sonus **P1M OC**)] sonum **P3Ma** sonitus **G1P2L2B ϕ** | obclusione (-em **P1**)] exclusione **Ma** | patiuntur (-ci- **P1**) **P1M**] patitur ***cett.*** eiciens pus *s. s.* **ϕ**

Haec ... dixisse *habet infra* **A** | Haec (Haec **P1**)] Hoc **G1CB** (Ḥ(Hoc?) **L1**) | enim] et **L1** autem **Mu** *om.* **G1P2L2BGe *ed.*G2** | sufficiat (-tiat **G1CP2**)] -ciant **Mu L2DOxGe *ed.*** | dixisse] *om.* **O** | si] si pus **BGe** | consistat] -ant **P1** consistat pus **D P3 m2** constat **MMuP3′ ϕ** | *post* thorace *habent* humor **O** pus **Ox** | ibidem] ibi **G1CP2BGe** | contineatur] -teneantur **P1** -etur **M** -entur ***ed.*** | *ad* ad ea *habent*.i. cum eis **ϕ** | dicta] pr(a)edicta **DOx** | praecedat (*post* pleuresis **Ox**)] -it **Ge** -unt **M** *s*cedant **P1** | pleuritis **P1** (-etis **AP2′** -ites **M**)] pleuresis ***cett.*** *cum* **P2** | nihil] et n. (nil **Ma**) **OG1MaDOxϕ** | *post* nihil *add.* quia **P3 m2** | manifestum] manifeste **G1** | spuentes **P1M**] spuens **AMuCP2L2B** spuat **OG1MaDϕ** spuatur **P3** spuentes ... confi*t*endum *om.* **Ox** | ipsum] ipsam **P1** | uiolenter] inuiolenter ***ed.*** | sputetur] putetur **P1** sputentur **M** | manifeste] -um **P1** | confi*t*endum] confidendum **P1 AC P2L2B** considerandum **M Mu G1** | pus] plus **P1** | est quod] est quia **P1** est qui **M** *om.* **O P3′MaDOx** (*add.* **P3 m2** *in marg.*) | continetur (-ten- **P1**)] non continetur **O P3′Ma**

[136] **in** Again, as in 2.7.2, for Greek περί; cf. also the next line in this section, 2.8.2 *in altera parte membri*.

[137] **ex grauedine ... fieri** I fear that *ex grauedine* translates ἐκ τοῦ βάρους as a single group. It seems that the translator has misunderstood the substantival infinitive. He is floundering, and things get worse as he moves into the second substantival infinitive clause (beginning περιρρέοντος αὐτοῦ, the participles being governed by ἐκ τοῦ ἀκούειν).

[138] **in altera parte membri** Latin *altera* surely indicates that our translator saw not στέρνων but ἑτέρων; *membri* must be for μέρος (perhaps mistaken as a genitive). Presumably, *in* is again for περί (cf. 2.7.2 and the preceding line in this section, 2.8.2 *in thorace*).

[139] **supercurrens** I understand *supercurrens* (sc. *pus*) as an object of *patiuntur* (just as in the Greek περιρρέοντος αὐτοῦ is governed by ἀκούειν). Of course, there is no warrant for *pus* in the archetype, but I am inclined to agree with the maker of ϕ that it is required.

[140] **ex ... euersionibus** One is torn between *ex*+ablative, which must have been in δ, and the accusative *subitaneas mutatas euersiones*, which given its distribution need have been only in γ and γ′. I favour the former because it matches more closely the Greek, where this is not a symptom but a cause, and where the phrase is introduced by a monosyllabic preposition (albeit ἐν in Puschmann's text!).

[141] **patiuntur** Here and at 2.8.3 *spuentes*, β has the plural, δ the singular. I stick with the plural, as in 2.7.4, 2.8.t., but without much conviction.

2.8.2 If, then, it is in the chest, it is clear both from many other signs and also from a sensation of heaviness which is felt to arise on the other side of the body-part(?), and, as (the pus) flows over, as a result of sudden disturbances, they often suffer sounds in their ears and blockage of the ears.

2.8.3 Suffice it to have said this much for the case when it is present in the chest and contained there. But if, in addition to what has been mentioned, pleurisy should precede, with the patients spitting nothing evident, but what there is being spat violently, it is plainly to be acknowledged that it is pus that is contained in the chest.

II, 151, 15–22 Puschmann

εἰ μὲν οὖν περὶ τὸν θώρακα, δῆλον ἐκ πολλῶν μὲν καὶ ἄλλων, ἔτι δὲ καὶ ἐκ τοῦ βάρους συναίσθησιν γίνεσθαι περὶ τὸ τῶν στέρνων μέρος καὶ περιρρέοντος αὐτοῦ ἐν ταῖς ἀθρόαις μεταστροφαῖς καὶ ψοφοῦντος ἀκούειν πολλάκις. (**2.8.3**). ταῦτα μὲν οὖν ἱκανὰ παραστῆσαι τὸ περιέχεσθαι ἐν τῷ θώρακι πῦον. εἰ δὲ πρὸς τοῖς εἰρημένοις προηγήσαιτο μὲν πλευρῖτις, μηδὲν δ' ἀξιόλογον ἀνεπτύσθη, τὸ δὲ πτυόμενον βιαίως γινόμενον, δῆλον ὅτι ὁμολογούμενον πῦόν ἐστι τὸ περιεχόμενον ἐν τῷ θώρακι.

[142] **consistat** The later tradition supplies variously *pus* or *humor*, but I leave *consistat* without a subject, partly because of the possibility that it was originally intended to mean 'establish, demonstrate' (παραστῆσαι); cf. the variant *constat*. Given that *consistere* is a favourite word of the translator, *constat* might indeed be the *lectio difficilior* and should not be ruled out.

[143] **ad ea** Again, as in 2.7.3, *ad* + accusative 'in addition to'; cf. the explanatory note '.i. cum eis' in ϕ.

[144] **spuentes** My tentative inclination at this stage is to take *spuentes* (as in β; cf. *spuens* in δ) as an absolute participle, either accusative as printed or, with a shift of word-boundary (suggested to me by Cloudy Fischer), ablative absolute with a singular patient as the unexpressed subject: *nihil manifestum spuente, sed hoc ipsum* .... The syntax of the Latin, then, parts company with that of the Greek. Greek ἀνεπτύσθη was perhaps mistaken for a form of the aorist passive participle.

One sympathizes, however, with the maker of θ for substituting the subjunctive *spuat* to match *praecedat* and *sputetur*. Indeed, ... *spu<t>ent[e] sed* ... may deserve serious consideration.

[145] **sputetur** Here the tradition is pleasingly unanimous that the translator used the subjunctive. There is unanimous agreement also that we have (the original iterative-intensive verb) *sputare* six words after the underived *spuere*. In the chapters on coughing at least there seems to be free variation between *sputo* (2.7.2, 2.7.4, 2.11.t.), *spuo* (2.2.3, 2.5.1, 2.9.2, 2.11.2, 2.11.3) and *exspuo* (2.2.4, 2.3.1). If *uiolenter* here seems an appropriate complement to the intensive form, *nihil* at 2.2.3 is surely not.

Puschmann's Greek text is odd here: πτυόμενον may have caused the corruption of γίνεται to γινόμενον.

[146] **manifeste** Here *manifeste* is a sentence-adverb (equivalent to *manifestum est quia* ...); cf. the slightly different use, again in diagnosis, at 2.7.3 'manifeste scito', and e.g. 2.204 'manifeste ex ipsis rebus declaratur passio' (II, 337, 31 τὰ προηγησάμενα πρὸς τούτοις αἴτια βεβαιοτέραν παραστήσει σοι τὴν διάγνωσιν).

[147] **confi*t*endum** All three variants have arguments in their favour. *confidendum* has manuscript support on both sides of the family. In Book 2, A (which here has *confidendum*) has much more frequently *considerare*, and it may be that we should read *considerandum* here. The archetype surely did not have *confitendum*, but I print it tentatively here (following the maker of θ followed by O), as at 1.52 and 2.1.4 and 3. pr. *confiteor* is unanimously attested and translates Greek ὁμολογέω. (Curiously, ὁμολογέω is not translated in a surprisingly large number of places, including II, 321, 4; 379, 4; 461, 3; 475, 28; 559, 7.)

2.9.t. De *fyma*[148] in pulmone consistente[149]

2.9.1 Quod si fyma meditauerit[150] fieri in pulmone, erit omnino[151] difficultas spirandi coangustatis praecordiis;[152] *n*unc quid*em* desubito contingit, sed adhuc[153] consueta agere ipsa consequitur actio, et, per partes[154] accrescens, laeditur.[155]

Tit. om. **P1 MaL2** | De] Signa de **Bϕ P3** (Signa *add.* **m3**) Si de **Ox** Signa si de **C** Signa si **M** | *fyma scripsi*] fimate **OP3** fýgmon **M** fymone **Ge** fimone **AG1** psýmone **P2** simone **Mu** flegmone **CBDOx ϕ** | in pulmone] pulmonis **C** | consistente] existente **BG1P3′ϕ** fiat **M** tussis fiat **C** fiat tussis *add.* **P3 m3**

Quod si] Quod **GeP3** (quod si **P3′**) | fyma **P1**] sima **Mu** fimam **A** fimon **Ox O** (*add.* .i. flegmō) fýgmon **M** flegmon **D** fýmonem **P2** fimonem **G1L2** flegmonem **CBϕ** flegmonem si **Ge** s(?)imata **P3** | meditauerit fieri (medetauerit fierit **P1** editauerit et fuerit **M**)] euenerit fieri ***cett.*** fuerit (-int **Ma**) **O P3Ma DOx** (fuerit *post* pulmone **O P3Ma**) | pulmone] -em **P1 L2** | omnino] omni modo **L2BGeG2L1** | spirandi] sperandi **A′** | coangustatis (-iatis **G2**)] coangustata **M** angustata **P1** que coangustatis (quē coangusta **P3′** (-tis *add.* **m3**)) **O P3MaD** | praecordiis] -ia **P1M** | *nunc* quid*em scripsi*] num quid **P1** num quod **M** non quidem **O G1P3MaD** nam quod **A** ñ quod **MuC** non quod **P2L2BOxGe** non quia **ϕ** | desubito] subito **C** | contingit **M O DOx**] -et **G1P3Ma** -at ***cett.*** | adhuc] adhuc si **Ge** *ante* adhuc *add. in marg.* dum **P3 m3** | agere ipsa] ipsa agere **Ox** | consequitur] -atur **L2BDGe** consequi ***ed.*** uidetur **Ma** | et] *om.* **Ge** | partes] -is **P1** | accrescens (adcr- **P1M** acr- **B**)] -entes **P3′Ge** | laeditur] -it **O G1CL2BP3Ge** -at **Ma**

[148] ***fyma*** The Greek term φῦμα is preserved (presumably 1st-declension feminine) in P1 in 2.9.1 (and cf. *sima* Mu and *fimam* A, as well as the learned *f/simata* in θ″ and *fimate* in the title in P3 and O). The word occurs in the Latin Oribasius (cited by the *ThLL*) and also in the Latin Galen, *Ad Glauc.* 2.1 'fima uero flegmone breuis et mollis id est que cito crescit et maturescit et saniem facit' [text of Montpellier 185] (= 11.77 Kühn ... πρὸς ἐκπύησιν ἐπειγόμενον; cf. Gar., *Pass.* 5.32); this reference, not in the *ThLL*, I owe to Cloudy Fischer.

The n-stem *fymo(n), onis* is also well attested in the tradition: it looks like a blend of *fyma* and *flegmo(n)* (cf. M's *fygmon*), but is perhaps already in δ, and deserves to be borne in mind.

[149] **consistente** It seems that δ had *consistente* (agreeing with Greek συστάντος) and that θ′ changed this to *existente* (on *consisto*, *existo*, cf. note on 2.7.4 *consistere*). The presence of *fiat* in M and P3 *ex corr.* suggests that it was in γ′. Its presence with the addition of *tussis* in C may be another link between C and P3 (cf. 4.7.5).

[150] **meditauerit** γ has preserved what must be the true reading, with *medito(r)* = Greek μελετῶμαι 'threaten', so that we should remove the negative supplied by Puschmann. In view of the simple *fueri(n)t* in O, θ″ and κ, it is likely that *meditauerit* was lost in θ or γ′. δ did its best to make sense of *meditauerit* with *euenerit*. Cf. Langslow, 'Alex. Trall.'.

[151] **omnino** *omnino* is common in the Latin Alexander, and translates a range of Greek intensifiers, including, apart from πάντως (here and e.g. 1.84 = I, 615, 7); παντοίως (e.g. 1.33 'Istud enim omnino iuuat' = I, 485, 8–9 αὕτη γὰρ παντοίως ὠφελεῖ; also 1.44 = I, 497, 9; 1.57 = I, 515, 15); πανταχόθεν (e.g. 1.33 'calefactis omnino' cf. I, 483, 24 θάλποντας πανταχόθεν); παντελῶς (e.g. 1.144 = II, 235, 15; cf. 1.123 'Si autem omnino laesae aures non audiant': II, 101, 1 παντελὴς βλάβη); πάντοτε (e.g. 2.29 = II, 263, 26); apparently also ἄγαν (1.56 = I, 515, 6); (and at 1.57 = I, 517, 25 *omnino* stands opposite τηνικαῦτα in Puschmann's text.)

[152] **difficultas spirandi coangustatis praecordiis** The order of the Greek words is reversed, and στενοχωρία translated with an absolute past participle, which could conceivably stand in a causal relation to the *difficultas spirandi*, but which I have translated as an ablative of attendant circumstances.

The reading of γ (*(co)angustata precordia*) could equally well be read as an absolute construction (feminine singular ablative or neuter plural or (with *-a* for *-am*) feminine singular accusative). Note the relative clause in O, Ma, P3 and D (presumably from θ) beginning with *que* before *coangustatis*.

2.9.t. Concerning a growth in the lung

2.9.1 But if a growth threatens to arise in the lung, there will be extreme difficulty in breathing, with constriction of the area of the chest: this sometimes happens suddenly, but also (sometimes?) it (the lung?) is able to perform its normal function, and is damaged as it (the tumour?) grows bit by bit.

II, 151, 23–153, 1 Puschmann

Περὶ φύματος ἐν τῷ πνεύμονι συστάντος
Εἴπερ εἴη φῦμα [μὴ] μελετηθὲν ἐν τῷ πνεύμονι, ἔσται μὲν πάντως στενοχωρία καὶ δύσπνοια ποτὲ μὲν ἀθρόως συμβαίνουσα, ποτὲ δὲ, τὰ συνήθη πράττοντος (πράττειν LM) αὐτοῦ δυναμένου, κατὰ μικρὸν (μέρος LM) αὐξανομένη.

[153] **nunc quidem** ... **sed adhuc** This is unsatisfactory. I prefer to hazard *nunc quidem* (Greek ποτὲ μέν) than to obelize *num quod* (vel sim.), but I acknowledge that I am leaning perilously on Puschmann's text. The variants *num quod* (M), *num quid* (P1) and *non quidem* (in O G1P3MaD, and hence probably in γ') are really very close to *nunc quidem*, especially given the following syllable *de-* (of *desubito*). I cannot exactly parallel *nunc quidem* for ποτὲ μέν in the Latin Alexander, but for ποτὲ μέν ... ποτὲ δέ A has at 1.79 *modo* ... *nunc* (I, 597, 26–599, 1); other versions include *quando quidem* ... *quando autem* (1.127 = II, 113, 22; cf. *quando* ... *quando* at 1.137 = II, 127, 3) and *interdum* ... *interdum* (2.177 = II, 209, 26; 2.265 = II, 559, 24; 2.269 = II, 569, 6). This is then answered rather lopsidedly by *sed adhuc* 'but also' (which suggests ἔτι δέ rather than ποτὲ δέ in the translator's Greek text).

[154] **per partes** The translator's text probably had κατὰ μέρος (like Greek mss. L and M here), which can perfectly well mean 'little by little'; cf. 2.5.4 with note ad loc., 2.11.7.

[155] **consueta agere** ... **laeditur** This is next to hopeless! The Greek at least is clear (although Puschmann surely needs to read πράττειν with L and M: τὰ συνήθη πράττειν αὐτοῦ δυναμένου 'while he (the patient) is able to carry out his normal business'). But for the Latin version we are reduced to emendation for *ipsa consequitur actio* — perhaps *ipse consequitur* [*actio*] — and we are still left with *accrescens*, which I have interpreted as an absolute participle with *fyma* as unexpressed subject, and *laeditur* (not in the Greek), which seems to require the lung or the patient as subject (unless it goes with *actio*).

2.9.2 Et spuunt nihil, neque soni aliquid[156] aut cencron[157] patiuntur. Neque enim contingere poterit[158] [nisi[159]] ex indigesto et necdum permixto *fymate*.[160]

Et] *om.* **P1** | spuunt] exspuunt **O** spuit **Ox** | spuunt nihil] nichil spuunt **P3Ma** | soni] sonum **P1M O Ma** | aliquid] aliquod **M** aliquem **OMa** aliqui **L2L1** | cencron **P3**] concron **Ma** centron ***cett.*** cetron **Mu** cendron **O** centro **A** centrum **P1** tenorum **M** *ad hoc uerbum habent* .i. punccionem **Ma** .i. punctionem **D** centron exponunt quidam punctiones **φ** | patiuntur] patitur **AMuC G1P2BOx** | enim] enim hoc **P3MaDGe** | poterit **Ma**] poterat **P1** potest ***cett.*** | *post* pot. *habent* patienti (pac- **Ma**) **O P3Ma DOx G2L1** | indigesto] -um (-deg- **P1**) **P1M** indigestione ***ed.*** | necdum] nedum **C** ***ed.*****L1** nondum **Ox** | permixto] permixtum (-mis- **P1**) et **P1M** | *fymate scripsi* (fimate **P3Ma φ** simate **Mu**)] fýmone **P2** fimone **O G1L2Ge** simone **B** flegmate **C** flegmone **DOx** refimato **A** fýmanus **M** firmanus **P1**

[156] **soni aliquid** Although *sonitus* is the regular word for ringing in the ears (cf. 2.6.1 above), A attests several examples of *sonus* in the chapters of Book 1 devoted to the condition (1.117ff.; and 1.110).

For *aliquid* + partitive genitive = Greek τι + adjective, cf. 2.40 'aliquid ... caloris' = II, 287, 6 τι θερμόν, 2.267 'aliquid frigdoris' = II, 561, 27 τι ψυκτικόν. It is noteworthy also that the form *aliquem* at any rate appears to be used by our translator(s) only as a pronoun, and not as an adjective as in *sonum aliquem* the reading of O and Ma.

[157] **cencron** The Latin variants suggest Greek κέγχρος, which means 'millet', rather than κέρχνος 'roughness, hoarseness', which is very suitably rendered with *raucor* in the very next section (2.10.1). LSJ, s. vv., suggests some confusion between the two Greek words, attesting κέρχνος 'millet' but not κέγχρος 'hoarseness'.

[158] **poterit** Cf. future δυνήσεται. Latin *poterit* is attested here only in Ma and indirectly in P1 *poterat*. If *poterit* was in γ′, Ma could have it from there via θ and θ″, while everywhere else it was corrected to *potest*. Alternatively, we ignore the Greek future and take it that P1 and Ma miscopied *potest*. I have not checked every example, but in A *poterit* stands for δυνήσεται at least at 2.157 = II, 461, 26; 2.254 = II, 529, 7 (cf. *possis* at 2.186 = II, 481, 15).

[159] **nisi** Another glaring discrepancy between the Latin version and Puschmann's text, perhaps connected with a corruption of ἔτι in the translator's Greek text.

[160] **et necdum permixto *fymate***: καὶ μηδέπω ἀποβεβλημένου τοῦ φλέγματος Both Greek and Latin versions are corrupt. If *fyma* is the right word in the Latin version, here the tradition is unanimous that it is masculine or neuter; contrast the feminine form I admitted in 2.9.t. The *-us* ending in M and P1 may reflect a Greek genitive singular ending, and given A's *-fimato* we should perhaps reckon with the presence of the Greek form *fimatos* in the archetype (the γ forms look like a cross between *fimatos* and *flegmonos*). Such a form is not likely to be introduced into the Latin tradition, but only corrected away. Pending the collection of more secure examples, however, I leave the suspiciously classical-looking *fymate* for the moment.

Latin *permixtus* is common in the Latin Alexander. Generally it translates a form of μείγνυμι (e.g. I, 449, 24 μικτήν; 455, 3 προσμήξας!; 479, 7 ἀναμεμῖχθαι) but at I, 467, 7 it renders συμπεπλεγμένη, a form easily confused with -βεβλημεν-.

The stem ἀποβεβλη- occurs only here in the Greek Alexander. The reading of Greek ms. M μεταβεβλημένου seems much preferable, as it can be paralleled in the context of a φλεγμονή being metabolized εἰς πῦον (II, 69, 7; 381, 21; 479, 27; 481, 4). This context could well fit a φῦμα (a species of φλεγμονή), which the Latin tradition seems to point to; this context also suggests the emendation φλεγμονῆς for φλέγματος (φλέγμα is quite out of place here).

2.9.2 And they spit nothing up, nor do they suffer any noise (in the ears) or hoarseness, for it cannot possibly occur while the tumour is immature and not yet thoroughly mixed.

II, 153, 2–4 Puschmann

καὶ οὔτε ἀναπτύουσιν οὐδὲν οὐδὲ ψόφον τινὰ οὐδὲ κέρχνον ὑπομένουσιν· οὔτε γὰρ συμβῆναι δυνήσεται ἔτι ἀπέπτου καὶ μηδέπω ἀποβεβλημένου (μετα- M) τοῦ φλέγματος.

2.10.t. Si tussis ex spissis et glutinosis[161] humoribus qui in pulmone[162] continentur generatur

2.10.1 Quando autem desubito qui laborant[163] sentiunt coangustata[164] praecordia se habere et absque febribus molestari et sit*i* mult*a*, s*ed*[165] habent etiam quendam raucorem[166] cum tusse, interea[167] et proiciunt humores manifestos[168] quam pinguissimos et glutinosos[169] qui circumtenentur in pulmone +– uel eius occupant cauernas –+ qui ibidem fluunt de capite aut ex alio aliquo[170] membro.

tit. om. **MaL2** *tamquam init. cap.* **P1** | qui ... generatur *om.* **OCP3** | qui ... continentur *om.* **D** | Si] Signa si **C** De **M** | tussis] -e **M** *om.* **C** | ex] qui ex **M** fiat ex **P3** sit ex **B** | spissis] pinguibus **OP3** | et glutinosis] gluttinosisque **A** | humoribus] humoribus fit **Ge** hu. sit **Ox** hu. fiat **OC** | qui] quod **P1** *om.* **M B** | pulmone] fleumone **P1** flegmone (fleğ. **P2**) **G1 P2** | continentur (-ten- **P1**) **P1 AMu G1P2Ox**] continetur uel **M** continetur et **ϕ** existentibus **B** | generatur] -etur **P1** -antur **G1** -entur **P2** *om.* **BOx**

Quando] Aliquando **ϕ** | desubito qui laborant] qui laborant desubito **Ox** | qui] que **P1** | laborant] -at **M** | sentiunt] -iant **P1** -it **M** | coangustata (quo- **P1**) **P1 A P3Ma**] coangusta **OMu** coangustantem **M** perangustata **G1CL2BL1** praeangustata **P2 G2*ed.*** praeangustiata **Ox** | praecordia se habere (abere **P1**)] se (*om.* **O**) habere p. **M O DOx** precordia **Ma** | absque] aliquibus **OMa** a quibus **P3′** absque aliquibus **P3DOx** | febribus] febre **G1** | molestari (*corr. ex* -ata **Ox**)] -are **P1** | et] et si **M** | sit*i* mult*a* *scripsi*] multa sitis **O** sitis nimia **Ma** sitis multa ***cett.*** *ante* multa *add. in marg.* non **P3 m2** | s*ed* *scripsimus*] sit ***cett.*** fit **Mu GeG2L1** *om.* **O** | habent] -et (abit **P1**) **P1M** et habent ***ed.*** | etiam] enim **Ox** *om.* **G1L2** | quendam] quemdam **O** quandam **Ma ϕ** | raucorem **O L2P3** (ruccorem **P1** rugura **M**)] ranc(h)orem ***cett.*** | *ante* cum *habent* et acrorem **P3DOxGe G2*ed.*** acrorem **Ma** | tusse] -i **DOx** -em **P1** | interea **P1M AMu P2**] interius ***cett.*** | humores manifestos] -is -us **P1** | quam] *om.* ***ed.*** ne dubites humores esse quam **P3 m2** | pinguissimos] -us **P1** plurimos **L** | qui] que **P1** | circumtenentur] circumligantur et tenentur **Mu** | pulmone] polmone **P1** | uel] *om.* **P1** | cauernas (cab- **M**)] et cauernas **Ge′** | qui] que **AMuP2** | fluunt] defluunt **M** | ex] *om.* **Ox** | alio aliquo] aliquo alio **L2Ox** aliquo altero **M P3MaD** altero aliquo **O**

[161] **spissis et glutinosis** For the collocation with *humores* in the context of coughing, cf. Orib., *Eup.* 4.78 p. 599 La 'Qui autem ex pinguis et gluttinosus humores tusses generantur' (4.77.7 p. 467, 21–2 διὰ πάχος ... καὶ γλίσχρον χυμόν). It is striking that the collocation (2.10.1) *pinguissimos et glutinosos* occurs just a few lines later in the younger Latin Oribasius (*pinguis et gluttinosus humores*). Note A's learned improvement of *et glutinosis* to *glutinosisque*.

[162] **in pulmone** It is at first sight striking that P1, G1 and P2 have *fleumon/flegmon*, but we have seen repeated confusion in P1 (cf. 2.7.1 and note ad loc.), and *flegmone* in G1 and P2 probably reflects only a single error (or marginal addition) in θ′.

[163] **laborant** The patient is singular in the Greek, but the Latin tradition is overwhelmingly in favour of the plural, witness *laborant* (except M), *sentiunt* (except M), *habent* (except γ), *proiciunt* (unanimous).

[164] **coangustata** Are the *p*- variants of the prefix (*per-*, *prae-*), which enter the tradition with θ′, to be explained palaeographically or as a result of anticipation of *praecordia*?

[165] **sit*i* multa, s*ed*** The Latin archetype must have had *sitis multa sit*. The very minor changes (undone thanks to the Greek text) yield a very different sense.

[166] **raucorem** Why was κέρχνον not so translated in 2.9.2? Was the translator thrown by Greek κέγχρον there?

[167] **interea** This use of *interea* (apparently only here in the Latin Alexander) is not recorded by the *OLD*, although Georges attributes it to Silius Italicus. Cf. Theod. Prisc., *Eup. faen.* 19, p. 22, 5.

[168] **manifestos** It is tempting to write *manifest*um, but the construction will not work, and we must accept that the Latin version as it stands resembles more a prognosis than a diagnosis.

[169] **pinguissimos et glutinosos** See the note on 2.10.t. *spissis et glutinosis*.

[170] **alio aliquo** I presume that, like M, γ′ (and hence θ) had *aliquo altero*. It seems that γ′ is often closer to M than to P1.

2.10.t. If coughing arises out of thick and glutinous humours which are contained in the lung

2.10.1 When the patients suddenly feel that the chest is constricted and troubled (although) without fever and without great thirst, but they have also a certain hoarseness with the cough, and from time to time bring up manifest humours, extremely thick and glutinous, which are contained in the lung or occupy its hollow spaces, and which flow there from the head or from some other part.

II, 153, 5–11 Puschmann

Περὶ γλίσχρων χυμῶν καὶ παχέων περιεχομένων ἐν τῷ πνεύμονι
Ὁπηνίκα δὲ ἀθρόως ὁ κάμνων αἴσθηται στενοχωρίας ἐκτὸς ὀχλήσεως πυρετοῦ καὶ δίψης πολλῆς, ἔχῃ δέ τινα κέρχνον μετὰ βηχὸς, ἔσθ' ὅτε δὲ καὶ ἀναγωγὴν ὑγροῦ, δῆλον, ὡς παχὺ καὶ γλίσχρον ἐστὶ τὸ περιεχόμενον ἐν τῷ πνεύμονι +– –+ καὶ συρρεῦσαν ἐκ τῆς κεφαλῆς ἢ ἐξ ἄλλου τινὸς μορίου.

2.10.2 Sit tibi manifestum ad cognitionem,[171] ex uuae irritatione et gargalionis[172] praecedenti, a[173] capitis uiti*o* consistere[174] superfluentem materiam in thorace.

2.10.3 Sic enim cognoscendae sunt[175] diuersitates et proprietates uniuscuiusque tussis, et quaecumque circa[176] thoracem et pulmonem passiones consistunt.[177]

Sit tibi manifestum **P1M AOMu**] et (*add.* **m3**) si tibi manifestum sit **P3** ut sit tibi manifestum **D** ut (*om.* **G1**) tibi (ibi **C**) manifestum sit ***cett.*** | ex] et **O P3′Ma** (et cum *in marg. corr. pro* ad cognitionem et **P3 m3**; *verba* scias ex *(v. inf. s. v.* uiti*o) referunt huc*) | uue] ube **P1** | irritatione] inritacionem **P1** | gargalionis] gurgulionis **P3Ma** ğgulionis **Mu** gurgostionis **O** | praecedenti a *scripsimus* (praecedentia ***plerique***)] praecedente **P3** -is (-es(?) **P1**) **P1M** praecedere **OMa** | uiti*o scripsimus*] uitia ***plerique*** uitia et **O P3′Ma** (scias ex *add. in marg. pro* et **P3 m2** *(v. supra s.v.* ex*)*) sui ad **M** | consistere] constringere **M** | superfluentem (fluentem **P1**) materiam **P1M O P3Ma**] -e -ia ***cett.*** | in thorace] *om.* **G1** | thorace] -em **AO Ox**

Sic] Si **Ox** | cognoscendae] cognuscendi **P1** | diuersitates] diuersitatum **M** inuersitatis **P1** | et] *om.* **P1M** | proprietates] propriaetas **P1** | thoracem] -e **P1M** | pulmonem] -e **M** -es **P1** | passiones consistunt] c. p. **DOx φ** *om.* **P3′** c. p. cum tussi. Sunt autem *add.* **P3 m2** | passiones] -is **P1M** | consistunt] contingant **P1** contingit **M** contingunt **Ma**

[171] **Sit** ... **ad cognitionem** Presumably, this is a jussive subjunctive for the Greek future perceived as a command. Normally, sentence-initial *sit* translates ἔστω (e.g. 1.57 = I, 519, 10; 1.81 = I, 601, 11; 2.21 = II, 249, 16), γινέσθω (2.38 = II, 283, 15). There is, however, a near-perfect parallel with the present passage at 1.94 'Sit autem tibi manifesta cognitio' = II, 31, 5 ἔσται δέ σοι δῆλον. Contrast *erit* for ἔσται at 1.86 'erit tibi manifesta cognitio' = II, 5, 20 ἔσται δῆλόν σοι.

The translator uses the phrase *manifesta cognitio* several times (above, and also at 2.186 *manifesta cognitio est* for the much more elaborate II, 481, 13–14 ἀκριβῆ τὴν διάγνωσιν καὶ ἀναμφίβολον ἔχειν ἀποδείκνυσιν), but *manifestum ad cognitionem* appears to occur only here, and looks like a one-off literal translation of φανερὸν εἰς διάγνωσιν, although a similar Latin construction translates something very different in Greek at 1.35 'Ad cognoscendum autem tibi manifestum est' = I, 487, 11 γνωρισθήσεται δέ σοι σαφέστερον.

[172] **gargalionis** A dissimilated form of Greek γαργαρέων (cf. Latin *gargareo*), which I take it was seen by our translator in his Greek text; γαργαρισμός (in Puschmann's text) means 'tickling'. Given its collocation with *uua*, it presumably refers to a wider area of the throat than just the uvula. Cf. André, *Anatomie*, 68–9, citing the Latin Oribasius and the Latin Hippocrates.

[173] **praecedenti a** 'Univerbation' of the preposition *a* with the preceding *praecedenti* (which agrees with *irritatione*) caused the simple change of *uitio* to *uitia* and instantly yielded an unintelligible text.

[174] **consistere** There is nothing corresponding in the Greek here to this favourite word of the translator, a formally imposing synonym of *esse*. Cf. note on 2.7.4 *consistere*.

[175] **Sic enim cognoscendae sunt** Cf. 2.2.5 'Sic enim erit cognoscenda'. Concluding *sic enim* occurs literally dozens of times in the Latin Alexander, introducing the end of diagnosis and therapy alike. The Greek at this point, however, leads us to expect rather a conclusion of the type *Sufficiant haec*, as at e.g. 1.103 = II, 57, 8.

[176] **circa** Above (2.7.2, 2.7.3 twice) we noted repeatedly *in* for περί. Now we have almost the converse in *circa* for κατά.

[177] **consistunt** With the variants (in γ and Ma) on the stem *conting-*, compare M's *constringere* for *consistere* in 2.10.2.

2.10.2 It should be clear to you, for the purpose of diagnosis, both from irritation of the uvula and from the earlier presence of swelling of the throat, that it is through the fault of the head that there is superfluous material in the thorax.

2.10.3 This, then, is how one is to diagnose the different forms and properties of each particular cough, and all the diseases which occur in the thorax and lung.

II, 153, 11–15 Puschmann

ἔσται δέ σοι φανερόν εἰς διάγνωσιν καὶ ἐκ τοῦ περὶ τὴν σταφυλὴν ἐρεθισμὸν καὶ γαργαρισμὸν προηγήσασθαί τινα, τὴν κεφαλὴν αἰτίαν εἶναι τῆς ἐπιρρεούσης ὕλης τῷ θώρακι. (**2.10.3**). ταῦτα ἀρκεῖ πρὸς τὸ διαγινώσκειν τὰς διαφόρους ἰδέας τῆς βηχὸς καὶ ὅσα κατὰ θώρακα ἢ πνεύμονα πάθη συνίστανται.

2.10.4 Sunt autem et alia de quibus in sequenti dicturi sumus,[178] ubi de ulceratione et ruptione uenarum et diabroseos[179] cogemur[180] scribere.

2.11.t. De lapide sputato[181]

2.11.1 Ego autem quod uidi necessarium existimaui non tacere, sed ut uobis exponam[182] quae uidi et miratus sum.

Sunt autem] *om.* **OP3′** | dicturi sumus] dicemus **OxGe ϕ** | ulceratione] -em **P1** ulcerato **Ox** | ruptione uenarum] u. r. **L2** | ruptione (-em **P1**)] corruptione **AG1** | diabroseos **P3D** (-broxeus **M** -brocius **P1**)] diabroceo **O** diabroseys **Ma** diabroseis (dya- **P2**) **G1CP2B** diabroceis **AMu** diabrosis **L2Ge** diabrosi (dya- ***ed.*** **L1**) **Ox ϕ** | cogemur scribere (cogimur scribere **O** cogimus scire uere **M**)] dicturi sumus **GeOx ϕ** dicturi sumus cogimur scribere **P3** dicturi sumus uel cogimur scribere **G1**

De lapide sputato] De latē sputato lapide **Mu** *om.* **P1M CP2Ma** (*del. (an ornatum?)* **B**)

autem] *om.* **C** | quod *s. s.* **L2** | uidi (uide **P1′**)] uidi et **O** iudicaui **C** | necessarium] neccarium **C** | existimaui] estimaui **Ox** putaui **M** | ut uobis] et uobis **M O P3′L1** de uobis ut **P1** uobis **DB** | quae **P1M AOMu P2P3Ox**] quod ***cett.***

[178] **dicturi sumus** The periphrastic future of *dico* occurs in all four times in Book 2, never in Book 1. Twice it renders a past tense in Puschmann's text, which may, if not accidental, hint at different versions of the work. Cf. 2.26 (II, 259, 3 εἰρήκαμεν!); 2.153 (II, 443, 15 ὡς εἶπον!); 2.240 (II, 507, 24 ῥηθήσεται).

The periphrastic future is otherwise attested at e.g. 1.31 'qui uomituri sunt' (I, 481, 2 τῶν ... ἐμούντων); 2.35 'et quando dormitum iturus est' (II, 275, 4 εἰς κοίτην); 2.67 'qui hydropici futuri sunt' (II, 393, 26 ὑδεριᾶν μέλλοντας); 2.238 'qui et accepturus est potionem' (nothing in Greek at II, 503, 23). It is evidently not dictated by a particular Greek form.

[179] **diabroseos** The Greek genitive (διαβρώσεως) was perhaps not understood and simply transcribed by the translator, being later made into an ablative by the Latin tradition, plural (e.g. *diabroseis*) or singular (*diabrosi*). The 'ablative singular' in O (*diabroceo*) may reflect knowledge of the Greek form in γ′. Might the variants with *-c-* (in P1 and η) reflect an original in Greek characters (with *-c-* for the lunate sigma)?

[180] **ubi ... cogemur** A reference to 2.158ff. (II, 187ff.). The classical use of the future after *ubi* is here very well attested (cf. *ubi* + present in a similar postponement at 1.60 'Reseruamus enim inibi hoc dicere ubi de fracturis conuenit loqui'; cf. I, 535, 5–6). In Book 1 at any rate, *ubi* 'when' with future reference is used by A only with the future perfect and always with reference to the doctor's requirement in therapy: 1.44, 1.123 'ubi uolueris'; 1.127 'ubi aestimaueris expedire'; 1.128 'ubi tibi necesse fuerit'; 1.131 'ubi necesse habueris'; 1.144 'ubi amplius fuerit opus'.

[181] **De lapide sputato** I translate this as an instance of the 'ab urbe condita' construction without at this point being able to give other, unequivocal examples of control of this construction in the Latin Alexander.

[182] **necessarium ... non tacere, sed ut ... exponam** The Latin Alexander attests both accusative + infinitive and *ut* + subjunctive after *necessarium*, accusative + infinitive e.g. at 1.85 (II, 5, 16–17); 1.138 (not in Greek, II, 127); 2.13 (II, 163, 17); 2.249 (not in Greek, II, 521, 9–10); *ut* + subjunctive at e.g. 1.27 (I, 475, 23); 1.103 (II, 55, 1). I have not found another passage where the two are used in successive clauses and this would be *variatio* of a different sort from that illustrated in 5.3.3 above. We could read *et exponam* (future indicative), but *et* does not have good manuscript support here.

2.10.4 There are others, too, of which we shall speak later on, when we are obliged to write about ulceration (or trauma?), rupture of the veins and *diabrosis*.

2.11.t. Concerning the spitting up of a stone

2.11.1 I have, however, thought it necessary not to keep quiet about what I observed, but to describe for you what I observed and was amazed at.

II, 153, 15–18 Puschmann

εἰσὶ δὲ καὶ ἄλλα, περὶ ὧν ὕστερον λεχθήσεται, ἔνθα καὶ περὶ ἑλκώσεως καὶ ῥήξεως καὶ διαβρώσεως ἀναγκαζόμεθα γράφειν. (**2.11.1**). ὃ δὲ ἐγὼ ἐθεασάμην, ἀναγκαῖον ἐνόμισα μὴ σιωπῆσαι, ἀλλὰ καὶ ὑμῖν ἐκθέσθαι· ἔδοξε γὰρ ἐμοὶ ξένον εἶναι καὶ θαυμαστόν·

2.11.2 Spuit quidam uir lapidem specialiter[183] et hoc[184] non forte[185] pinguem humorem et glutinosum, sed existentem[186] lapidem, nec asperum sed satis lenem et durum, et resistentem fortiter tactui, ita ut cadens in terra sonum faceret.

2.11.3 Iste uir per multum tempus[187] molestias[188] sustinens de tusse non poterat fortiter extussire,[189] donec lapidem spueret.

2.11.4 Vsus est[190] etiam et diaeta temperata et humida magis, et[191] infrigdatus est mediocriter.

spuit] expuit **D** | quidam] quidem **ϕ** | uir] *om.* **Ox** | specialiter] specialem **C** | et ... glutinosum **P1M AMuC P2B**] et hoc non fortem et pinguem humorem et glutinosum **DGe ϕ** et hoc fortem non ex pingui humore et glutinoso **Ox** non ut lapis fortem sed ex pingui humore et glutinoso **O** et non fortem et pinguem et glutinosum humorem existentem **P3** ex non forti et pingui et glutinoso humore **Ma** et non forte et pingui humore et glutinoso **L2** et ex forti et ex pingui humore et glutinoso **G1** | sed existentem lapidem *om.* **O** *add. in marg.* **P3 m2** | sed] sit **P1** *om.* **G1L2 P3′Ma** | existentem lapidem] -e -e **C** -e -em **M G1L2** *om.* **P3′** | nec asperum] necessarium **M** nec ipsum lenem (lenem *add.* **m2**) **P3** sed asperum **CP2L2B** nec **G1** | sed] sit **P1** et **MC** nec **P2L2Ox** *om.* **G1** | satis lenem et durum] durum nec satis lenem **C** | lenem] leuem **P2** asperum **P3** | et] nec **G1** | resistentem fortiter tactui] f. t. r. **Ge** | resistentem] -nte **P3** -ns **P1M** | fortiter tactui] t. f. **P2** | tactui] tactu **M** ***ed.*** actaui **P1** ad tactum **DOx** | ita ut] ut aut **M** ut **OMaD** | in terra **P1M AO P3L2Ma DOx**] in terram ***cett.*** | sonum **P1M MuC G1P2L2B**] sonus **O** sonitum ***cett.*** | faceret] -iat **P1M**

uir] ubi(?) **Ox** *om.* **P3′Ma** *add.* **P3 m2** uir qui **M** | per] *om.* **DOx** | multum tempus] multo (-um **P1**) tempore **P1M DOx** multa tempora **O** | molestias] -iam **MO** | sustinens] patiens **Ge** sustinuit **G1** sustinuerat **DOx** pertulit **Mu** | de tusse *quasi tit.* **P1** *corr. ex* tussu **Mu** | non] et non **P1M DOx** | non poterat fortiter extussire] *om.* **G1L2Ge′** | poterat] *corr. ex* oportet **Mu** | extussire] tussire **Ox** | lapidem] *om.* **C** | spueret] expuerit **P1** ex(s)pueret **O G1L2B P3MaGeϕ**

Vsus] Iussum **M** | est] est ei **M** *om.* **G1CP2L2BGe** | etiam] autem **ϕ** | et] est **G1** *om.* **OxGe** | diaeta temperata et humida] diaetam -am et -am **P1** | magis, et] magis **P1 C** magis dari et **M** | infrigdatus est mediocriter] m. i. e. **C** i. m. e. **Ge** | infrigdatus] infrigidatus **P1** ***ed.*****L1** | mediocriter] medicriter **O**

[183] **specialiter** Neither *specialis* nor *specialiter* appears to occur elsewhere in the Latin Alexander. I have assumed the classical sense (the adverb seems to be attested first in Cels. 5.24.4). *species* is a plausible translation of ἰδέα, but beyond that I cannot relate the Latin to the Greek. The translator may not have seen how ἀκριβῶς is to be taken in this context. At 2.236 (= II, 503, 6) ἀκριβῶς is rendered appropriately enough *diligenter*, but it is striking that the word is not translated or mistranslated at II, 515, 28; 527, 30; 549, 17.

[184] **et hoc** Latin *et hoc* suggests that the translator's text contained (adverbial) καὶ τοῦτο before οὐχὶ παχὺν; cf. 2.2.4.

[185] **forte** This is neither a form of the adjective *fortis* 'strong' nor the derived adverb (which would anyway be *fortiter*: cf. 2.11.23) but the adverb *forte* 'by chance, perhaps' almost bleached of meaning and functioning as a particle serving to reinforce the negative. In Books 1 and 2 ms. A has *forte* ten times, always after a negative, as here: seven times *nisi forte* for εἰ/ἐάν μή, three times *ne forte* for μή. I take *non forte* here, then, to be for the strong negative οὐχί (only here in the Greek Alexander).

[186] **existentem** It is tempting to propose *existenter*, to match Greek ὄντως morphologically. Alas, the two other occurrences of ὄντως in the Greek Alexander (II, 155, 13; 265, 3) are not translated in the Latin version; curiously, both are in the immediate context of a strong endorsement of Archigenes, whom Alexander greatly admired and frequently cites. According to the *ThLL*, s.v. 'exsisto', 1875, 84ff., this adjectival use presents a unique example of *existens* meaning 'fere i. q. uerus'; on the weaker use of *exsisto* = *sum*, see note 63 above. On *lēuis* for levis (in the next line), see Löfstedt, *Coniectanea*, 79–84.

2.11.2 A man spat up a stone, specifically that is to say, not just some thick and glutinous humour but actually a stone, not rough but quite smooth and hard, and very firm to the touch, so that it made a noise when dropped on the ground.

2.11.3 This man, having endured annoyance from coughing for a long time, could not strongly cough out until he spat up the stone.

2.11.4 He used also a balanced and rather moist diet, and he was moderately cooled.

II, 153, 19–24 Puschmann

ἔπτυσέ τις ἀνὴρ λίθον τὴν ἰδέαν ἀκριβῶς, οὐχὶ παχὺν χυμὸν καὶ γλίσχρον, ἀλλ' ὄντως (ὅλως M) λίθον, οὐ τραχὺν, ἀλλὰ καὶ πάνυ λεῖον καὶ σκληρὸν καὶ ἀντίτυπον, ὥστε καὶ κτύπον ποιεῖν ῥιπτόμενον τῇ γῇ. (**2.11.3**). οὗτος ὁ ἀνὴρ πολὺν χρόνον ὀχληθεὶς ὑπὸ τῆς βηχὸς οὐκ ἠδυνήθη τοῦ βήσσειν ἰσχυρῶς ἀπαλλαγῆναι, ἕως ὅτου τὸν λίθον ἀνέπτυσεν. (**2.11.4**). ἐχρώμην δὲ καὶ διαίτῃ εὐκράτῳ καὶ ὑγραινούσῃ καὶ μᾶλλον ψυχούσῃ μετρίως·

[187] **per multum tempus** It is thinkable that κ and O found *per multo tempore* in θ (from γ′): κ dropped the preposition, while O changed *multo tempore* to *multa tempora*. The instinct of the maker of κ regarding the usage of the Latin Alexander was correct. I have found only one other instance of *per multum tempus*, namely at 2.177 = II, 209, 24 ἐπὶ πλείονα χρόνον, while *multo tempore* is common for a variety of Greek expressions: cf. e.g. 1.24 'Quod si habeat iam multo tempore passionem' = I, 473, 6 ἐπὶ τῶν ἤδη χρονίων θερμῶν δυσκρασιῶν; 2.12 'quamuis satis multo tempore reumatizarent' = II, 161, 1 καίτοι πολὺν χρόνον ῥευματισθέντας; 2.73 = II, 405, 7 πλείονα χρόνον; 2.100 (Philumenus); 2.214 = II, 359, 2 ἐπὶ πλείονα χρόνον.

[188] **molestias** The singular *molestia* seems in fact to be commoner than the plural (in A in Book 1 by 13:5), but nearly always in the phrase *sine/absque molestia*.

[189] **fortiter extussire** The archetype must have contained *extussire*. Presumably it was taken by the Latin tradition to mean (absolute) 'to cough out': that is to say, situated in the windpipe or at its bifurcation, the stone would have prevented strong coughing. This idea, which I owe to Cloudy Fischer, is preferable to the transitive alternative 'to bring (something) up by strong coughing', as the latter creates a tautology with the next clause (*donec lapidem spueret*). As the Latin has nothing corresponding to Greek ἀπαλλαγῆναι, I am inclined to suspect that a word has been lost, but this could easily be another fault of the translator.

For *fortiter* = ἰσχυρῶς, cf. e.g. 1.30 = I, 479, 10; 1.33 = I, 483, 15 (-ῶς M 2203); 1.59 = I, 527, 23.

[190] **Vsus est** Note the 3rd person (the patient) in the Latin for the 1st person (the doctor/author: ἐχρώμην) in the Greek. I cannot parallel this. Contrast 2.268 *Vsus sum* = II, 567, 9. It is perhaps tempting to see in M's *iussum* a trace of an original *usus sum*, but the subject of *infrigdatus est* (in all mss.) can only be the patient, so that the archetype must have had *usus est*, and M's *iussum* must be for *usus*.

[191] **magis, et** M has *magis dari et*, the *dari* being supplied to make sense of the corrupt *iussum est ei* (for *usus* . . .) at the start of the sentence. The Latin *humida magis et infrigdatus est mediocriter* makes better sense than Puschmann's Greek text, and suggests that we should transpose καὶ μᾶλλον to read καὶ ὑγραινούσῃ μᾶλλον καὶ ψυχούσῃ μετρίως.

2.11.5 Erat enim sollicitus nimis[192] et tenuis habitudine, ut etiam existimaretur pthisicus[193] esse, et postea[194] proiecit lapidem, non post multos dies ut pthisici solent ita defunctus est.[195]

2.11.6 +– Gk II, 155, 2–22 –+ +– Redeamus[196] igitur et de curis aliqua breuiter dicere non omittamus. –+

enim] et nemis **P1** | sollicitus] -as **L** | tenuis] -i **CP2B** -uus **M** | habitudine] abitudinem **P1** | existimaretur (existimatur **Mu′**)] -ent **P3′** estimaretur **OxGe** | pthisicus (pty- **M P2 P3Ma** ty- **CD** pti- ***cett.***)] tussicum **P1** | proiecit] proicit **P1M** | lapidem] *om.* **D** | non **P1M O D**] et non ***cett.*** | post] *om.* **P1** | multos] -us **P1** | ut] et ut **O** ita ut **Mu** | pthisici (pty- **M Ma** ty- **CD** pti- ***cett.***)] tussici **P1** | ita] et ita **M** *om.* **Mu Ox** | defunctus (defumtus **P1**)] defectus **Mu** | est] s(unt) **Mu′**

Redeamus] Videamus **P1** Regrediamur **O** | *post* igitur *habent* ad tussem (-im **Ox**) **DOx** | et] *om.* **M** | curis (**P3 m2**) aliqua] curas (cura **M**) aliquas **P1M** cura aliqua **OP3** cura aliquid (aliqual **P3′**) **P3′Ma** | breuiter dicere] d. b. **G1** | breuiter] *om.* **M A** | dicere] expedire **Ox** | omittamus (-mit- **P1**)] obmittamus (-mit- **Ge**) **P3L2 Ge** | *post* omittamus *habent uerba* ut non alibi adiutoria requirantur (*v. 2. 11. 8 inf.*) **P3′Ma**

[192] **sollicitus nimis** For *sollicitus* = φροντιστικός, cf. 1.76 = I, 593, 6; 2.69 = II, 399, 23; 2.252 = II, 523, 29. LSJ cites for φροντιστικός in the sense 'nervous, worried' only Gal. 10.538.

There is nothing in Puschmann's text corresponding to *nimis* (we would expect e.g. Greek ἄγαν, πάνυ or σφόδρα; cf. note 53 above).

[193] **pthisicus** Note the prevalence of variants with hypercorrect *y*. Presumably, P1's *tussicum, tussici* is prompted by the main subject of this chapter, coughing.

[194] **postea** I tentatively take *postea* to be the equivalent of *postquam*, as often in Late Latin, including in the Latin Oribasius (Mørland, *Oribasius*, 171; Hofmann and Szantyr, 599, with further references). I cannot find a parallel in ms. A, but that may merely reflect careful correction (as with the addition of *et* before *non* here).

[195] **defunctus est** The Latin of 2.11.5–8 is in so many respects quite different from the Greek. The death in the Latin version of this patient, who survives in the Greek, is one of the most disastrous mistranslations encountered so far.

[196] **Redeamus** Typically, after omitting a section of the Greek original, the translator inserts a transitional sentence of his own.

P1's *Videamus* for *Redeamus* might indicate either that a capital was missing in his exemplar or that he was taking dictation. At all events, he attests a further subjunctive form.

2.11.5 For he was excessively anxious and of a slender physical condition, so that he was even judged to be a consumptive, and after he threw up the stone, a few days later, as consumptives usually do, he died.

2.11.6 Let us then resume, and not omit to say something about treatments.

II, 153, 24–155, 2 Puschmann

ἦν γὰρ καὶ φροντιστικὸς καὶ λεπτὸς τὴν ἕξιν, ὥστε καὶ ἐοικέναι αὐτὸν τοῖς φθινώδεσι. καὶ εἰ μὴ τούτοις ἐχρησάμην, οἶμαι ὅτι ἂν ἀπώλετο παραπλησίως τοῖς φθόην νοσήσασι.

2.11.7 Ad autem facile inueniend*um*,[197] per partes ad tussem adiutoria et[198] expedientia et a multis probata[199] scribam.

2.11.8 Vnde[200] in sequenti generaliter curas et ipsas differentias uobis exponam, ut non alibi indigentes adiutoria requiratis.

Ad ... scribam] *om.* **Ma** | Ad autem facile inueniend*um scripsi*] ad autem facile inuenienda (-as **P1**) **P1 P2′** ad inuenienda autem facile **A** ad hec autem facile inuenienda **MuCP2** ad facile autem inuenienda sunt **M** ad hec autem facile inuenienda sunt **G1L2B** ad hec enim facile inuenienda sunt **Ge P3 m2** *in marg.* ad hec omnia facile inuenienda sunt **Ox φ** ut facile inueniantur (*uix leg.*) **O** ut autem facile inueniantur **D** | per partes] *post* adiutoria **Ox** *post* describam **D** | per] *om.* **O** | partes] -is **P1** | adiutoria] *ante* ad tussem **G1** | et$_1$] *om.* **P3DOxGe φ** | expedientia] expet- **P1** exper- **A** | et$_2$] *om.* **M** | a] *om.* **C** | probata] -as **P1** | scribam] describam **ACD** desicca[--] **O** scribam *hic om. et ante* curas (*2. 11. 8*) *transpos.* **P3OxGe φ**

Vnde - exponam] *in fine post* requirantur **Ma** | in sequenti (-e **P1**)] inconsequenti **P3Ma** | generaliter] *om.* **Ox** | curas] -am **M** -a **P1** scribam curas **P3Oxφ** (scribam *add. in marg.* **P3 m3**) | ipsas differentias] d. i. **C** | ipsas] ipsarum **Ge** | differentias] deff- **P1** | ut - requiratis *add. in marg.* **P3 m2** | indigentes] -ia **O** *om.* **P3′Ma** | requiratis **AC P3 m2 Ox**] -atur **M** requirantur (-quer- **P1**) **P1OP3′Ma** -ant ***cett.***

[197] **Ad autem facile inueniend*um*** This is more in hope than expectation! At least there are numerous parallels for *ad* + gerund: cf. e.g. 1.35 'ad cognoscendum'; 1.60 'difficiles ... ad excitandum' (I, 531, 3 δυσδιέγερτοι); 1.70 'iera multis dedi ad purgandum' (I, 555, 24 ἐγὼ καὶ τῇ ἱερᾷ καθῆρα). I suppose a slavish imitation of the Greek word-order and an erroneous pause after *inueniendum* (εὑρίσκειν). The change of *inueniendum* to *inuenienda*, to agree with *adiutoria*(?), might have prompted the introduction of *haec* ('for the purpose of finding them (cataphoric) easily, I shall write down ...') — although the introduction of *sunt* would also have prompted the addition of *haec*, in order to make sense of *Ad*. *Sunt* is in M and apparently θ′ (G1B), which did not know γ′ (although G1 may have had separate, indirect access to γ′), and could therefore be original, the first of two main verbs in this sentence, the second being *scribam*. On the other hand, *sunt* is not in η nor in P1 (unless it is reflected in the -*s* of P1 *inueniendas*).

[198] **et expedientia et ... probata** The first *et* is not in the Greek but is well supported in the Latin tradition, and again suggests a respectable level of Latinity in the original translation.

[199] **a multis probata** The phrase *a multis probata* is apparently not in the Greek, unless it reflects a very corrupt Greek version of ὑπὸ τῆς διαγνώσεως ὑπαγορευομένην. Forms of *probo*, *probatus* are common in the Latin Alexander, often where Puschmann's text has nothing corresponding. They often answer Greek πεῖρα or a related form (e.g. 2.25 = II, 255, 22 πεπείραται; 2.46 = II, 307, 3 πολλὴν πεῖραν δέδωκεν), but sometimes translate other words (e.g. 2.12 = II, 163, 14 δόκιμα).

[200] **Vnde** *unde* is surprisingly frequent in the Latin Alexander, both in relative clauses and in indirect questions. For its (late) use as a sentence-connective (= *quamobrem*) at the end of a chapter, cf. 2.132 (Philagrius) 'Quod si ea quae diximus diligentius non adhibeantur, in scyron conuertetur: unde nunc a nobis erit dicendum'; 2.238 (at the end of a recipe) 'Deponit enim bene sine molestia et acutum est nimis, unde magis securus id dabis'. Sundelin, 26 cites two examples from Theod. Prisc. (1.7, 16 p. 17, 12; 3.5, 13 p. 233, 9); for references to its use also in Gaius, Tertullian and the *Didasc. Apost.*, and further literature, see Hofmann and Szantyr, 209.

2.11.7 For ease of reference, I shall describe one by one the remedies for coughing, (remedies) both quick-acting and widely approved.

2.11.8 And from there I shall next explain the different kinds of treatments to you in a general way, so that you will not need to look elsewhere for remedies.

II, 155, 22–8 Puschmann

πρὸς δὲ τὸ εὐχερῶς εὑρίσκειν τὰς κατὰ μέρος ὕλας τῶν βηχικῶν βοηθημάτων καὶ ἁρμόζειν δύνασθαι πρὸς τὴν ὑπὸ τῆς διαγνώσεως ὑπαγορευομένην διάθεσιν, (**2.11.8**) ἀκόλουθον +– ἐνόμισα μετὰ τὰς διαγνώσεις –+ καὶ τὴν καθόλου ἀγωγὴν καὶ τὰς διαφορὰς ὑμιν̂ ἐκθέσθαι τῶν βοηθημάτων +– μετὰ τῆς ἀκριβοῦς αὐτῶν συσταθμίας, –+ ὥστε μὴ παρ' ἑτέρου δεῖσθαι μανθάνειν, +– ἀλλ' ἐντεῦθεν ἀναλέγεσθαι τὸ ζητούμενον. –+

APPENDIX: A MORE DETAILED OVERVIEW OF THE CONTENTS OF THE LATIN ALEXANDER (COMPARING THE EARLY PRINTING WITH SELECT MAINSTREAM MANUSCRIPTS)

The following tables offer a much more detailed overview of the contents of the Latin Alexander, based on the divisions and sub-divisions employed in Table 2.1, pp. 15–16 above. They were originally intended merely to show to the interested reader the precise contents of the early printing, in accessible form, chapter by chapter. It subsequently seemed worthwhile to offer, in just a few additional pages, a survey of the work in the earlier branches of the tradition, γ, η and ε.

The left-hand column reproduces the chapter-numbers and chapter-titles in running text of the 1504 printing (*ed.*), with notes reporting collation with one or both of its closest congeners, G2 and L1. The other columns report divergences from *ed.* to be found in some of the most important mainstream manuscripts (P1, M, A and P2 for Book 1; P1 and A only for Book 2; all except P3, L2 and B for Book 3). Failing indication otherwise, the point of comparison is always the information reported for *ed.* in the left-hand column. In addition, the following conventions are used:

1. In the notes, all book-and-chapter references are to *ed.*;
2. Arabic numerals are used throughout in order to save space, although they are in fact used only in G2, *ed.* and L1 (and presumably in ϕ);
3. Shading indicates the absence of chapter(s) or part(s) thereof present in *ed.*;
4. A dot indicates the presence of chapter(s) or part(s) thereof present in *ed.*; if chapters are numbered in a given manuscript,[1] a dot indicates that the number is illegible or missing;
5. If a single chapter in *ed.* is subdivided in a manuscript, the cell corresponding to that chapter is normally subdivided; conversely, if two or more separate chapters in *ed.* are treated as a single chapter in a manuscript, the cells corresponding to that chapter are merged into one.

[1] Of those manuscripts in which the chapters are numbered, G2 and L1 (the daughters of ϕ) and M and A nearly always have prominent chapter-titles and -numbers. P1 has nearly all chapter-numbers and some titles in red. Often, however, the space left for the title is empty. A dot indicates that the number is illegible or missing. P1 is particularly prone to take the first words of the chapter into the title, or, conversely, to begin the chapter with the last words of the title. O has chapter-numbers and -titles in capitals, Mu in red. D has chapter-titles, initials and, sporadically, numbers. P2 has titles and some numbers, although after 1.29 numbers are rare. In each case, a dot indicates that the number is illegible or missing.

G1, C, Ox, Ma and Ge have no chapter-numbers. G1 has chapter-titles and -initials; a few chapters are subdivided. C has many chapter-titles in red, but often titles are omitted and chapters 'run together' (indicated in the table by omitting the walls between cells), the key visual clue to the start of a chapter then being the ornate initial alternately in blue, red and green. Ma has some chapter-titles sketched in but not written out properly. It has fine initials; a few chapters are subdivided. Ox and Ge have chapter-titles and -initials.

Book 1: (1) Diseases of the hair and scalp (I, 441–65[2] Puschm.)

Alex. Trall. Lat. *ed.* (G2)	P1 (M[3])	A	P2
1 De allopitia et ophiasi	1	1	• no t.
2 Signa ex quo humore allopitia generata fit	2 ... humore generata sit	2 ... humore generata fit	2 as P1
3 Cura ad tineam capitis	3 Curatio ...	3 Curatio ...	3 Curatio ...
4 De simplicibus medicamentis	4	4	•
5 De compositis medicamentis ad tineam capitis	5 De compositis medicamentis (ad tinea capitis M)	5	5 De compositis medicamentis • Item aliud (1.5 line 7)
6 De capillis cadentibus	6 ... cadentibus curatio	6[4]	6
7 Ad capillos cadentes ut non cadant nec furfures nascantur	7 Item de capillis ut non cadant et furfures non nascantur (M as A)	7 ... cadentes et caluos	7 as A • Item ad capillos cadentes (1.7 line 3)
8 Ad capillos ut citius crescant	8 ... ut crescant	8 ... ut crescant	8 ... ut crescant
9 Ad capillos denigrandos	9 as A (... nigrandum M)	9 Ad capillos nigros	9 Ad capillos nigrandos
10 Ad capillos nigros faciendos qui cani sunt	• as A (without Item), but in normal text	• Item ad nigros capillos faciendos probatum[5]	• Item probatum, but in normal text
11 Ad rubeos capillos tingendos et flauos faciendos	10[6] (M has 1. 12. t. here)	10	10 ... intinguendos ...
12 Ad capillos nigros tingendos et flauos faciendos	11 as A (corr. ex Ad c. n. f. faciendos) (1st 5 words of ch. om.)	11 Vt capillos nigros flauos facias	11 as A (without flauos)
13 Ad capillos auro similes faciendos	12 (M as P2)	12[7]	12 Vt capillos auro similes facias
14 Ad capillos albos faciendos	13 no t. Vt capillos aluos facias M	13	13
15 Ad ptiriaseos, i. furfures	14 no t. (M as *ed.*)	14 Ad pitiriaseos	14 Ad pturaseos
16 Ad pediculos et lendines	15[8] M as *ed.*	15 ... et lentes	15 ... et lendes
17 Ad psidracia et exantimata in capite facta	16 M as *ed.*	16	16 ... facta in capite

[2] Note that the Greek chapters corresponding to Latin 1.7–9 are in Greek ms. Mf only.
[3] I compare M especially where the title is missing from P1, which occurs very frequently after 1.12. Failing indication to the contrary, however, the manuscript reported is P1.
[4] 1.6–13 are in the first instance deliberately omitted in A: see p. 40 n. 9.
[5] This title corresponds to the first phrase of 2.10 in *ed.*
[6] In P1 (though not in M) this chapter ends with 1.12.t. as in A.
[7] The first phrase of 1.13 'Vt capillos aureo facias colore' is not in P1M A P2.
[8] On 1.16–17 in P1, see, p. 50 n. 37.

Book 1: *Continued*

Alex. Trall. Lat. *ed.* (G2)	**P1 (M)**	**A**	**P2**
18 Ad ulcera in capite scrissa et rubea; ch. begins Modica ulcera assimilantia . . .	17 M . . . spissa et rubra; ch. begins Modice adsimilantes . . .[9]	17 . . . spissa et rubra modica assimilantia titinulas ex quibus tabes quaedam defluit	1<7> . . . spissa et rubea
19 De acore signis	18 M De acori signa	18	18
20 Curatio achorarum	19 M Curatio acorum	19	19

Book 1: (2) Headache: *cephalargia, cephalea* and *emigranium* (I, 465–509 Puschm.)

Alex. Trall. Lat. *ed.* (G2)	**P1 (M)**	**A**	**P2**
21 De cephalargia capitis	20 M as A	20 De cephalargia	20 as A
22 Signa si ex nimio solis ardore dolor capitis factus fuerit	21 M as A, ending capitis factus fuerit dolor	21 . . . ex solis ardore factus fuerit capitis dolor	• as A
23 Curatio si de sole doleat caput hominibus	22 M as *ed.*, without hominibus	22 . . . de sole caput doleat	• as A
24 Curatio calide distemperantie et diuturni doloris capitis	23 M . . . diuturni capitis doloris facti	23 . . . distemperantie capitis et diuturni doloris	23 as A
25 Si de nimio epatis calore caput dolet	24 M De nimio epatis calore distemperan() cephalar() generan() dolo()	24 . . . calore cephalargia generatur	24 as A, but epatis dolore
26 Si de frigida epatis distemperantia caput doleat	25 M De frigida distemperantia facta cephalargia	25 . . . frigida distemperantia epatis doleat caput	25 as A
27 Curatio frigide distemperantie	26 M as *ed.*	26	26 in marg.
28 Si male habente stomacho caput doloribus affligatur	27 M Si de stomacho caput dolet; ch. begins Si male habes in stomacho	27	• . . . dolore . . .
29 Curatio si ex colerico humore dolor capitis efficitur	28 M as *ed.*	28 Si ex col. hum. capitis efficiatur dolor	28 in marg., as A, but ending capitis dolor fuerit
30 Si ex pinguibus et frigidis humoribus dolor capitis factus fuerit	29 M as A	29 Si ex pinguibus capitis factus fuerit dolor	29 Si ex pingui-bus humoribus capitis dolor est
31 Curatio si caput doleat ex febribus	30 M as A	30 . . . si febrientibus caput doleat	• Cura si ex febre caput doleat

9 P1 has no t., but chapter begins 'Modica adsimulante'.

Book 1: ***Continued***

Alex. Trall. Lat. ***ed.*** **(G2)**	**P1 (M)**	**A**	**P2**
3<2> Curatio si ex uino caput doleat	31 M Si ex ... doleat ut facilius sanus sit	31 Si ex ...	• as A
3<3> Si ex percussura caput doleat	32 M Si ex percussione caput doluerit	32 Si ex percussu caput dolet	•
34 De cephalea .i. dolore capitis	33 M De cephalea (1st 3 words of ch. om. P1)	<33>	•
35 Signa si ex e<n> fraxi caput doleat	34 (corr. ex 35 P1) M Si de infraxin caput doleat	34 Si ex infraxin caput doleat signa	• as A, without signa
36 Signa si ex flegmone in capite fiat cephalea .i. capitis dolor	35 M Signa si flegmon in capite fit; ch. begins Sephalis id est dolor	35 (om. capitis)	• ... capite fiat dolor
37 Signa si ex uentositate fiat capitis dolor	36	36	•
38 Signa si ex acredine humorum dolor capitis fiat	37 M as A	37 ... capitis fiat dolor	• ... humorum fiat
39 Signa si ex calore fuerit dolor aut distemperantia capitis facta	38 M ... ex colerico humore distemperantia fuerit	38 ... calore fuerit facta distemperantia	• ... calore fuerit
40 Curatio cephalargicorum	39 M Curatio cephalicis	39 Curatio cephalicorum	39 as A
41 Curatio si ex colerico humore dolor capitis fiat	40 M Si ex ...	40 ... humore fiat capitis dolor (1st 4 words of ch. om.)	• ... humore fiat dolor
42 Ad capitis purgationem irrinum .i. capitis purgatorium	41 M ch. begins Etrinum	41 ... inrinon ...	•
43 De cerotis ad capitis dolorem et trociscis anodinis	42 M De cerotis et trociscis ad capitis dolorem; ch. begins Ergo anodinis[10]	42	• ... dolorem de trociscis anodinis
44 Curatio quibus ex qualitatis distemperantia dolores sunt	43... doloris fiant	<43> ... dolores fiunt	• ... dol() fiunt
45 De emigraneo dolore	44 M as A	44 ... emigranii ...	• 1. 46 t. here
46 Si patiatur caput ex stomacho et exinde emigraneus dolor fiat	45 as A	45 Si compatiatur ... exinde emigranii surgant dolores	• 1. 47. t. here

[10] P1 has no t., but chapter begins 'Et trociscis anotenis'.

Book 1: ***Continued***

Alex. Trall. Lat. ***ed.*** **(G2)**	**P1 (M)**	**A**	**P2**
47 Si ex frigido humore in stomacho existente emigraneus dolor fiat	46 as A (om. in)	46 ... stomacho consistente emigranium fiat	• no t.
48 De uomitu et catartico et cataputiis	• but in normal text	• De uomitu et catharticis catapotiis	• as A
49 Si de colerico humore fit emigranea passio	47 M ... humore fiunt emigranea passio	47 ... humore fiat emigranium	• as A
50 Crisina locale ad dolores ex frigido dolore emigraneo	48 M Crisina localis ex frigido humore ad emigranii dolorem	48 Chrisma localis ... frigido humore emigranii	• as A
51 Quibus ex colerico humore fiunt emigranee passiones	49	49 ... emigranice ...	• ... emigran() dol()

Book 1: (3) *Phrenesis* (I, 509–27 Puschm.)

Alex. Trall. Lat. ***ed.*** **(G2)**	**P1 (M)**	**A**	**P2**
52 De frenesi	50 M as A	50 De frenetica passione	• as A
53 Que causa est frenetice	51 M ... freneticis	51	•
54 Signa future frenetice	52 M as *ed.*	52	•
55 Nothe frenetice signa	53 M Signa non uere freneticie	53 Note frenetitie signa	•
56 De his quibus iam diuturna frenesis est uentura signa	54 M De his quibus diu futura est frenesis signa	54 Signa quibus diuturna est frenesis	• as A
57[11] Curatio freneticorum	55 M as *ed.*	55	• Curatio frenesis
58 De cibis in frenesi	56 M De cibis	56	• De cibis

Book 1: (4) *Lethargus* (I, 527–35 Puschm.)

Alex. Trall. Lat. ***ed.*** **(G2)**	**P1 (M)**	**A**	**P2**
59 De litargico.i. obliuioso	5<7> M De lytargo ...	57 De lytargo	De litargico
60 Curatio litargicorum	58 M as *ed.*	58	Curatio

[11] The last six words of this chapter are not in *ed.* (*saut du même au même*).

Book 1: (5) Epilepsy (I, 535–67, 575 Puschm.)

Alex. Trall. Lat. *ed.* (G2)	P1 (M)	A	P2
61 De epileptia	59 M De epylempsia	59	•
62 Signa epilepsie	60 M Signa epylempsie	60	•
63 Cura<tio> epileptie	61	61 Curatio e.	• Curatio e.
64 De apozimis et cathaputiis dandis	62	62 De apozimis	• De apozimatibus
65 De catarticis	63	63	•
66 De apoflegmatismis	64	64	•
67 De uomitu	65	65	•
68 Si de stomacho epilepsia fiat	<66>	66 ... fiat epylempsia	•
69 Si ex aliquo membro fiat epilepsia	67	6<7> De diuturna epilempsie passione (= 70.t. *ed.*)	•
70 De diuturna passione epilepsie	68	68 ... epylempsie passione	• ... epilempsie passione
71 De phisicis ligaturis ad epilepticos	69	69	• De phisicis et ligaturis
72 Quomodo cognosces epilepticos	72.t. in text	70 Item de ligaturis	• Post paroxismum factum[12] quomodo ...
• Aliud ad hoc ipsum			• Aliud ad hoc ipsum
			• <T>heodorus
73 De ligaturis Archigenis	70	• Item de ligaturis	• De ligaturis
74 Quid cauendum est epilepticis	71	71	•

Book 1: (6) *Melancholia* (I, 591–617 Puschm.)

Alex. Trall. Lat. *ed.* (G2)	P1 (M)	A	P2
75 De melancolia	72	72	•
76 Signa si ex plenitudine sanguinis fiat melancolia	73	73	•
77 De cura (Curatio G2) melancolie	74	74 Curatio m.	• Curatio m.
78 Si ex colerico humore melancolia aut mania fuerit facta	75	75	•

[12] These are the last three words of 1.71 in *ed.* They are underlined in G2!

Book 1: *Continued*

Alex. Trall. Lat. *ed.* (G2)	P1 (M)	A	P2
79 Si ex acredine et mordicatione colerica aut ex qualitate sanguinis melancolia fiat	76 Signa qui ex . . .	76 Signa si ex acredine et mordico colerico aut . . .	•
8<0> Curatio si ex acredine aut humore colerico passio fuerit generata	77	<77>	•
81 De cibo dando menomenis uel melancolicis	78	78	•
	• Carnes autem	• De fructibus	
82 Signa si ex melancolico sanguine facta fuerit mel<a>ncolia	78	79	•
83 Curatio melancolie	79	80	•
84 De (Curatio de G2) armenico litu	80[13] Dacio Armineu lito	81 Datio armenico liti	• De armenio litu

Book 1: (7) Eye-diseases (II, 3–69 Puschm.)

Alex. Trall. Lat. *ed.* (G2)	P1 (M)	A	P2
85 Incipit de oculorum passionibus	81 M as P2	82 De o. p.	• . . . ad oc. passiones
86 Signa quomodo (quando G2) sanguineus humor flegmonem facit	82 M Signa quando . . .	83 Signa quando . . .	• Signa quando . . .
87 Curatio flegmonis de sanguine facti	83 Curatio flegmonem sanguineis	84	•
88 De colliriis mitigatiuis in dolore aurium (doloribus oculorum G2) ex sanguineo humore factis	84 De coleria mitigatiua (rest of t. begins ch.)	85 . . . in doloribus oculorum . . .	• . . . in doloribus ex . . .
89 De colliriis apocrusticis q(uae) monoymera uocantur	85 Collirium apocrusticum (rest of t. begins ch.)	86	• Colliria
90 Si ex colerico et acro humore fiant dolores in oculis	86 Signa ex colerico humore fiant dolores	87 Signa si . . . fiant dolores	• Signa si . . . fiant dolores

13 In P1 this chapter begins with the last six words of 1.83.

Book 1: ***Continued***

Alex. Trall. Lat. *ed.* (G2)	P1 (M)	A	P2
91 Curatio hiis qui de colerico et acro humore laborant	87	88 Curatio eorum qui . . .	• Curatio eorum qui . . .
92 Signa anfraxis in oculis facte	8<8>	89	•
93 Curatio anfraxis si sola facta fuerit in oculis	89	90	•
94 De mulsa in constipatis (conspissatis G2) poris curatio	90 . . . poris	91 Curatio de . . . conspissatis poris	• as A
95 Signa qui flobothomari opus habent et qui catarticis purgari	91 no t.	92 . . . catartico purgari	• as A
96 De ulceratione oculorum si simul cum flegmone fuerit	92	93 De ulceratione si . . .	• De ulcere si . . .
97 Collirium ad cicatrices uel albugines tollendas	93	94 Colliria . . .	• Colliria . . .
98 Colliria mordicantia ad calliginem oculorum	94 as A	95 Colliria mordicantia ad caligines oculorum	• as A
99 De ydrocollirio et exidrocolliriis facientibus ad ampliopiam	95	96 De ygrocollirio et exyrocolliriis	• De ygrocollirio et ygrocolliriis (!)
100 Ad nictilopas .i. eos qui post transmutatum solem non uident	96 no t.	97 Ad nectalopas	• Ad nictalopas
101 Ad tingendas albugines et leucomata tingenda	97 no t., but ch. begins Ad leucomata tingenda satis bonum	98 Collirium ad t. a. oculorum et ad l. satis bonum	• Ad t. a. oculorum ad l. t.
	98 as A	99 Collirium dracomaticum	
102 Xirocollirium et ydrocollirium que faciunt ad sicosim et ad putredines ulcerum et ypopias et myocephala	99 no t., but ch. begins Qui faciunt . . .	100	100 (t. includes the first sentence to carnes)
103 De mulsa	100	101	101
104 Ad staphilomata	101	102	•
105 Ad ptirias et sicosim	102 (t. om. P1′)	103	•
106 De ryadis	103	104 Ad driadas	• Ad riadas
107 Ad egylops	104	105	•

Book 1: (8) Ear-diseases, including *parotis* (II, 71–125 Puschm.)

Alex. Trall. Lat. *ed.* (G2)	**P1 (M)**	**A**	**P2**
108 De passionibus aurium	105	106 Ad aurium passiones effectas	• as A
109 Signa si ex anfraxi aut de sanguine dolores fiant	106	107 ... aut de flegmone dolores ...	• ... aut flegmone dolores ...
110 Curatio si ex anfraxi aut humoribus aut spiritibus (spiritu G2) dolores fiant	107 M ... si infraxin ab humoribus spiritus fiunt doloris	108 ... humoribus uel spiritu fiant dolores	•
111 De aurium dolore qui ex frigoris causa fit	108	109 ... doloribus ... fiunt	• ... doloribus ... frigidis causis fiunt
112 Si aures ex nimio aeris calore et acro humore doluerint	109 (with 119 t.!)	110 ... calore doluerint	• as A
113 Si in aure interius flegmon fuerit factus (cum dolore G2)	110	111	• ... factus cum dolore
114 Curatio flegmonis	111	112	•
115 Cura ad aurium ulcera siue apostemata	112	113 Ad aurium ...	• as A
116 Ad oppressas et fractas aures ex ruinali percussione	113 (Ex r. p. begins the ch.)	114 ... ex ruina uel ...	•
117 De tinnitu uel sonitu aurium	114	115	•
118 Ad eos quorum sordibus repletur auris	115 no t.	116 ... quorum aures sordibus replentur	• Ad aures sordibus repletas
119 Si in aure fuerit aliquid ingressum	116 no t.	117 ... ingressum siue faba siue lapillus	• as A
120 Ad uermes si in auribus fiant	117 no t.	118 ... aure ...	• as A
121 Si aures ex catarro indoluerint	118 no t.	119 Si ex catarro aures doluerint	• Si ex catarro aures ...
122 De fluxu (Ad fluxum G2) sanguinis de auribus[14]	119 no t.	120 Si ex auribus sanguis fluat	• as A
123 Ad aures surdas	120 no t.	121	•[15]
124 De parotidis	121 no t.	122[16]	•
125 Curatio si ex plenitudine sanguinis fiant parotide	122	123	•

[14] This chapter begins very differently in *ed.* compared with P1 A P2.
[15] The third sentence 'Quibusdam ... ordinanda sunt' *add. inf. manu alia* P2.
[16] In A this chapter begins 'Parotide sunt similes glandulis que circa aures nasci solent' (not in *ed.* P2).

Book 1: ***Continued***

Alex. Trall. Lat. *ed.* (G2)	**P1 (M)**	**A**	**P2**
126 Curatio in quibus parotide sunt scirotidis tumoris	123	124 . . . scirodis humoris	• . . . parotide cum scyrodis tumore
127 Signa si in pus conuertantur parotide et cura	124	125	•
128 Curatio si ex colerico humore fiant parotide	125 . . . reuma fiant . . .	126 . . . colerico reumate fiant . . .	• Si . . . reumate . . .
129 Si ex flegmatico humore parotide fiant	126	127 . . . parotide fuerint facte	• as A
130 De dieta	127	128	•

Book 1: (9) Nose, face and teeth (not in the Greek)

Alex. Trall. Lat. *ed.* (G2)	**P1 (M)**	**A**	**P2**
131 De narium passione	128	129 . . . passionibus	129 as A
132 Ad sanguinis fluxum de naribus	129	130	•
133 De liuore in facie	130	131 Ad liuorem de facie tollendum	131
134 De dentium causis id est passionibus. Galienus de dentium passionibus	131 De dencium causatione Galieni	132 De dentium passionibus. Galienus de dentium passionibus	132 as A
135. De dentium dolore cura (Ad dentium dolores G2)	(135 t. in text)	• Ad dentium dolorem	• Ad dentium dolores

Book 1: (10) *Synanche* (II, 125–45 Puschm.)

Alex. Trall. Lat. *ed.* (G2)	**P1 (M)**	**A**	**P2**
136 De squinance uel sinance (De sinance G2)	132 De senances	133 Ad sinancem	134 Ad sinances
137 Curatio sinancis	133	134	135 Cura s.
138 De simplicibus adiutoriis	•	•	•
139 De confectione dyamoron uel aliis medicamentis ad sinancem congruis[17]	134	135	136

[17] This chapter begins 'Dyamoron simplicem ad sinancem hoc modo conficis' *ed.*, 'Diamoron simplex' P1 A (*om.* P2).

Book 1: *Continued*

Alex. Trall. Lat. *ed.* (G2)	**P1 (M)**	**A**	**P2**
140 De flobothomia et catartico ac uentosis sinancis	135 no t.	136 ... ac uentosis	137 as A
141 De hiis qui extrinsecus sunt adhibenda in fomentationibus et cathaplasmatibus[18]	136 no t.	137 De fom. et cat. que extrinsecus sunt adhibenda atque dieta	• as A
142 De dieta sinanticorum	(142. t. in text)	•	•

Book 1: (11) *Pleuritis* (II, 229–43 Puschm.)

Alex. Trall. Lat. *ed.* (G2)	**P1 (M)**	**A**	**P2**
143 De signis pleureticorum	137 no t.	138 De pleureticis[19]	139 De pleureticis
144 De cura pleureticorum	138 Curatio pletoricis	139 Curatio pleureticorum	140 as A
145 De cibis dandis sinanticis (pleureticis G2)	139 no t.	140 De dieta pleureticorum	141 Dieta pleureticorum
146 De uentris fluxu in pl<e>uresi	140	141 ... fluxu pleuresis	•
147 De lateris dolore qui sine febre fit	141	142 Ad lateris dolorem qui sine febribus fit	• Ad laterum dolorem qui sine febribus fit
148 De catartico pleureticis dando	142	143	•
149 De cathapuciis pleureticis dandis[20]	143 De cataputias	144 De catapotiis	•

Book 2: (1) Coughing (II, 147–67, 185 Puschm.)

Alex. Trall. Lat. *ed.* (G2L1)	**P1**	**A**
1 De tussi	1 no t.	1
2 De tussis cognitione quae de calida distemperantia generatur	2 no t.	2
3 De tussi si ex frigida distemperantia oritur	3 no t.	3 De tusse quae ex ... fit
4 De tussi si ex sicca aut humida distemperantia fuerit facta	4 no t.	4

[18] This chapter begins 'Fomentationes autem et cathaplasmata' *ed.* (*om.* A P2).
[19] In the first sentence of this chapter A omits 'acutissimus dolor lateris'.
[20] At the end of this chapter: purgant *ed.* facient purgationem P1 A P2.

Book 2: *Continued*

Alex. Trall. Lat. *ed.* (G2L1)	P1	A
5 De tussi si ex humoribus fiat	5 no t.	5
6 De tussi si ex capite fluat humor	6 no t.	6
7 Si de capite in pulmonem fluat humor	7 no t.	7 Signa si . . . fluat
8 Signa si [ex] tussientibus pus in thorace fluat et humor	8 no t.	8
9 Signa de flegmone in pulmone existente	9 no t.	9 De fimone . . . consistente
10 Si tussis ex spissis et glutinosis fit humoribus qui in pulmone continetur et generatur	10 no t. but ch. begins with 10. t., ending . . . quod in fleumone contenentur generetur	10 . . . spissis gluttinosisque humoribus qui in pulmone continentur generatur
11 De lapide sputato		•
12 Medicamenta ad tussim quibus uti oportet	11 no t.	11
13 De dyacodion confectione	12 no t.	12 De diacodion

Book 2: (2) Diseases of the digestive tract (II, 245–313 Puschm.)

Alex. Trall. Lat. *ed.* (G2L1)	P1	A
14 Ad stomachi diuersas passiones uel accidentia quae cardiacam uocant aliqui	13 Ad stom. diu. pass.; ch. begins Stomachum quem antiqui cartian nominabant	13 . . . quae antiqui cardian nominabant
15 De stomachi frigida distemperantia	14 no t. (1st word of ch. om.)	14
16 De stomachi cinorodoxeos	15 no t. (1st 4 words of ch. om.)	15 t. includes 1st sentence of ch.[21]
17 Si de calida distemperantia fuerit cynorodoxeos	16 no t.	16
18 Curatio si ex frigido conti<n>gat cynorodoxeos	17	17 . . . ex frigdore . . .
19 Curatio calide distemperantie cynorodoxeos	18	18
20 Curatio si ex imbecillitate uirtutis cateltice fiat cinorodoxeos	19	19 . . . ex imbecilla uirtute . . .
21 Curatio si ex frigore imbecillis fiat cateltica uirtus	20 (imbecillis om.)	20
22 Curatio si ex calore nimio fuerit imbecilla cateltica uirtus	21 . . . nimium inuicella fiat . . .	21
23 De bolismo	22 De bulemis (1st word of ch. om.)	22 De bolimis

[21] The chapter thus begins 'Quoniam quidem . . .', which suggests that the first sentence in *ed.* did indeed originally belong to the title.

Book 2: ***Continued***

Alex. Trall. Lat. ***ed.*** **(G2L1)**	**P1**	**A**
24 De anorexia id est fastidio stomachi	23 ... id est fastidium	23 ... id est fastidio
25 Si de colerico humore fastidium fiat	24 Quomodo oportit facere uomicam; ch. begins Quibus resedit tenuis et colericus humor in stomacho	24 Quomodo oportet fieri uomicam quibus residet tenuis sed colericus humor in stomacho
26 Si de spissis et glutinosis humoribus fastidium fiat	25 Si de gl. et sp. hum. fiat f. (1st 11 lines only due to the loss of a folio)	25
27 Si de calida distemperantia facta fuerit absque humore de solo calore anorexia		26
<2>8 Si de nimio frigore distemperantia sine humore generauit fastidium		27
29 De siti nimia		28 De siti et unde praecedat et curatio eius
30 Ad eos qui habent ardorem in stomacho et nimis sitiunt		29
31 Ad sitim cathaputie		30
32 De coleribus nigris in stomacho existentibus cum inflatione	(from line 3)	31 ... consistentibus cum inflammatione
33 Confectio ad stomachum frigidum medicaminis dyaporon	32 no t. (1st 3 words of ch. om.; ch. begins Qui facit ...)	32 Confectio medicaminis diaporon quod facit ad anatropas stomachi et ciliacos et disintericos (= 1st sentence of cap. in *ed.*)
34 De epithimate ad stomachum reumatizantem	33 no t. (1st 4 words of ch. om.; ch. begins Et in febribus ...)	33 Epitima ad stomachum reumatizantem et in febribus et sine febribus et ciliacos et quibus stomachus compatitur et reiciunt cibos (= 1st sentence of cap. in *ed.*)
35 Antidotum ad stomachum frigidum	34[22] no t.	34
36 De cardiaca passione	35 no t.	35
37 Curatio cardiace		
38 De nausea et uomitu	36 no t.	36
39 Signa qualis humor aut quo loco fluit aut in quo continetur loco	37 no t.	37 ... humor aut de quo ...
40 Si melancolicus aut colericus humor uomitum excitet	38[23] no t., but ch. begins with 2.40.t., ending ... uomicam excetit	38 Curatio si ... uomicam excitet

[22] The last sentence of this chapter is much shorter in P1 than in *ed.* and A: 'Dabis ieiuno et post cibum cocl. i.'
[23] P1 omits the last sentence of this chapter ('Sic enim ... curationem').

Book 2: *Continued*

Alex. Trall. Lat. *ed.* (G2L1)	**P1**	**A**
41 Curatio si ex flegmate repletus stomachus nauseam facit	39 no t.	39
42 Curatio si ex oroydis et tenuis humor in stomacho imbibitus fuerit	40 no t. (1st sentence of ch. om., as A)	40[24] Curatio si orodis ...
43 De curatione stomachi et fl<e>gmonibus	41 no t. (last 7 words of ch. om.)	41[25] De flegmone stomachi
44 De cerotis et epithimatibus galieni	•	•
45 Vnctiones stomathice que fiunt ad frigorem stomachi	42 no t.	42 Vnctiones que faciunt ad infrigdatum stomachum
46 Ad frigidum stomacum embalmata	43 Ad frigdatum stomachum; ch. begins Inlabata	43 Ad infrigdatum stomachum inbamata
47 De cura uiscerum	• no t.	44 De duricia uiscerum
48 De acida eructatione stomachi	44 no t.	45 De acido ructu stomachi
49 De amaritudine oris	46 no t.	46
50 De hiis qui satis <spuunt> et humidum habent stomachum	47 no t.	47

Book 2: (3) Cholera (II, 321–35 Puschm.)

Alex. Trall. Lat. *ed.* (G2L1)	**P1**	**A**
51 De colerica passione	48 no t.	48 De colericis passionibus
52 Curatio si ex plenitudine indigestorum ciborum colerica passio fuerit generata	49 no t.	49[26] ... indigestorum humorum colerica passio generatur
53 Curatio si ex qualitate uiciosa stomachi colerica passio generetur	50 no t.	50 ... uitiosi ...
54 Si ex colerum plenitudine colerica passio generetur	51 no t.	51
55 Curatio	•	
56 Curatio ad eos quibus paruus fit uomitus aut uentris fluxus	52 no t.	52 Ad eos ... uomitus aut solutio

[24] First sentence of chapter not in A.
[25] A omits last two words of chapter.
[26] This chapter is not in A′.

Book 2: (4) Diseases of the liver (II, 379–413 Puschm.)

Alex. Trall. Lat. *ed.* (G2L1)	**P1**	**A**
57 De epatis flegmone	53 no t.	53
58 Signa si in cirta epatis flegmon fuerit	54 no t.	54 . . . in cirta magis quam alibi fiat
59 Signa si in sima epatis fuerit inflammatio	55 no t.; ch. begins Si autem in sima . . .	55
60 Signa si in musculis epatis flegmon fuerit	56 no t.	56
61 Curatio de flegmone epatis	57 no t.	57 . . . de inflammatione . . .
62 De potionibus et apozimatibus	•	• De potionibus
63 Signa anfraxis epatis	58 no t.	58
64 Curatio anfraxis epatis	59[27] no t.	59
65 De scyrosi epatis	60 no t.	
66 De epithimatibus et cathaplasmatibus ad flegmonem et ad anfraxim et ad scyrosim	60 no t.	60 De c. et e. . . . et ad scyron
67 De potionibus et antidotis ad epatis passiones	61 no t.	61
68 De athonia epatis et epatica dissinteria	62 no t., but ch. begins Epatica desenteria	62
69 Signa calide distemperantie epatis	63 no t.	63
70 Signa frigide distemperantie	64 (corr. ex 65) t. only, immed. followed by 2.71.t.	64 . . . distemperantie epatis
71 De sicca distemperantia epatis	sicca dis. immed. after 2.70.t.; ch. begins Sicciorem corpus	65 . . . distemperantia
72 De distemperantia humida epatis	• De hum. dis.	
73 Curatio calide distemperantie epatis	65 (corr. ex 66)	66
	• De pescibus . . . accipere	
74 Curatio epatice dissinterie de frigida epatis distemperantia	66 as A, but ending . . . temperate	67 . . . epatice distemperantie de frigida distemperantia generate
75 De potionibus et epithimatibus ad epaticas distemperantias	67 De p. et cataplū	68 De p. et cataplasmatibus
76 Antidotum gifi ad frigidas distemperantias	68 Ad frigidam epatis distemperantia; ch. begins Ad dissintericas passionis	69 Ad frigidam epatis distemperantiam ad dyssintericas passiones
77 De embroca et cathaplasmate	• as A, but in normal text	• Expediens embroca ad frigidam epatis distemperantiam
78 Cura de athonia epatis	• Curacio attonie epatis	• Curationi epatis

27 After *adhiberi*, at end of 2.164 *ed.*, P1 has 'De cataplum et epitimata ad fleumonem ad infraxim ad sciron dicimus igitur ad singulas passionis qualia' (= 2.66.t. + 1st 7 words of 2.66!).

Book 2: (5) Philumenus, on diseases of the stomach and intestines (not in the Greek)

Alex. Trall. Lat. *ed.* (G2L1)	**P1**	**A**
79 De reumate uentris Filominis	69 De reuma ...	70
80 De dissinteria reumatica	70	71
81 Signa dissinterice passionis Philomini[28]	71 Signa desin terae passionis; ch. begins Filomini	72
82 De dissinterica passione	• Curatio desenteriae	• Curatio dysinterie
83 De lacte dando	72	73
84 De potionibus ad epaticam dissinteriam		
85 De embroca et cathaplasmate ad calidam distemperantiam	last sentence only	last sentence only
86 De cibo dissintericorum	73[29] (corr. ex 75)	74
87 De fastidio		
88 De leguminibus	•	•
89 De ptisanis	• but in normal text	• De tipsanis
90 De oleribus	•	•
91 De piscibus	•	•
92 De carnibus	•	•
93 De quadrupedibus carnibus	• De quatropedibus	
94 De pomis	•	•
95 De potionibus simplicibus ad uentrem stringendum	74 (corr. ex 76) De p. ch. begins Sim. ad uentrem constringende	75 ... constringendum
96 De falsa opinione indoctorum medicorum	75 no t., but ch. begins Ad dissentericus	76 De trociscis diuersis ad dysintericos
97 De trociscis	• no t.	
98[30] Enema ad dissintericos et dolores nimios uel inflammationes	• Ad dissintericus; ch. begins Ad doloris ...	77 ... ad dysintericorum dolores ...
99 De ciliacis Philomini	76 no t., but ch. begins Flaminum	78
100 Signa ciliacorum	• no t.	•
	• no t.	• Curatio ciliacorum
101 De cronica ciliacorum passione	• no t.	• De cronia ciliacorum
102 De tenasmone	77 no t.	79 De tenismo
103 Curatio	• no t.	•

[28] In this chapter febres ... corodes *om. ed.* P1 (*saut du même au même*); et defectione ... uomitus efficitur *om. ed.*

[29] This chapter ends 'ubi cocta fuerit' in P1.

[30] The last sentence of this chapter in *ed.* repeats the text of 2.71. It is not in P1 or A.

Book 2: (6) Philagrius, on diseases of the spleen (not in the Greek)

Alex. Trall. Lat. *ed.* (G2L1)	**P1**	**A**
104 Ad splenem Philagrius	78 no t.	80
105 Signa frigide distemperantie splenis	79 no t. (last 7 words of ch. om.)	81 Signa spl. f. d. (last 7 words of ch. om.)
106 De calida distemperantia splenis	80 no t., but ch. begins Splenis	82
107 Curatio calide et sicce distemperantie splenis	81 no t.	• . . . distemperantie
108 Curatio frigide et humide distemperantie splenis	82 no t.	83 . . . distemperantie
109 Curatio calide et humide distemperantie	85	84
110 De simplici distemperantia	85	85
111 Curatio humide distemperantie	86	86
112 Curatio sicce distemperantie	87	87
113 Curatio frigide distemperantie	88	88
114 Curatio calide distemperantie	89	•
115 De uentositate splenis	90	89
116 Curatio uentositatis	•	•
117 Signa flegmonis splenis si de solo sanguine fiat	91 Signa fleumonis splenis; ch. begins Si de sanguinem solo fiat	90 Signa si flegmon splenis de . . .
118 Signa si flegmon de colerico humore fiat in splene	92 . . . si inflammatio . . . fiat; ch. begins In splene	91 . . . si inflammatio . . .
119 Signa si flegmon ex melancolico humore in splene fit generatus	no. illeg.; t. as in A, but ending generatur humore	92 . . . si inflammatio in splene de m. h. generatur
120 Signa si flegmon ex humore flegmatico in splene fuerit generatus	94 . . . si in splen inflammatio de flegma fuerit generata	93 . . . si inflammatio in splene de flegmate fuerit generata
121 Curatio flegmonis in splene generati	95	94
122 De epilatibus	•	•
123 De fomentationibus	•	•
	• as A (2.123 line 20)	• Ad nimiam factam inflammationem (2.123 line 20)
124 De clisteri	•	•
125 De cibo	•	•
126 De statu	•	•

Book 2: *Continued*

Alex. Trall. Lat. *ed.* (G2L1)	**P1**	**A**
127 De catartico aut apozimate uel inunctionibus	• De catartico aut apozima	• De cathartico et apozima
		• De iniectionibus (2.127 line 6)
128 De catarticis potionibus	• Putionis (= 4th word of 2.128)	
129 De cathaplasmate faciendo	•	•
130[31] De carnibus	•	•
	• De auibus	
131 De potionibus	•	• De epitimatibus (*sic*)
132 De epithimatibus	• De aepitimas	•
133 De scyron splenis	• Sinna de scyronsplenis	95 Signa scyron splenis
134 Curatio scyron splenis	•	•
135 De cibo	• De ciuis	• De cibis
	• De auibus	
136 De potionibus	•	•
137 De sanguine tollendo	•	•
138 De potione tonotica spleneticis	•	97 (*sic*)
139 De epithimate	• De aephithimas	98 De epitimatibus
140 Malagma Amithonis	• malagma ameta onus, but in normal text	• Malagma Amitaonis
	• Item alia epithima (2.140 line 8)[32]	• Item aliud epitima (2.140 line 8)
141 Confectio epitimatis atonotici ad splen confortandum	•	•
	• Item epithima (2.141 line 7)	
142 Curatio si ex uentositate tenditur aut inflatur splen	• . . . inflammatur	99
143 Galieni dicta de splenis scyros et uentositate	• Galeni de . . .	• Galieni de . . .
144 Epithima epatis et splenis	• Epithima aepatis; ch. begins Spleniticis	• Epitima epaticis et spleneticis
145 Epithima ypotirion		• Epitima eupatorion
146 Epitima dyaspermaton		
	• Item aliut Ep. d. (2.146 line 5)	
	• 2.147.t. (2.146 line 10)[33]	
147 De potionibus ad splenem	• De putione	
14<8> De trociscis	•	•
149 Item epithima	•	•
150 De tusse	100	•

[31] The second sentence of this chapter ('Dandi autem sunt cibi pisces aspratiles' P1A) is not in *ed.*
[32] At 2.140 line 16 P1 breaks off in the middle of the recipe, has a heading *De aephitimas*, and repeats 2.139 and 2.140 entire!
[33] This section ends with the first three words of 2.147 'commemorationem iterum faciemus'.

Book 2: (7) Dropsy (II, 439–61 Puschm.)

Alex. Trall. Lat. *ed.* (G2L1)	P1	A
151 Causa que est ydropicie Alexandri	101 Causa aedropiciae alexandriae	100 Causa ydropicie Alexandri
152 Signa	102 Signa ydropicae	101 Signa ydropicie
153 Curatio ydropicie	103	102
	2.154.t. (2.153 line 10)	
154 Curatio anasarce ydropicie[34]	• De cataplasma	• De cataplasmatibus
155 De ydrope asclite et tympanite	104[35] De ydropem ascitem et tempanitem	103 De ydropicis ascite timpanite
156 De dieta ydropicorum	• Cyuorum qualitas (2.156 line 4)	•
	105 De oleribus (2.156 line 10)	
157 Ad eos qui cum febre ydropisim patiuntur curatio	105 t. as A; ch. begins Curatio	105 … febre ydropem patiuntur

Book 2: (8) Those spitting blood (II, 187–209 Puschm.)

Alex. Trall. Lat. *ed.* (G2L1)	P1	A
158 Ad emoptoicos	106	106
159 Signa dyarixis	107	107
160 Signa dyabrosis	107	108
161 Signa anastomaseos	108	109
162 Vt scias ex quibus locis fluat sanguis	109 t. as A, but ending … fuit sanguis	110 Signa ut cognoscas ex …
163 Curatio rixis in emoptoicis	110 Curatio rixin; ch. begins Inmoptoicus	111 Curatio rixin emoptoicis
164 De dieta emoptoicorum	• De ciuis	• De cibis
165 Curatio ad rixin passionem	111 Putionis ad rexin passionem	112 Potiones ad rixin
166 De embrocis et epithimatibus	• as A	• Curatio ad rixin de embrocis et epitimatibus uel emplastris
167 De quattuor medicaminibus ad rixim		
168 Curatio dyabrosis emoptoicis	112 Curatio ad …	113
169 De cibo	• as A	• De ciborum obseruantia
170 Ad eos qui ex tristicia aut sollicitudine aut ex abstinentia sanguinem expuunt	•	•

34 2.154.t. is also at 2.153 line 10 in *ed.*, but in normal text.

35 This chapter begins with the last three words of 2.154 'iuuat autem optime'.

Book 2: ***Continued***

Alex. Trall. Lat. ***ed.*** **(G2L1)**	**P1**	**A**
171 Signa si de capite fluit acredo	113 as A	114 Si de catarro sanguinem expuunt
172 Si de acribus humoribus passio fiat		
173 De lapide ematite	· but in normal text	·
174 De bolo armenico	·	·
175 Que sunt adiutoria extrinsecus adhibenda	·	·
176 De hiis que sunt cauenda	· but in normal text	114 Si de catarro sanguinem expuunt (*sic*)
177 De lacte dando	· De lactibus	· De lacte

Book 2: (9) Diseases of the kidneys, bladder and genitals (II, 463–501 Puschm.)

Alex. Trall. Lat. ***ed.*** **(G2L1)**	**P1**	**A**
178 De nefreticis quibus lapides in renibus nascuntur	114 Ad nefriticus . . .	115 Ad nefreticos . . .
179 Signa nefreticorum	· but in normal text	·
180 Curatio nefreticorum	115	116
181 De extrinsecis adiutoriis id est fomentationibus et saccellis	· as A	· De fom. et sacc.
182 De cerotis et cathaplasmatibus	·	·
	sed de ircinum sanguinem (cf. A), but in normal text (2.182 line 6)	· De hirci sanguine (2.182 line 6)
183 De potionibus	·	·
		· Potiones confecte uel antidota (2.183 line 19)
184 Curatio de flegmone cum inflammatione facto in renibus	· as A	· De sanguine tollendo
185 Signa si inflammatio in renibus ex plenitudine humorum fiat	116 as A (De fleumone . . . factio)	117 De flegmone.i. inflammatione in renibus facta
	· as A, but in normal text	· Quae sunt extrinsecus adhibenda (2.185 line 43)
186 Curatio inflammationis in pus conuerse	117 as A, but ch. begins Signa sunt haec	118 Si inflammatio in renibus pus faciat signa sunt hec
187 De hiis qui pus per urinam faciunt	118 as A	119 Curatio inflammationis in pus conuerse (= 2.186.t.!)
188 De trociscis et antidotis ad renum et uesice ulcera		

Book 2: *Continued*

Alex. Trall. Lat. *ed.* (G2L1)	**P1**	**A**
189 Signa acredinis in urinis de stranguria	119 Ad straguiria	120 Ad stranguiria
190 Curatio calide distemperantie	• as A, but generate om. (1st 4 words of ch. om.)	• Curatio stranguiriae de calida distemperantia generate
191 Curatio frigide distemperantie de stranguria	• as A, but ending . . . facta fuerit	• Curatio stranguirie de frigida distemperantia facte
192 De dissuria	120 De disiria est enim et cum dolori est et sine dolore[36]	121
193 Curatio dissurie	•	122
194 Curatio si in uesica lapides fiant	121 as A	123 . . . lapides fuerint
195 Signa lithiaseos	122	124
196 Curatio	• but in normal text	•
197 Si uesica scabiosa sit	123 as A	125 Signa si uesica scabra sit
198 Curatio eiusdem	• Curatio	• Curatio
199 Signa dyabetis	124	126
200 Curatio dyabetis	• Curatio	• Curatio
201 Signa gonorree	125 Signa de gorria	127 Signa de gonorria
*<2>02 Curatio gonorree	• Curatio	• Curatio
203 De priapismo	126 as A	128 Ad priapismum

Book 2: (10) Colic (II, 335–77 Puschm.)

Alex. Trall. Lat. *ed.* (G2L1)	**P1**	**A**
204 Colica passio que fit ex frigido et flegmatico humore	127 as A (but with . . . ex frigdorem et . . .)	129 De coli passione que . . .
205 De dieta	•	•
206 De balneis	•	•
207 De fomentationibus	•	•
208 De cathaputiis	•	•
209 De encatismatibus ad coli dolorem	• but in normal text	• De incatismatibus
	De ephitimas (2.209 line 6)	
210 De iniectionibus	• De enectationibus	•
2<1>1 De simplicibus potionibus ad colicum dolorem	• as A (but ending . . . flegma fit)	• Potiones ad coli dolores qui de flegmate fiunt
212 De tyriaca	• but in normal text	•
213 De philonio antidoto	• but in normal text	•
	• Antidotus Marcelli (2.213 line 4)	

[36] i.e. with part of the first sentence of 2.192.

Book 2: *Continued*

Alex. Trall. Lat. *ed.* (G2L1)	**P1**	**A**
214 De narcoticis antidotis	• but in normal text	• De antidotis
215 De uomitu colicis faciendo	•	•
216 De sinapismo et dropace	• De sinapismu et dropaces	• De sinapismis et dropacibus
217 De exercitatione	•	•
	• De uno in alio loco (!) (2.217 line 5)	
218 De uentosa colica	• as A	• De uentositate
219 Si de stercore duro anfraxis faciat coli dolores	128 as A	130 … infraxin f[r]acta coli patiatur dolorem
220 De cathaputiis	•	•
221 Signa si de colerico humore colica fuerit passio generata	129 as A (but om. humore)	131 … humore colus fuerit generatus
222 Curatio si de colerico humore colica fuerit passio generata	• as A, but in normal text	• … humore generetur colica passio
223 De balneis	• but in normal text	•
224 De exercitationibus	• as A	• De exercitatione
225 De catartico dando	• De catartica danda	• De purgatione uentris et de c. d.
226 Cura de colica passione si de flegmone fuerit	130 as A	132 Colus si cum inflammatione consurgat in intestinis
227 De cibis dandis	•	•
228 De cathaplasmate	•	•
229 De cerotis	•	• De ceroto
230 De balneis	• De balneum	•
231 De uino dando	• but in normal text	•
232 De phisicis ligaturis	131 as A	133 De fisicis et ligaturis et potionibus et caracteribus ad colum
233[37] De caracteribus		
234[38] De lapide medicon		

Book 2: (11) Gout (II, 501–75 Puschm.)

Alex. Trall. Lat. *ed.* (G2L1)	**P1**	**A**
235 De podagra	132	134
236 De podagre causis		
237 Signa si de colerico humore podagra fuerit generata	132	135
238 Curatio podagre calide de coleribus adhibenda	133 as A, but ch. begins Catartica	136 … coleribus cathartica[39]

[37] In P1 and A, the first recipe of 2.233 comes between the second and third recipe in 2.234.
[38] *ed.* repeats last sentence of 2.232 at end of 2.234.
[39] A lacks the ingredients of the last recipe in 2.238.

Book 2: *Continued*

Alex. Trall. Lat. *ed.* (G2L1)	**P1**	**A**
239 Podagricis que sunt extrinsecus adhibenda	• but in normal text	•
240 De embrocis	•	•
241 De dieta	•	•
242 De balneis[40]	•	•
243 Que oportet podagricis extrinsecus adhibere ad dolorem mitigandum et calorem extinguendum	• as A, but in normal text • De pusca (!) (2.243 line 26)	• Que oportet podagricis extrinsecus adhiberi
244 Confectio dyaltee caceltice	•	• Confectio dialteas calastici
245 De <e>mplastris	• exinplus ficinis (cf. A), but in normal text	• Exemplar fenicis
246 De linimentis	• but in normal text	•
247 Signa si de flegmatico humore podagra generetur	134 as A	137 ... podagra fuerit generata
248 Curatio flegmatice podagre	• as A (but om. si)	• Curatio si de flegmatico humore podagra generatur
249 De catarticis	•	•
250 Oximel Iuliani catarticum	• ch. begins Catarticus	•
251 De cathaputiis dandis	• De catapudias	•
252 De antidoto dyacorallion	• De antidotus; ch. begins Podagricis • Antidotus (2.252 line 28)	• De antidotis podagricis aptis
253 Item de antidoto Trachii		
254 De potionibus	• De catapl. (2.254 line 22)	
255 De localibus curis ad eos qui de frigidis humoribus doloribus exagitantur	• as A	• ... de frigido humore ...
256 De calefacientibus potenter[41]	• as A, but in normal text	• Item aliud cataplasma
2<57> De balneis	• as A	• De balneo
258 De unguentis dyaforeticis	• as A	• De unguentis
259 Ad eos qui in pedibus de flegmatico humore nimios habent tumores	135 ... habent humoris	138
260 Psilotrum podagricis	•	•
261 Curatio podagre ex sanguine generate	136 as A, but ending ... generata podagra	139 Si ex sanguine fuerint generata

[40] Before *Propoma*: inprimis ... εὔκρατον *om. ed.*
[41] At the end of this chapter 'Anodinum enim est' is not in *ed.*

Book 2: ***Continued***

Alex. Trall. Lat. ***ed.*** **(G2L1)**	**P1**	**A**
262 De localibus curis	• but in normal text	•
263 Ad porros hoc est si in nodis tumores fuerint et lapides	137 . . . nudus tuberus fecerit aut lapidis	140 . . . nodis tuberes fecerit
264 De antidotis	• De antidotus	• De antidoto
265 Ad porros	• as A	• De cerotis ad poros
266 De anodinis antidotis et catarticis dandis	138	141
267 Catarticum de hermodactilis		
	139 as A (2.267 line 16)	142 Catarticum de hermodactilo (2.267 line 16)
268 De cathaputiis	140 De cataputias	143
269 Potio de coronopodium	141 Putionis de coronopodio	144 Potiones de coronopodio et diamiro
	142 Antidotus podagricus (2.269 line 20)	145 Antidotum de coronopodio (2.269 line 20)
270 De antidoto alio podagricis dando per totum annum	• but in normal text	• Item antidotum aliud
271 De localibus adiutoriis mitigatiuis	143	146

Book 3: Prologue (I, 289 Puschm.) and (1) *Ephemerae febres* (I, 291–311 Puschm.)

Alex. Trall. Lat. *ed.* (G2L1)	**γ (P1 M)**	**η (A O[42] Mu) C**	**G1**	**P2[43]**	**P3 (Ma)[44]**	**D**	**Ge**	**Ox**
Proemium libri tertii[45]	Prologus	as γ	no t.	as γ	no t.	no t.	no t.	no t.
1. De effimeris febribus	2	2	•	•	•	•	Signa . . .	Signa . . .
2. Cause[46] effimerarum	3	3	•	•	no t.	•	•	•
3. Curatio si ex nimio calore[47] febriunt	4	4	•	•	• no t.[48]	•	•	•
4. Curatio ad eos qui ex labore febriunt	5	5	•	•	. . . ex calore	•	•	•
5. De hiis qui ex indigestione ciborum febriunt[49]	6	6	•	•	no t.	•	•	•
6. Curatio calide distemperantie	7	7	•	•	•	5. t.	•	[50]vv. 1–22 only
7. Ad eos qui de frigida distemperantia corruptis cibis acidum ructant	8	8	•	•	•	6. t.	•	
8. Curatio frigide distemperantie ex indigestione facte	9	9	•	•	•	7. t.	•	
9. De effimeris febribus ex anfraxi factis	10	10	•	•	[51]	8. t.	•	from v. 21 only

42 O has no chapter-numbers and no titles, save only 3.3, which has both.
43 P2 has no chapter-numbers, and the chapter-initials are not written in after 3. Prol. The chapter-titles in P2 are uncannily close to those of *ed.*
44 I add a few notes on Ma, which has no chapter-titles but (except for 3.65) fine chapter-initials: chapter (sub-)divisions in Ma agree with those in G1 and (save 3.3) P3.
45 *ante Prol.* Incipit . . . de febribus singulis P1 . . . de singulis febribus AOMu . . . de diuersitate febrium C . . . de effimeris febribus Ox . . . de febribus DGe *post Prol.* Incipit . . . inprimis de effemeras feb() M
46 Cura M Curatio *cett.*
47 labore P1M AC G1 P3 dolore Mu calore P2 D Ox Ge
48 P3 has a chapter-initial at 'Si enim antequam . . .'
49 At the end of this chapter 'Oportet igitur . . . adhibere curationem' is in G2L1 but not in *ed.*
50 Due to the loss of a folio; cf. p. 48.
51 *Fin. cap. add. in marg. manu alia.*

Book 3: (2) Fevers from corruption (I, 311–27 Puschm.)

Alex. Trall. Lat. *ed.* (G2L1)	**γ (P1 M)**	**η (A O Mu) C**	**G1**	**P2**	**P3 (Ma)**	**D**	**Ge**	**Ox**
10. Ad eos qui ex putridis humoribus febriunt	11	11	•	•	•	9. t.	•	•
11. Signa sino[do]che febris ex putredine facte	12	12	•	•	•	10. t.	•	•
12. Signa sinoche febris	13[52]	13	•	•	•	12. t.	•	•
13. Curatio sinoche febris	14	14	•	•	•	12. t.	•	Curatio
	De dieta ad humectandum	as γ[53] <u>O ends</u>[54]		•[55]	De dieta	13. t.		
14. De inflammatione erisipilatoydos[56]	15	15	•	•	•	•	•[57]	
15. Signa de hiis qui habent causon et erisipilatoydes inflammationes	16	16	•	•	•	•	•	•
16. Signa de uero et non uero causon	17	17	•	•	•	•	•	•
17. Curatio causonis	18	18	•	•	•[58]	•	•	Curatio
18. Ad eos qui in stomacho nimium habent ardorem	19	19	•	•	•	•	•	
19. Signa si ex putredine sanguinis fuerit facta febris[59]	20	20[60]	•	•	•	•	•	
20. De dieta febricitantium[61]	21	21	•	•	•	•	•	•
	De balneo	as γ	•	•[62]	no t.	21. t.	as Ox	•[63]

[52] *ad fin.* tunc eis . . . fieri cognitionem *om.* P1

[53] *hunc tit. necnon et uerba* Aqua igitur frigida danda est *om.* C, *qui 3.14. tit. in cap. 3.13 post uerba* non calefaciat *posuit. Hinc usque ad 3.19.t. tit. quemque cum praecedenti cap. habet* C.

[54] O breaks off two lines from the end of 3.13.

[55] *subtit.* Aqua igitur danda est frigida P2

[56] erisip. *om.* A. *nouissimum uerbum cap.* (*iussimus*) *om.* P1M P3. *In fine cap. add.* erisipilatodes (pilatodes A) inflammatio AMu.

[57] Ge′ as Ox (running straight on without 3.14.t., *add. in marg.* Ge).

[58] Cognosci autem *usque ad fin. cap. add. inf. manu alia* P3.

[59] *In fine cap. uersus* Vidi enim aliquem . . . et cerota *om. ed. habent* G2L1.

[60] De aqua danda in causonide C

[61] *post* qui leuius febriunt *uerba* Oximellis uero fugiendus qui fortiter omnino febriunt *om. ed.* P3′ *habent* G2L1.

[62] *post uerba* omnino infrigdant *subtit.* Item de febrientibus P2

[63] *tit.* Curatio ardorem nimium patientibus Ox Ge

Book 3: (3) *Syncope* in fevers (I, 329–37 Puschm.)

Alex. Trall. Lat. *ed.* (G2L1)	**γ (P1 M)**	**η (A Mu C)**	**G1**	**P2**	**P3 (Ma)**	**D**	**Ge**	**Ox**
21. De sincopi in febribus	22	22	•	•	•	•[64]	•	•
22. Curatio si ex putredine fiat[65]	23	23	•	•	•	•	•	•
23. Signa si de colerico et tenui humore sincopes patiuntur	24	24	•	•	•	•	•	•
24. Curatio sincoporum ex plenitudine factorum	25	25	•	•	•	•	•	Curatio
- De uino	De uino dando	as γ[66]	as γ	•	as γ	•	•	•[67]
- Item de balneo et cibo	De balneo	as γ	as γ	•	as γ	as γ	•	as γ
25. De colerica passione	26	26[68]	•	•	•	•	•	•
26. Curatio si ex colerico et tenui humore sincopis fiat	27	27	•	•	•	•	•	Curatio
	De uino dando	as γ[69]	•	no t.	as γ	De uino	•	

[64] De febrium sinthomatibus D
[65] Curatio] Cognitio *cett.* | putredine] plenitudine C D Ox Ge
[66] *non habet* C.
[67] De uino quibus debet dari Ox Ge
[68] Last sentence *om.* Mu
[69] *non habet* C.

Book 3: (4) Fainting (I, 337–47 Puschm.)

Alex. Trall. Lat. *ed.* (G2L1)	**γ (P1 M)**	**η (A Mu C)**	**G1**	**P2**	**P3 (Ma)**	**D**	**Ge**	**Ox**
27. De angustiis et malfactionibus	28	28[70]	•	•	•	•	•	•
28. De hiis[71] qui subito euacuati angustias patiuntur	29	29	•	•	t. quasi init. cap.[72]	•	•	•
29. Quibus de[73]plenitudine angustiantur	30	30	•	•	•	•	•	•
30. Ad eas que ex matrice angustiantur	31	31	•	•	•	•	•	•
31. Ad eos qui ex defectu stomachi angustiantur	32	32	•	•	•	•	•	•
32. Ad eos qui de causon angustiantur	33	33	•	•	•	•	•[74]	•
33. Ad eos qui de frigido stomacho angustiantur	34	34 (t. om. C)	•	•	•	•	•	•
34. Ad eos qui de pessimo humore in stomacho mordicationes patiuntur	35	35A ends[75]	•	•	•	•	•	•[76]
35. Si ex flegmate in stomacho[77] angustias patiuntur	36	36	•	•	•	•		
36. De dieta ad eos qui ex flegmate in stomacho angustiantur[78]	37	37[79]	•	•	no t.	•	•	no t.

70 3.28.t. here and repeated at head of next chapter AMu.
71 De his omnibus (hominibus M) P1M AMu P3′
72 *Fin. cap. add. in marg. manu alia* P3.
73 Qui ex G2L1 D
74 3.32.t. *et init. cap. om.* Ge′, *add. in marg.*
75 A breaks off in 3.34, v. 4, although most of the column is blank.
76 Ox and Ge run together 3.34 and 3.35.
77 in stomacho *om.* P1M P3′
78 Dieta ad flegma repletis M De dieta flegmate repletorum G1 De dieta *om.* D
79 3.36 solent . . . 3.37 et frica *om.* Mu

Book 3: *Continued*

Alex. Trall. Lat. *ed.* (G2L1)	**γ (P1 M)**	**η (A Mu C)**	**G1**	**P2**	**P3 (Ma)**	**D**	**Ge**	**Ox**
37. Ad eos qui ex calore angustiantur	38	38	•	•	•	•	•	•
38. Ad eros qui ex inflammatione angustiantur	39	39 (t. *om.* Mu C)	•	•	•	•	•	•
39. Ad eos qui de siccitate uel inanitione sincopim patiuntur	40	40 (39 Mu[80])	•[81]	as G1; so too Ma	no t.[82]	•	•	•
40. Si de anfraxi in dominio corporis existente angustiantur	41	41	•	•	•	•	•	•
41. Signa anfraxis	42	42	•	•	•	•	•	•
42. Ad eos qui de incisione uulnerum uel effusione puris angustiantur	43	43	•	•	•	•	•	•
43. Ad eos qui ex tristicia aut gaudio aut dolore angustiantur	44	44	•	•	•	•	•	•
44. Ad eos qui de ylei dolore aut coli angustiantur	45	45	•	•	•	•	•	•
45. Ad eos qui imbecilli uirtute facta angustiantur	46	46	•	•	•[83]	•	•	•

[80] *hinc usque ad cap. 57 eandem numerationem atque ed. habet* Mu.
[81] After *nutries* words are missing; then *signa* (*supersinas ed.*) *passionis*; then *modice uino* to end of chapter is missing in G1 P2 Ma D Ge Ox.
[82] *Fin. cap. add. in marg. manu alia* P3.
[83] But t. and first sentence are very different; so, too, Ma.

Book 3: (5) *Hecticae febres* (I, 349–69 Puschm.)

Alex. Trall. Lat. *ed.* (G2 L1)	**γ (P1 M)**	**η (Mu C)**	**G1**	**P2**	**P3 (Ma)**	**D**	**Ge**	**Ox**
46. De ethicis febribus	47	46 (t. om. C)[84]	•[85]	•	•	•	om. Ge/[86]	•
47. De marasmode	48	47	•	•	•	•	•	•
48. Quomodo oportet cognosci et discerni ab effimera ethicam febrem[87]	49	48	•	•	•	•	•	•
49. Quomodo discernenda est ethica a putrida	50[88]	49	•	•	•	cf. γ	cf. γ	cf. γ
50. *Quomodo* diiudicamus sinochum ab ethica	51	50	•	•	•	•	•	•
51. Signa ethice febris	52	51	•	•	Signa.	•	•	•
52. Signa ethice *quando* transmutatur in marasmoydem	53	52[89]	•	•	De signis.	•	•	•
53. Curatio ethice febris	54	53	•	•	•	•	•	•
54. Quibus non oportet dari potum aque frigide	55	54	•	•	•	•	•	•
55. *Quando* oportet aquam frigidam dari[90]	56	55	•	•	•	•	•	56. t.

84 *3.45 et 3.46 quasi cap. unum scribit* C.
85 *hic habet 3.46.t. super 3.45.t.* G1.
86 3.46.t. and the whole chapter is added in the margin in Ge.
87 Quomodo oportet discerni ethicam ab effimera G2L1 *fin. cap. add. in marg. manu alia* P3.
88 Quomodo oportit determinare ictica febre. Ab eo quem ex putridinem fit P1 *et sim.* M D Ox Ge
89 *uerba* fortiori ... non curatur *ad finem cap. transpos.* Mu.
90 Si quando cum inflammationes sunt ignita (= *initium capituli ed.*) P1 *et sim.* M *tit. incipit* Quando cum inflammatione ... C G1 P2 Ge Que nunc inflammatione ... D

Book 3: *Continued*

Alex. Trall. Lat. *ed.* (G2 L1)	**γ (P1 M)**	**η (Mu C)**	**G1**	**P2**	**P3 (Ma)**	**D**	**Ge**	**Ox**
56. Si[91] transmutata sit ethica febris in marasmode	57	56	•	•	•	•	•	57. t.
57. *Quomodo* curari oportet ethicam in {a}qua non pot(est) aqua frigida dari	58	57[92]	•	•[93]	cf. C	•	•	1st 4 words of 57. t.
58. De embrocis et dieta ad febres ethicas[94]	59	59	•	•[95]	•	•	•	•
De domo			De domo et aere		as G1	•	•[96]	
59. De balneo[97]		•	•	•	•	•	•	•
60. De lacte dando ethicis[98]		De lacte	as η	no t.	as η	•	•	as η
61. De uino[99]		•[100]	•	•	•	•	•	•
62. Ad eos qui in marasmodem de sincopo transeunt[101]	60	60	•	•	•	•[102]	•	•

91 Si iam P1M Mu C D Ge
92 aliquando autem mollius *usque ad fin. cap. om.* C P3′ *add. P3 manu alia.*
93 aliquando *usque ad fin. cap. suppl. in marg.* m2.
94 De inbrocas ad icticus P1 *et sim.* M De dieta et embrocis ad ethicas febres Ox Ge
95 *bis uersus aliquot suppl. in marg.* m2.
96 De loco praeparando Ge
97 59.t. *om.* L1; more elaborate in D.
98 De lactibus P1M
99 Quibus dandum sit uinum D; *ad fin. cap.* uinum dare inimicus igitur eis dare uinum P1 *et sim.* M Mu
100 *subtit. om.* C.
101 Ad eos qui de sincopus marasmodis paciuntur P1 *et sim.* M
102 From here to the end, D is very hard to read on the microfilm.

Book 3: ***Continued***

Alex. Trall. Lat. ***ed.*** **(G2 L1)**	**γ (P1 M)**	**η (Mu C)**	**G1**	**P2**	**P3 (Ma)**	**D**	**Ge**	**Ox**
63. De testiculis gallorum[103] qui parastate dicuntur	61 <u>P1 ends</u>[104]	61	•	•	•[105]	•	•	•
64. De pomis	62[106]	62[107]	•	•	•	•	•	•
65. De marasmode febre perfectius existente[108]	63	63[109]	•	•	•	•	•	•
66. Lixoperita epithimata et embroce et emplastra febrientibus Martyrii medici[110]	64	•	Cf. M		t. = De. (*sic*!); <u>P3 ends</u> v. 8; 3. 66 is not in Ma			
	65[111]		Cf. M; om. last 2 vv. of ch.					

[103] gallorum *om.* P1M P3
[104] P1 breaks off in 3.63, v. 1.
[105] Last sentence (from *cadat* to the end) very different; so, too, Ma.
[106] *ad fin. uerba* sed neque alii ciui dati qualitates uel quantitates ipsum et tempore et ordine et modis usus quia omnia emendata cautius uobis tradidimus *habet* M.
[107] *3.63 et 3.64 quasi unum cap. scribit* C.
[108] De marasmon M *litt. init. cap. ornatam om.* Ma.
[109] *post* inchoantem marasmon *uerba* et nondum omnino per desiccata sterea existimet aliquis se ad curationem suscipere tumoris interdicta condicione *habet* Mu *deinde spatium ante cap. ultimum.*
[110] Lyxiperitus pannus et embrocas febrientibus M *et sim.* G1 De efimeris et hecticis et marasmodis febribus lithoperita epitimata et embroce febrientibus litoperitum epithima Martirii medici Mu Lyxoperitō. Ad febres lixoperito epytha Mauri medici C
[111] *post 3.66, v. 8 tit.* Lyxiperitus et inbrocas Galieni ad febres *habet* M De epithimate Gal. G1.

INDEX OF LATIN WORDS, PHRASES AND CONSTRUCTIONS

*(This index includes Latin words in Greek letters, and Greek words which are used as if they were Latin. An asterisk * indicates an unattested word or form.)*

INDEX OF GREEK WORDS, PHRASES AND CONSTRUCTIONS

*(An asterisk * indicates an unattested word or form.)*

INDEX OF NAMES AND SUBJECTS

(The works contained in the manuscripts described in Chapter 3 are indexed only selectively.)

INDEX OF PASSAGES DISCUSSED

(This index includes only those passages which are quoted and commented on, not those which are merely listed. References in bold are to passages quoted in extenso *or otherwise receiving special treatment. For the conventions used in references, see p. xiv.)*

INDEX OF MANUSCRIPTS

(*This index includes* (s.v. 'ed.') *the early, 1504, printing of the Latin Alexander. Other sigla used in the present work (Puschmann's and Zipser's for Greek mss., mine for Latin mss.) are given in bold after the respective catalogue numbers. Page numbers in bold refer to principal descriptions or extensive quotations. Mainstream and excerpting mss. of the Latin Alexander are listed on pp. 38–9.*)

(A) Greek Manuscripts

(B) Lost Greek Copies (postulated by Zipser)

(C) Latin Manuscripts

(D) Lost Latin Copies (postulated in Chapter 4; cf. the stemma, **Plate XII**)